T0202346

Voluntarily Stopping Eating and Drinking

Voluntarily Stopping Eating and Drinking

A Compassionate, Widely Available Option for Hastening Death

Edited by

TIMOTHY E. QUILL, MD

PAUL T. MENZEL, PHD

THADDEUS M. POPE, JD, PHD

JUDITH K. SCHWARZ, PHD, RN

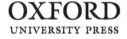

OXFORD

UNIVERSITY PRESS

OXFORD
UNIVERSITY PRESS

Oxford University Press is a department of the University of Oxford. It furthers
the University's objective of excellence in research, scholarship, and education
by publishing worldwide. Oxford is a registered trade mark of Oxford University
Press in the UK and certain other countries.

Published in the United States of America by Oxford University Press
198 Madison Avenue, New York, NY 10016, United States of America.

Library of Congress Cataloging-in-Publication Data
Names: Quill, Timothy E., editor. | Menzel, Paul T., 1942– editor. |
Pope, Thaddeus M., editor. | Schwarz, Judith (Nurse), editor.
Title: Voluntarily stopping eating and drinking : a compassionate, widely
available option for hastening death / edited by Timothy E. Quill,
Paul T. Menzel, Thaddeus M. Pope, Judith K. Schwarz.
Description: New York, NY : Oxford University Press, [2021] |
Includes bibliographical references and index.
Identifiers: LCCN 2021002997 (print) | LCCN 2021002998 (ebook) |
ISBN 9780190080730 (hardback) | ISBN 9780190080761 (epub) |
ISBN 9780190080747
Subjects: MESH: Euthanasia, Active, Voluntary | Starvation |
Dehydration | Right to Die
Classification: LCC R726 (print) | LCC R726 (ebook) | NLM WB 65 |
DDC 179.7—dc23
LC record available at https://lccn.loc.gov/2021002997
LC ebook record available at https://lccn.loc.gov/2021002998

DOI: 10.1093/med/9780190080730.001.0001

5 7 9 8 6

Printed by Integrated Books International, United States of America

To the patients, families, caregivers, and clinicians whose stories we shared in this book, and to countless other patients, friends, and family members who have needed and wanted both excellent palliative care and a wider range of end-of-life choices.

—Timothy E. Quill

To Bonnie, for her constant love and stimulating support, and in memory of my nephew, Paul Frederick Helm.

—Paul T. Menzel

For Linda and Phineas. And Reina, Larry, Nedra, Lessandra, Nathaniel, Matthias, Cameron, Clayton, and Tucker. I hope none of us ever need this book. But some probably will.

—Thaddeus M. Pope

To my friend Joan, the first person who asked me to help facilitate a peaceful death, over 20 years ago. I knew very little then, and she began my education in understanding how hard it can be to die well, and about some of the clinical challenges of VSED. To my patiently supportive and loving family members, particularly Jessi and Jason who, along with several very good friends, have indulged my passion for choice at the end of life and participated in endless discussions of the complexities involved.

—Judith K. Schwarz

How quiet
It is in this sick room
Where on the bed
A silent woman lies between two lovers –
Life and Death . . . .

—Langston Hughes, "Sick Room" (1926)

Contents

Foreword

Why should I agree to write a foreword for a book about two of my least favorite things: dying, and abjuring eating and drinking? No one escapes death; I understand this incontrovertible fact. Whatever our wishes, in the face of our most determined, even desperate, efforts, the outcome is not at our discretion.

Dying is another matter. Many of us can have a say in the manner and, perhaps, the timing of our dying. How should we feel about this? In *The Myth of Sisyphus*, Albert Camus begins by naming suicide as "the one truly serious philosophical problem." Later in that essay he offers this counsel: "It is essential to die unreconciled and not of one's own free will" (p. 55). Camus, we should remember, was only 46 when his publisher's car flew off an icy road in rural France in January, 1960, killing him immediately. The idea that the technologies and institutions of medicine might one day exercise undue control over the circumstances of dying was likely foreign to him.

There are some readers, I am sure, who prefer to "die unreconciled and not of one's own free will." But there are also many people, equally thoughtful and sincere, who embrace life as fiercely as Camus, acknowledge the inevitability of death as he also did, yet desire fervently to escape avoidable suffering and the affronts to dignity that so often accompany dying.

But giving up food and drink? My mother's parents came to America from the Abruzzo, a region of Italy known for its natural beauty, its mountains—and, in the early twentieth century, its poverty. Whatever hardships they'd endured, by the time my father—from an impoverished Irish American family—appeared, they welcomed him warmly and did what good families do: they fed him. My father, who'd had to compete with his siblings for the often-meager offerings at the table, told us many years later that until he met my mother, he didn't realize that food had taste. For my Italian grandparents, food was a tangible, daily expression of solidarity and love. Which makes the prospect of forgoing all eating and drinking resonantly poignant. If indeed food equals love, more or less, then surely denying someone food reveals love's absence; so, at least, it may feel to us at first glance.

Voluntarily Stopping Eating and Drinking: A Compassionate, Widely Available Option for Hastening Death invites the reader to think more calmly and deeply. Its attentiveness to clinical realities, law, ethics, and institutional constraints illuminate the decisions made by the multiple actors involved in each of the cases that form the connective tissue of the book. I often found myself wanting to argue with the authors (of the chapters on ethics, mostly). But at the same time, I admired their clarity and courage. Even readers who may disagree with some of their analyses will come away enlightened, their perspectives broadened.

This is an important book destined to shape practice, policy, and discourse on dying. It will be an important resource for clinicians, ethicists, lawyers, administrators, and policymakers, along with individuals and families weighing their options as life's end looms into view. *Voluntarily Stopping Eating and Drinking* is likely to shape public and private conversations about our options as death draws near.

Thomas H. Murray, PhD
President Emeritus, The Hastings Center

Preface

In the 21st century, people in the developed world are living longer. They hope that they will have a healthy longer life and then die relatively quickly and peacefully. But frequently that does not happen. While people on average are living healthy a *little* longer, they tend to live sick for a *lot* longer. And at the end of being sick before dying, they and their families are frequently faced with daunting decisions about whether to keep going with life-prolonging medical treatments or whether to try finding more meaningful and forthright ways to die more easily and quickly. To make matters even more complex, about half these patients no longer have the capacity to make decisions for themselves. So, families or clinicians must decide and act on their behalf, if the suffering associated with such situations is going to be avoided or minimized.

In this context, many people are searching for more and better options to hasten death. There are two main groups. First, there are those who are currently suffering unacceptably. Second, there are those who want to preempt the last phase of the dying process and thereby avoid potential suffering or unacceptable deterioration in their future.

Voluntarily Stopping Eating and Drinking (VSED) is a lesser known, available option for persons who are looking for an escape from these situations by hastening their death at a time of their own choosing. For some, the possibility of directing the stopping of their eating and drinking in the future may allow them to continue living without fear that they might eventually become trapped in an unacceptable condition without the potential for escape. Others who are looking for an escape *right now* might be able to initiate VSED without needing permission or assistance from others, and without having to worry about breaking the law.

In that sense, VSED is different from other "last resort" options such as Medical Aid in Dying (MAID) which is currently legal in only eleven states and the District of Columbia in the United States, and in fourteen jurisdictions elsewhere in the world. VSED is theoretically a possibility for almost anyone with decision-making capacity who has decided that continued living is no longer acceptable. Stopping eating and drinking may also be potentially accessible to those who have lost decision-making capacity but earlier made their preferences for this option extremely clear through a detailed advance directive.

VSED is not only more widely available but also a much more compassionate way to hasten death than is widely appreciated. Despite its wide accessibility legally, VSED is frequently portrayed as a "dismal choice" and dismissed as "starvation."[1] This is distinctly misleading. Dying by starvation and dehydration in normal circumstances is indeed a terrible process. But for persons near the end of life who are determined to end life on their own terms, the process of dying by VSED can be relatively comfortable and peaceful, particularly if they have good palliative support. Properly pursued and supported, VSED needs to be recognized as a much more viable option than it currently is.

This book begins with an overview of VSED. The Introduction defines the process and puts it in the context of caring for seriously ill patients, including potential options for hastening death. Part I of the book (comprising the first six chapters) then focuses on VSED by people with decision-making capacity. In Chapter 1 we present four real clinical cases of patients with decision-making capacity who seriously considered and then initiated VSED, concluding each case with a brief list of its notable characteristics and issues raised.

Chapter 2 explores the clinical aspects of VSED in much more detail, including how the process played out in each of the initial four cases. A main advantage of VSED is that it gives power and control directly to the initiating person. But the process is also associated with predictable difficulties including dry mouth, thirst, eventual weakness, and sometimes confusion toward the very end. Fortunately, these challenges can be anticipated and usually managed with careful advance planning and skilled assistance from clinicians and caregivers. VSED typically lasts 10 to 14 days from initiation to death provided one is disciplined about not drinking. The initiating person is usually alert and capable of meaningful interaction with family and friends for most of the time but will usually become very weak and much less responsive toward the end. Chapter 2 gives state-of-the-art clinical instructions and

---

[1] For example, a *New York Times* editorial supporting the legalization of MAID refers to VSED as one of only two "dismal choices" available to those living in jurisdictions where MAID is not available. Some "manage to get a lethal dose of drugs . . . under the table . . . . Others are advised to starve themselves to death" (New York Times 2016).

practical ideas about how to implement VSED if appropriate and desired, including strategies for managing some of its predictable challenges.

Chapters 3, 4, and 5 in Part I explore the associated ethical, legal, and institutional aspects of VSED for patients with decision-making capacity, returning regularly to the practical issues raised in the initial four case presentations and in the clinical chapter. Part I closes (in Chapter 6) with a summary of "best practices, enduring challenges, and opportunities" raised by VSED when it is initiated by patients with decision-making capacity.

Part II of the book (comprising Chapters 7 to 12) has the same general structure as Part I, but it explores the more controversial option of stopping eating and drinking for persons who have lost decision-making capacity before initiating the process. In this situation, decisions about implementation must be based on the person's previously articulated Advance Directive for Stopping Eating and Drinking (AD for SED).

Many patients who still have decision-making capacity would not want to continue living in a future of unacceptable suffering or deterioration, and for some that would include situations in which they will have lost decision-making capacity from a condition like progressive dementia. But they would also prefer not to act preemptively while they still have capacity to do so, because they are still finding their life meaningful and are not suffering in ways that are unacceptable. Can they postpone the decision to hasten death by stopping eating and drinking until their capacity is lost, but still be assured they can access this escape by empowering others to act later on their behalf?

Like Part I, Part II begins (in Chapter 7) with four cases. Each focuses on a person at a different stage of losing decision-making capacity who made it clear the future conditions in which they did not want to continue living if capacity were fully lost. Each case presentation includes "notable characteristics" and "issues raised" to be addressed in subsequent chapters.

Chapter 8 explores the clinical aspects of Stopping Eating and Drinking by Advance Directive (SED by AD). It recommends that all patients who value a hastened death by an intervention like SED by AD if they lose decision-making capacity should initiate extensive advance care planning. They should include a detailed instructional advance directive, naming and fully informing a health care proxy, and ideally even providing a videotaped advance directive statement about their preferences with regard to eating and drinking in the context of future loss of decision-making capacity. The clearer and more specific a person can be in advance of losing decision-making capacity about one's genuine wishes in this domain, the more likely it is that those preferences can be actualized in the future.

Part II explores three main options with regard to empowering surrogate decision-makers to limit future provision or withholding of food and fluids if a person loses decision-making capacity:

1. **Withhold all feeding (both self-feeding and assisted feeding).** Otherwise provide maximum comfort measures (moistening mouth, pain relief, sedation for any agitation).
2. **Withhold all assisted feeding, and facilitate only comfort oriented self-feeding.** Provide easy access to foods that the patient appears to enjoy in amounts as much or as little as the person willingly eats by his or her own hand.
3. **Provide comfort-oriented assisted feeding if needed,** but only in amounts that clearly contribute to the patient's immediate comfort.

Chapters 9, 10, and 11 explore the ethical, legal, and institutional aspects of SED by AD, as well as the less controversial option of "comfort feeding only" when it does and does not include direct caregiver assistance. Part II closes (in Chapter 12) with a summary of "best practices, enduring challenges, and opportunities" posed by SED by AD, or receiving comfort-oriented feeding only in one of its two forms presented above, once decision-making capacity is lost.

Appendices available in the final part of this book are divided into six general categories, most of which will include citations or easily accessible links to materials of interest:

Appendix A: Recommended Elements of an Advance Directive for Stopping Eating and Drinking (AD for SED)

Appendix B: Sample Advance Directives for Stopping Eating and Drinking

Appendix C: Cause of Death on Death Certificates with VSED or SED by AD

Appendix D: Position Statements and Clinical Guidance

Appendix E: Personal Narratives

Appendix F: Glossary

We anticipate this book will be useful to a wide range of readers, including but not limited to:

- Patients and family members looking to explore the full range of end-of-life options for themselves or for someone they love. This might be for possible use in their current situation, or in the future with particular emphasis on VSED if they have decision-making capacity and on SED by AD if decision-making capacity is currently or may soon be lost.
- Clinicians of all kinds (doctors, nurses, nurse practitioners, physician assistants, social workers, nutritionists, chaplains) who care for seriously ill patients and want to be aware of all possible options for responding to unacceptable suffering or deterioration.
- Ethicists, lawyers, theologians, scholars, clinicians, patients, and family members interested in exploring the possibility of stopping eating and drinking at the end of life in a multidimensional way.
- Anyone, mortal as we all are, who wants to think through a wide range of approaches to the end of one's own life, or the end of their loved ones' lives.

We hope you enjoy the book and are stimulated and challenged by it. VSED and SED by AD are not simple options. But they sometimes provide the most viable approach available to remedy what is or might become an untenable situation for a given individual. They are sometimes critically important pieces of the challenging puzzle of finding meaningful, achievable options for hastening death in response to unacceptable current or future conditions.

Reference

New York Times. 2016. "Aid in Dying Movement Advances" (editorial). *New York Times*, October 10, 2016, A20.

Acknowledgments

Many people and organizations have been instrumental in inspiring and supporting us in writing and editing this book. We especially thank all the contributing chapter and case authors and co-authors. They have provided material and perspective that the four of us could not, and they carefully attended to developing their contributions specifically for this book.

We are indebted to those who hosted and sponsored the conference, "Hastening Death by Voluntarily Stopping Eating and Drinking: Clinical, Legal, Ethical, Religious, and Family Perspectives," in October of 2016 at Seattle University School of Law. It was there that the four of us first all met. The conference itself would likely not have happened had concerted interest in VSED not been shown several years earlier by Robb Miller, then Executive Director of Compassion and Choices, Washington (now End of Life Washington); conversations with him and others, including Erin Mae Glass and Lisa Brodoff, eventually led to the planning of a conference hosted by Seattle University School of Law. We are indebted to Dean Annette Clarke and others there for their support.

The four of us have gained greatly from working with each other. The collaboration required for a volume as integrated as this one is extensive and demanding. Each of us is grateful for all that the others contributed and for making the whole experience enjoyable.

Finally, we thank Oxford University Press, especially Editor Lucy Randall and her Assistant, Hannah Doyle, as well as Poonguzhali Ramasamy, Carol Neiman, and two anonymous reviewers.

Timothy E. Quill:
Thanks to the University of Rochester Medical Center for creating an environment that supports both excellent technical medical care as well as a profoundly caring environment as exemplified in its integrated biopsychosocial model. Our administration (Kathy Parinello and Ray Mayewski) and the Department of Medicine (Paul Levy) have been very supportive of our palliative care programs (now led by co-author Rob Horowitz) not because they are good for the bottom line, but because they are central to delivering the

best possible care for seriously ill patients and their families. My interdisci-plinary palliative care teammates, including nursing aides, social workers, nurses, nurse practitioners, physicians, administrators, and researchers, bring this comprehensive practice to the bedside every day. Together we have become so much more effective than we could be as individuals. Finally, to my wife Penny and daughters Carrie, Megan, and Crissy for their ongoing support and love, and for their outstanding work as clinicians caring for seri-ously ill patients and as advocates for more comprehensive care for all those in need.

Paul T. Menzel:

My fascination with many of the questions that motivate this book origi-nated in teaching biomedical ethics over many decades at Pacific Lutheran University—particularly some of the writings of Norman L. Cantor, John Robertson and Rebecca Dresser, and Nancy K. Rhoden. My first close ac-quaintance with actual VSED was its unflinching preemptive use by Jeptha Carrell, as conveyed to me in subsequent conversations with his wife Demaris. Colette Chandler-Cramer extended and sharpened my under-standing with her clinical experience, providing invaluable material for my first publication on using advance directives to withhold food and fluid by mouth, co-authored with her. Bonnie Steinbock enabled me to see a critically important approach to handling the "then-self vs. now-self" problem cre-ated when previous directives and the current apparent wishes of a person in advancing dementia conflict. And Dena Davis, my co-author of Chapter 9, has greatly expanded my understanding of the complexity of using ADs to halt oral feeding in severe dementia.

Thaddeus M. Pope:

Judith Schwarz and Stanley Terman have opened ivory tower windows, pointed me toward the trenches, and directed my scholarly attention to practical issues that are materially relevant for seriously ill individuals. I am grateful for the 2009–2010 partnership with Lindsey Anderson (Imbrogno) to produce our first major VSED article. By inviting me to speak with their members, Compassion & Choices, Final Exit Network, and other organ-izations gave me hundreds of Socratic questioners who helped refine my thinking. But I most appreciate individuals like Phyllis Shacter who have shared how my VSED scholarship helped their family members. I hope that this book guides and supports many more.

Judith K. Schwarz:
I am grateful to the many patients and their family members I have been privileged to support over the years, some of whose experiences are included in this volume. I continue to learn so much from them, and thank them for their willingness to share their stories with others who benefited from hearing about their experiences. I greatly value the relationships I have had with skilled hospice and palliative care clinicians over the years, the depths of their knowledge, and their willingness to share their expertise with me. My colleagues at End of Life Choices New York—Ayana Woods, David Leven, and Lillian Mehran—have provided much support and collaboration. They were instrumental in helping to develop our "dementia directive," one of the first advance directives to stop eating and drinking in the country, downloaded from our website by hundreds of people. Each brings an important contribution to our efforts to expand choice, improve end-of-life care, and gain access to medical aid in dying in New York State.

Contributors

Editors

Paul T. Menzel, PhD, is Professor of Philosophy emeritus, Pacific Lutheran University. He has published widely on moral questions in health economics and health policy, including *Strong Medicine: The Ethical Rationing of Health Care*, and (as co-editor) *Prevention vs. Treatment: What's the Right Balance?* Most recently, he has written on end-of-life issues, including advance directives for dementia and voluntarily stopping eating and drinking. He has been a visiting scholar at Kennedy Institute of Ethics, Rockefeller Center-Bellagio, Brocher Foundation, Chinese University of Hong Kong, and Monash University.

Thaddeus M. Pope, JD, PhD, is Professor of Law at Mitchell Hamline School of Law in Saint Paul, Minnesota. He has over 200 publications in leading medical journals, law reviews, bar journals, nursing journals, bioethics journals, and book chapters. He coauthors the 1500-page *The Right to Die: The Law of End-of-Life Decision Making* and runs the popular *Medical Futility Blog*. Pope has co-authored clinical practice guidelines for medical aid in dying and major policy statements on critical care ethics for professional medical societies. Apart from his scholarship, Pope has served as a legal consultant and expert witness in court cases involving end-of-life treatment.

Timothy E. Quill, MD, is Professor of Medicine, Psychiatry, Medical Humanities, and Nursing at the University of Rochester School of Medicine, where he was the founding director of their Palliative Care Division. He was a board member and a past president of the American Academy of Hospice and Palliative Medicine. He was the lead physician plaintiff in a U.S. Supreme Court Case *Quill v. Vacco* testing the legal permissibility of physician-assisted death. Quill has been a practicing palliative care physician, an author/editor of seven previous books, multiple peer-reviewed articles in major medical journals, and a regular lecturer and commentator on medical decision-making, physician–patient relationships, palliative care, and end-of-life issues.

Judith K. Schwarz, PhD, RN, is Clinical Director of End of Life Choices New York and was the East Coast Clinical Coordinator for Compassion & Choices. She has counseled many hundreds of patients suffering from incurable and progressive or terminal illnesses and their families about end-of-life options. She publishes regularly in nursing and palliative care journals. For years her work has focused on voluntarily stopping eating and drinking as an option to achieve a peaceful, patient-controlled death. More recently she began responding to requests for assistance from patients diagnosed with an early stage of dementia. With colleagues in other disciplines she developed the End of Life Choices New York "Dementia Directive" that has been completed by hundreds of individuals.

Other Chapter Authors

Dena S. Davis, JD, PhD, holds the Endowed Presidential Chair in Health—Humanities & Social Sciences at Lehigh University, and is Professor Emerita at Cleveland-Marshall College of Law. Davis has been a Visiting Scholar at the National Human Genome Research Institute, Arizona State University, the Brocher Foundation, and the Hastings Center. Her most recent book is *Genetic Dilemmas: Reproductive Technology, Parental Choices, and Children's Futures.* She has been a Fulbright scholar in India, Indonesia, Israel, Italy, and Sweden. She has served on the Board of the American Academy of Religion and the American Society of Bioethics and Humanities, and is a Trustee of Emerson College.

David A. Gruenewald, MD, is Medical Director of the Palliative Care and Hospice Service at the Department of Veterans Affairs Puget Sound Healthcare System, Seattle, WA. He is also Associate Professor of Medicine in the Division of Gerontology and Geriatric Medicine, Department of Medicine at the University of Washington School of Medicine. He is a practicing palliative medicine physician and geriatrician and has authored multiple peer-reviewed articles on palliative medicine and geriatrics topics, including voluntarily stopping eating and drinking in institutional long-term care settings.

V. J. Periyakoil, MD, is Associate Professor of Medicine, Stanford University School of Medicine, and Director of the Palliative Care Education & Training and Hospice & Palliative Medicine Fellowship Programs at Stanford. She serves as Senior Associate Editor of the *Journal of Palliative Medicine* and Associate Editor, the *Journal of the American Geriatrics Society.* She is a member and founding chair of numerous national professional committees in geriatrics, ethnogeriatrics, and palliative medicine. In the clinical realm, she serves as the Associate Director of Palliative Care Services at the VA Palo Alto Health Care Center.

Other Case Authors

Margaret P. Battin, MFA, PhD, is Distinguished Professor of Philosophy and Medical Ethics at the University of Utah. She has authored, co-authored, edited, or co-edited some 20 books, including *Drugs and Justice* and *The Patient as Victim and Vector: Ethics and Infectious Disease*; two collections on end-of-life issues, *The Least Worst Death,* and *Ending Life*; and a comprehensive sourcebook, *The Ethics of Suicide: Historical Sources.* She is currently completing *Sex & Consequences: A Thought Experiment for Saving the Planet and Living in What-If Land,* on real-world thought experiments. She has been named one of the "Mothers of Bioethics."

Robert K. Horowitz, MD, is the Gosnell Distinguished Professor in Palliative Care and Chief of the Palliative Care Division at the University of Rochester Medical Center. He worked for many years as an emergency physician and as director of the URMC Adult Cystic Fibrosis Program. In addition, he teaches clinicians, trainees, and community members about facilitating difficult conversations, advance care planning, and a range of "palliative care" issues, and authors occasional scholarly contributions in these realms.

Ty Markham is a long-time educator and licensed clinical psychologist. A passionate environmentalist, she founded and chaired a nonprofit environmental organization in Utah for many years. She continues as a board member and is also serving on the board of another nonprofit organization, "Scenic Utah." Now semi-retired, Ty runs a seasonal wellness retreat/bed & breakfast business near one of Utah's red rock national parks, where her favorite pastime is hiking with family and friends.

Stanley A. Terman, PhD, MD, a bioethicist and board-certified psychiatrist in Sausalito, CA, introduced general readers to VSED in 2007 with *The BEST WAY to Say Goodbye: A Legal Peaceful Choice at the End of Life.* He has continued to dedicate his career to help those who fear future prolonged dying in advanced dementia and loved ones searching for ways to help their relatives who have already reached advanced dementia. His two protocols, "Strategic Advance Care Planning" and "NOW Care Planning," use My Way Cards*—a patient decision aid that illustrates and describes about 50 conditions—that asks, "Would this condition cause you enough suffering to want to die?" Dr. Terman is currently writing on how some flaws in current advance directives can be overcome by using the criterion "severe enough suffering."

Introduction

Voluntarily stopping eating and drinking, also known by its acronym VSED, is a practice in which a currently or prospectively seriously ill patient makes an intentional decision to hasten her own death by completely stopping the intake of all fluids and food. Although the process may appear grim at first glance, most people who initiate VSED find it tolerable and meaningful provided they work with an experienced, skillful clinician partner. VSED provides an opportunity to achieve a relatively peaceful, personally controlled death for those who seek an escape from the prospect of unacceptable suffering or deterioration in their present condition or foreseeable future. We begin by putting the practice in its broad context.

I.1. Patient and Caregiving Context

When people first learn they have a serious illness, they and their families usually first go to a health care setting where they get an accurate diagnosis and prognosis, and where they will have access to hopefully effective medical treatment. At that transition point, they formally become "patients" while continuing to be "persons." Since most persons exploring VSED are also patients, we will use these terms interchangeably while emphasizing that the patient's "personhood" is always in the center of the discussion (Cassel 1982).

Depending on their prior personal or family experiences with illness and death, many patients begin to wonder how they must adapt because of the challenges posed by their illness. Some may begin to consider the "what ifs" regarding how much suffering and debility they are willing to endure in the future. Many patients worry about these issues privately in silence, fearing that openly discussing their concerns will further frighten them as well as their families. Others may be interested in discussing what kinds of end-of-life options they might have should their suffering and quality of life become unacceptable to them.

Patients and their families often have pressing questions and concerns in four domains as they face serious, potentially fatal illness. (1) How can I be sure I am getting the best possible medical treatment for my disease? (2) How can I make the most of my situation given my new circumstances? (3) Is it time to focus all my energy on enhancing my quality of life? (4) What are my options to achieve a peaceful death, if the suffering or deterioration associated with my illness becomes more than I can or want to bear despite skilled efforts to treat and palliate my condition? Clinicians can potentially open the door to discussion in any or all of these four domains.

1. **How can I be sure I am getting the best medical treatment for my disease?** Our Western health care system is best equipped to address this domain. Our primary care system in the United States is currently fragile and unevenly available, but for most persons who get sick enough, it is relatively easy to find subspecialists and systems ready and willing to provide state-of-the-science, disease-directed treatment for most kinds of serious illnesses, both common and rare. Yet, depending on the illness with which a person is stricken, our medical treatments may be complex, burdensome, and not uniformly effective. Furthermore, some patients and their families may struggle with new limitations and suffering caused by their diseases and associated treatments.

2. **How can I make the most of my situation given my new circumstances?** Our current health care system is often much less clear about who will address this second domain, the palliation-focused prong of treatment. If the patient is lucky enough to have a primary care provider who already knows her personally and is willing to take on the role, then that may be the best option here. However, in the modern era, the presence of a personally committed primary care provider already engaged in the patient's world is often the exception rather than the rule. Next in line to serve this function might be the patient's new disease-specific specialist.

This second domain of care would include palliative care in the broadest sense of the practice, defined as addressing the biological, psychological, social, and spiritual dimensions of a patient's illness (Quill et al. 2019). As summarized in Box I.1, when and if the disease progresses and biological treatments become less effective, the psychological, social, and spiritual dimensions of the patient's illness may provide the biggest opportunity to address patient and family suffering and anguish. They must be explored to assist with meaningful medical decision-making. The specialty of palliative care has emerged to help address these dimensions, sometimes assisting and

---

Box I.1 Dimensions of Potential Suffering

Physical—pain, shortness of breath, confusion, weakness, nausea, vomiting....

Psychosocial—family distress, economic, caregiving challenges, living situation....

Existential—"Why me?" "How did this happen?" "Who am I now?"....

Spiritual—"How could a caring God let this happen?" "Why do bad things happen to good people?"....

---

backing up the already existing medical providers and treatment teams and other times taking on a primary treatment role in addressing and relieving the many potential sources of the patient's suffering.

3. Is it time to focus all my energy on enhancing my quality of life? Many seriously ill patients eventually reach a point when continued treatment of their underlying disease becomes relatively ineffective and/or overly burdensome, and no longer makes sense to them medically or personally. This painful transition point requires that they accept that disease-directed therapy is no longer working, and that the main effective treatments that clinicians have to offer are intended to improve the patient's quality of life. The bulk of treatment is then directed to maintaining the patient's comfort and dignity and to making the most of the time that remains.

Fortunately, hospice care helps address this challenging phase of a patient's illness with a sophisticated system of care, usually provided in a patient's own home but also potentially available in hospitals and nursing facilities. Its goal is to provide expert palliation and support for both patient and family toward the end of the patient's life. Of course, the initial transition to hospice may be psychologically very painful for patients and their families, as they must give up their hopes and dreams of cure or remission and a longer life through disease-directed treatment (Casarett and Quill 2007). Once patients and their families (and sometimes their treating doctors) work through this painful acceptance of the limits of medical treatment aimed at curing or stopping the progression of the disease, most eventually become appreciative of all that hospice can provide in terms of patient and family support and assistance with symptom-directed care.

Working together, these professionals can usually help the patient and family relieve much of the suffering associated with serious medical illnesses

(McCann et al. 1994). Nevertheless, at some point in this process, some patients or their family members may want to address the fourth question posed below.

4. What options do I have to achieve a peaceful escape through death if the suffering and prospective quality of life with my illness becomes more than I want to bear despite the best palliative efforts? Many seriously ill patients think privately about this question at differing points in their illness, but fear to bring it up with their medical providers because of worry they might be labeled "suicidal" or "weak." They may also fear that if they share these concerns with their medical providers, they might be perceived as "giving up" and will no longer be offered the full range of disease-directed treatments.

This fourth question may reflect the intention to hypothetically explore potential death-hastening options if suffering becomes unacceptably severe *in the future* while continuing current disease-directed and/or palliative treatment *in the present*. Alternatively, it may be asking about potential options for escaping suffering *right now* because the patient is feeling dissatisfied or even desperate about his or her current circumstance. We explore many of the clinical, ethical, legal, and institutional options for addressing both versions of the question in subsequent chapters and illustrate them with a wide range of clinical examples.

The seriously ill person, her family, and her clinicians must also think through their own personal moral boundaries, limits, and acceptable possibilities under such circumstances. There is widespread agreement about hospice being "standard of care" for such situations (provided the patient is terminally ill and finds that approach acceptable), but some may prefer other, more definitive "last resort" options that are less well known under the patient's current circumstances.

I.2. "Last Resort" Options

Hospice care is the standard of care for patients with an average overall prognosis of six months or less if the disease follows its usual course, and who have agreed to forgo further disease-directed therapy and accept only comfort-oriented treatments (Lynn 2001). Hospice patients generally agree not to start any new life-prolonging therapies and not to continue any disease-directed therapies they may have been receiving unless those are also contributing to their comfort and dignity.

If a patient who has not already been receiving best possible treatments asks about any available means for hastening death in their current clinical situation, a referral to a palliative care specialist or to a hospice program would almost always be in order first to ensure that all standard treatments to enhance comfort and dignity are considered if not tried. Even if a requesting patient is already receiving some form of hospice or palliative care, a request for a hastened death should not only be met by careful listening and exploration, but also by a re-evaluation and redoubling of efforts to address the causes of the underlying unacceptable suffering.

How should one move forward if a patient currently receiving the best possible hospice care asks about means for achieving death "now" rather than waiting for "nature to take its course"? Of course, all such patients should have a careful biopsychosocial and spiritual evaluation of the "why now" of this question. All efforts should first be made to assure that the patient is indeed receiving skillfully delivered palliation and support.

But what should these patients be offered when they are receiving skillful palliation while still requesting assistance in hastening death, and that request is genuine and consistent with their life story, medical situation, and personal values? What follows is a brief description of the options for hastening death under such difficult circumstances. (See Table I.1 for a summary list of the basic definitions of these options.)

Withholding or Withdrawing Life-Sustaining Treatment

The first place one looks in this domain would be the major treatments such as mechanical ventilators (breathing machines) and dialysis treatments (kidney replacement therapy), but this might also include implanted cardiac devices or any other specialized, potentially life-prolonging treatment for their condition. A second would be very basic life-extending treatments such as antibiotics for pneumonia.

Fully informed patients have a right to refuse all such treatments provided they have decision-making capacity, even if their desire and intention is to die sooner rather than later. Surrogate decision makers are also permitted to make these decisions on behalf of an incapacitated patient provided they believe it is what the patient would want under the current circumstances or what they believe is in the patient's best interests. Across most (but not

Table I.1 Definitions of Death-Hastening Measures to Address Current or Future Unacceptable Suffering or Deterioration

Withholding and Withdrawing Treatment

Life-Sustaining Treatment	Not starting, or stopping once started, potentially life-sustaining treatments (mechanical ventilator, cardiopulmonary resuscitation, antibiotics, etc.) with a patient not expected to survive without such measures.
Artificial Hydration and Nutrition	Not starting, or stopping once started, artificial hydration and nutrition (provided intravenously or directly through a feeding tube) with a patient who is unable to eat or drink enough to likely sustain herself in the near future.

Stopping Eating and Drinking (SED)

Voluntarily SED (VSED)	Complete cessation of all oral intake by a decisionally capable person who is physically able to eat and drink, with the intention of hastening his or her own death.
SED by Advance Directive (SED by AD)	Not providing any food or fluids to a person who has lost decision-making capacity based on the person's advance directive clearly stating that she would want this done in her current circumstances.
Withholding Manually Assisted Feeding by Mouth	Not assisting a person to eat or drink who is unable to self-feed because of coexisting medical problems, based on clear knowledge of his current (if still capacitated) or prior wishes (if capacity has been lost).

Palliative Sedation (PS)

Proportionate PS (PPS)	Providing gradually increasing amounts of sedation as needed to relieve the suffering of a seriously ill patient (relatively common practice) with the goal of maintaining alertness if possible. The process might end up with palliative sedation to unconsciousness if and only if lesser degrees of sedation are inadequate to provide relief.
PS to Unconsciousness (PSU)	Providing sedation to unconsciousness (PSU) is one step in response to severe, acute suffering that is usually from a medical emergency that cannot be otherwise mitigated. PSU should be relatively rare.

Lethal Medications

Medical Aid in Dying (MAID)*	Clinician-provided, but patient self-administered lethal medication. MAID is also known as "physician-assisted death," "physician aid-in-dying," or "aid in dying." It is also sometimes called "physician-assisted suicide," though this is not a preferred label because of the association of "suicide" with mental illness.
Euthanasia	Clinician-provided, and also clinician-administered lethal medication at the request of a seriously ill, decisionally capable patient at a time of the patient's choosing (also called Voluntary Active Euthanasia).
Euthanasia by Advance Directive	Clinician-provided, and also clinician-administered lethal medication to a seriously ill patient without decision-making capacity based on a clearly expressed prior request from the patient.

*In Canada, the term MAID also includes the practice of Euthanasia as defined above. In almost all other jurisdictions, MAID is defined more narrowly as above, and we have chosen that definition in this book.

all) Western religions and cultures there is widespread agreement about the permissibility of stopping life-sustaining therapy even with the intent of hastening death, and it is almost always legally permitted.

Withholding and Withdrawing Artificial Hydration and Nutrition

Some ethicists and some religions (e.g., Orthodox Jewish) separate artificial hydration and nutrition through feedings tubes as basic or fundamental life-sustaining treatment that is part of basic human caring, and not a medical treatment that can be withdrawn or withheld. If a person from such a tradition was unable to speak for herself about her wishes under such circumstances and had not make her preferences clear in this domain in the past, the family and clinical team should consider meeting with faith leaders from the patient's tradition to try to understand the meaning of such acts from that tradition.

Voluntarily Stopping Eating and Drinking (VSED)

With VSED, the patient hastens her death by completely stopping the intake of all fluids and food. Clinicians should be fully involved in the initial patient evaluation and in ensuring informed consent. Clinicians should also commit to providing intensive symptom management and support throughout the VSED process from initiation until the patient's death. Otherwise, in terms of direct implementation, VSED is almost completely under a patient's own control. VSED is different from comfort-oriented feeding in important ways (Quill et al. 2018; Horowitz, Sussman, and Quill 2016). First and foremost, the patient pursuing VSED usually is suppressing the natural drive to eat and drink with the intention of achieving an earlier death.

Once VSED is initiated, the drive to eat diminishes relatively quickly as the patient becomes ketotic (the ketones generated in this circumstance are a byproduct of the body trying to generate fuel when there is no calorie intake, and they tend to negate the subjective sensation of hunger). As VSED progresses, however, the now dehydrating patient often becomes profoundly thirsty, a symptom that can be very challenging to manage, requiring patient discipline and palliative care guidance and support. VSED usually takes about 10–14 days from initiation to death depending both on the patient's state of hydration at the outset and on how successfully she can adhere to not swallowing any liquids. VSED by seriously ill patients with full decision-making capacity is the subject of the first half of this book.

Stopping Eating and Drinking by Advance Directive (SED by AD)

While VSED is for patients with decision-making capacity, stopping eating and drinking by advance directive allows patients to leave instructions now that if and when she later loses decision-making capacity and reaches a spec-ified level of deterioration or discomfort, she wants food and fluids withheld as a means of hastening her death. The application of instructions for SED by AD would be initiated by designated surrogate decision makers who had previously been specifically empowered to do this by the previously capaci-tated patient for a later time when the pre-specified triggering circumstances are met.

SED by AD remains significantly more controversial than standard VSED, given the absence of decision-making capacity and lack of contemporaneous consent by the patient. The clinical, ethical, legal, and institutional aspects of AD for SED on behalf of a seriously ill patient who has lost capacity but had previously expressed clear consent for the process are the subject of the second half of this book.

Withholding Manually Assisted Feeding by Mouth

Withholding manually assisted feeding by mouth is a special case of SED where a patient has become dependent on caregiver-assisted eating and drinking by mouth, usually because of a chronically debilitating condition such as end stage Parkinson's disease, amyotrophic lateral sclerosis (ALS), or end stage dementia. If the patient had full decision-making capacity (ALS, typically), then this decision to stop eating and drinking would be very sim-ilar to a usual VSED decision as outlined above. If decision-making capacity had been lost, as in end stage dementia, then the decision would be similar to SED by AD, requiring a clear prior articulation of the person's preferences about having assistance with eating and drinking continued or stopped if decision-making capacity is lost in the future.

Proportionate Palliative Sedation (PPS)

With proportionate palliative sedation, the clinician provides sedatives to help the patient escape the conscious experience of unacceptable suffering that has been inadequately responsive to unrestrained use of usual palliative treatments (Cherny and Portenoy 1994; Lo and Rubenfeld 2005). The level of sedation should be proportionate to that needed to adequately relieve the patient's suffering—not more and not less. In cases where suffering is particularly severe, sedation may need to be progressively increased to a level that renders the patient unconscious, but only if lesser levels of sedation were inadequate.

PPS is relatively common in US hospice and palliative care programs, but with considerable variability in how frequently and how aggressively it is utilized. Proportionate sedation usually does not hasten death, and hastening death is generally not its intent, though in circumstances where sedation to unconsciousness is required to relieve severe suffering, death may be somewhat hastened because patients can no longer eat and drink.

Palliative Sedation to Unconsciousness (PSU)

Although unconsciousness may rarely be the end point of PPS, it is the intended end point for PSU, which is reserved for relatively rare palliative care emergencies (e.g., a patient with neck cancer whose tumor is eroding into his carotid artery and he is actively and traumatically bleeding to death). These cases must be addressed emergently, as delay is usually traumatic for patient, family, and staff. There is considerable variation among palliative care and hospice programs in terms of how frequently PSU is implemented and what are the appropriate indications (Quill, Lo, and Brock 1997; Jansen and Sulmasy 2002; Cherny and Portenoy 1994; Rietjens et al. 2008). We advise careful review of these cases to ensure that the decision to initiate PSU is based on clear indications.

Medical Aid in Dying (MAID)

Medical aid in dying occurs when a terminally ill patient with decision-making capacity requests and then receives a prescription for a dose of medication to achieve a desired death to escape a current or future situation that is associated or potentially associated with unacceptable suffering or deterioration. The clinician provides a qualifying patient with a prescription for a lethal medication in response to the patient's specific request. The patient may then take the medication by her own hand at a time of her own choosing. Or she may be reassured by the possibility, but then choose not to take it at all (Quill, Lo, and Brock 1997; Quill, Lee, and Nunn 2000).

In some jurisdictions, waiting periods up to twenty days are required between the patient's initial request and receipt of the prescription. The clinician is morally responsible as an assistant, but the patient must independently take the medication by his or her own hand to complete the process. In the United States, MAID is currently legal in ten US states and the District of Columbia. MAID is also legal in three Australian states, all of Canada, Columbia, New Zealand, and five Western European countries (Netherlands, Belgium, Luxembourg, Spain, and Switzerland).[1]

Euthanasia

Euthanasia is like MAID in that the patient is provided a lethal medication at her own explicit request. But with euthanasia, the clinician directly administers the lethal medication intravenously to the patient at a time of the patient's choosing. In euthanasia the clinician is both an accomplice and the final actor, albeit at the patient's explicit request. In jurisdictions where both MAID and euthanasia are legally available (like Canada and the Netherlands), patients choose euthanasia much more frequently than MAID (Health Canada 2019). There is some evidence that clinicians find assisting patients with euthanasia more psychologically burdensome than MAID (Abohaimed et al. 2019).

Euthanasia by Advance Directive

In most jurisdictions where euthanasia is legally permitted, it is reserved for those with contemporaneous decision-making capacity. However,

---

[1] In the United States, the term "Medical Aid in Dying" (MAID) includes only clinician-assisted, *patient* delivered death. Other jurisdictions additionally permit clinician-assisted, *clinician* delivered death (euthanasia); in those jurisdictions, the latter is overwhelmingly preferred by patients and clinicians (Health Canada 2019). We use "MAID" in this book exclusively in the narrow definition: clinician-assisted, *patient* delivered death.

the Netherlands, Belgium, Columbia, and Luxembourg allow euthanasia based on a clearly articulated advance directive for those who have lost decision-making capacity but made it clear that they would want euthanasia to be implemented under what is now their current condition (Canada Department of Justice 2016). Having lost the important anchor of contemporaneous consent, this practice remains very controversial and is not legally permitted elsewhere (Miller, Dresser, and Kim 2019).

Table I.2 summarizes each of the death-accelerating measures reviewed above. It distinguishes them according to the cause of death, final actor, and decision-making capacity requirements.

Table I.2 Distinguishing Features of Death-Hastening Measures to Address Unacceptable Current or Future Suffering or Deterioration

Death-Hastening Measure	Cause of Death	Final Actor	Capacity at Initiation
Withholding and Withdrawing Treatment			
Life-Sustaining Treatment (LST)	Absence of LST	Clinician and/ or Patient	Yes or No
Artificial Nutrition/Hydration	Dehydration	Clinician and/ or Patient	Yes or No
Stopping Eating and Drinking (SED)			
Voluntarily SED (VSED)	Dehydration	Patient	Yes
SED by Advance Directive (SED by AD)	Dehydration	Clinician or Other Caregivers	No
Withholding Manually Assisted Feeding by Mouth	Dehydration	Clinician or Other Caregivers	Yes or No
Palliative Sedation (PS)			
Proportionate PS (PPS)	Sedation and Dehydration (May not cause)	Clinician	Yes or No
PS to Unconsciousness (PSU)	Sedation and Dehydration	Clinician	Yes or No
Lethal Medications			
Medical Aid in Dying (MAID)	Lethal Drug	Patient	Yes
Euthanasia	Lethal Drug	Clinician	Yes
Euthanasia by Advance Directive	Lethal Drug	Clinician	No

I.3. Advantages and Challenges

If VSED (and SED by AD) had little if any advantage relative to the other death-hastening measures outlined above, there would be little point in writing this book. VSED does, however, have some distinct attractions once people understand that the process can be a relatively peaceful and comfortable path to death when accompanied by appropriate palliative support.

VSED has five advantages over MAID and euthanasia:

1. VSED is legal in virtually all jurisdictions, whereas MAID and euthanasia are illegal in the majority of countries worldwide and the majority of states in the United States.
2. Even where legal, MAID and euthanasia are often restricted to conditions with a "terminal" prognosis (likely death within six months). The liberty to pursue VSED, by contrast, has virtually no such prognostic restrictions. It can therefore be a realistic option for people with slowly progressive disease (e.g., most progressive dementias, including Alzheimer's).
3. VSED can often provide a faster path than MAID or euthanasia, where qualifying for eligibility and receiving an actual prescription may take considerably longer than VSED's typical 10- to 14-day timeline.
4. While it is wise to have clinician and family partners throughout the process, VSED is almost entirely within a patient's own personal control.
5. Because VSED requires considerable patient resolve and will power to carry through to completion, potential doubts about the patient's consent are minimized.

VSED also has two advantages over even refusing life-sustaining treatment.

1. VSED is not dependent on a circumstance of needing lifesaving or life-sustaining treatment, providing the opportunity to hasten death when there is no lifesaving treatment for the patient to refuse.
2. Even when there is life-sustaining treatment to refuse, VSED is sometimes a faster and more comfortable route to death. Refusing lifesaving treatment (e.g., stopping medical treatment for congestive heart failure) might involve weeks or even months of suffering that can potentially be difficult to adequately palliate.

Nonetheless, despite these advantages, VSED, and especially SED by AD, confront distinct challenges in many dimensions. Some of these challenges are actual barriers, and others are potential problems that can be managed or negotiated with competent care or advice. VSED is most straightforward when it is initiated by seriously ill patients who have full decision-making capacity. This possibility is explored in detail from clinical, ethical, legal, and policy perspectives in Part I of this book. The process of stopping eating and drinking might also be initiated on behalf of incapacitated patients who have let it be known with clearly articulated advance directives (ADs for SED) that they would want this option if and when they subsequently lose capacity, but then can no longer consent in "real time." Such a decision might be supported by a "Ulysses Contract" (introduced and defined in Chapter 10, Section 10.9). This unique advance directive would be completed while the person still had decision-making capacity, clearly stating that she would want food, drink, and other non-palliative treatment withheld once decision-making capacity is lost, even if then she still seems to enjoy eating and drinking. Such an advance directive would provide substantial evidence about the now incapacitated patient's prior wishes in this domain, but it is not without the clinical, ethical, legal, and policy challenges to be explored in Part II of this book.

We hope this book addresses the opportunities and challenges of both of these practices in sufficiently thorough detail but also in an accessible manner, so that a wide audience of clinicians, counselors, patients, family members, attorneys, institutional administrators, and other interested parties can become familiar with what they need to know about VSED and about SED by AD as realistic options.

Of course, these options for many individual reasons are not "for everyone," especially because they require a great deal of personal determination, resolve, support by others, and advance planning. We hope this book enlightens the reader about the possibilities of both VSED and SED by AD. But this book should never be read as urging people to hasten death this way, or at all. That choice is strictly an individual prerogative.

I.4. Basic Plan for This Book

This book is divided into two major parts. Part I is devoted to the standard practice of voluntarily stopping eating and drinking for patients with decision-making capacity (VSED). Part II explores the possibility of allowing advance directives for stopping eating and drinking (AD for SED), completed when a patient has decision-making capacity and activated later by clinicians and family members when the patient's decision-making capacity has been lost (SED by AD).

The two parts of the book have similar structures. They begin with several detailed presentations of real patients who engaged in variations of VSED or SED by AD, as recollected and experienced by the treating clinicians, family members, or friends. At the end of each case, the editors identify a series of challenges and questions raised by the case for consideration in the subsequent chapters. Four subsequent chapters within each part focus on clinical and cultural issues (Tim E. Quill, Judith K. Schwarz, and V. J. Periyakoil), ethical issues (Paul T. Menzel and Dena Davis), legal issues (Thaddeus M. Pope), and institutional issues (David Gruenewald).

The final chapter in each of the two parts of the book identifies key summary points divided into three sub-categories:

Best Practices, including characteristics of patients for whom VSED or AD for SED are likely to be successful in achieving a peaceful, dignified death. They also identify markers for when VSED is more likely to be more successful or more problematic in comparison with other more standard palliative care or last-resort approaches.

Enduring Challenges, including symptom management during the process (especially for thirst and delirium) as well as the challenges posed by an aging population, a growing incidence of dementing illness, and increasing cultural diversity where practices like VSED may prove more problematic.

Opportunities that VSED and AD for SED may provide in people's search for a wider range of meaningful end-of-life options amidst changing law and evolving clinical practice.

Bibliographies of references used by the authors preparing individual chapters focusing on the clinical, ethical, legal, cultural, and institutional aspects of VSED and SED by AD close each of the chapters in the book. In addition, a wide range of additional resources and links to related websites are available in the Appendices.

References

Abohaimed, Shaikhah Salah, Basma Matar, Hussain Al-Shimali, Khalid Al-Thalji, Omar Al-Othman, Yasmin Zurba, and Nasra Shah. 2019. "Attitudes of Physicians towards Different Types of Euthanasia in Kuwait." *Medical Principles and Practice* 28: 199–207.

Canada Department of Justice. 2016. "Legislative Background: Medical Assistance in Dying." https://www.justice.gc.ca/eng/rp-pr/other-autre/index.html.

Casarett, David J., and Timothy E. Quill. 2007. "'I'm not ready for hospice': Strategies for Timely and Effective Hospice Discussions." *Annals of Internal Medicine* 146, no. 6: 443–449.

Cassel, Eric J. 1982. "The Nature of Suffering and the Goals of Medicine." *New England Journal of Medicine* 306, no. 11: 639–645.

Cherny, Nathan I., and Russel K. Portenoy. 1994. "Sedation in the Management of Refractory Symptoms: Guidelines for Evaluation and Treatment." *Journal of Palliative Care* 10, no. 2: 31–38.

Health Canada. 2019. "Fourth Interim Report on Medical Assistance in Dying in Canada." https://www.canada.ca/en/health-canada/services/publications/health-system-services/medical-assistance-dying-interim-report-april-2019.html.

Horowitz, Robert, Bernard Sussman, and Timothy Quill. 2016. "VSED Narratives: Exploring Complexity." *Narrative Inquiry in Bioethics* 6, no. 2: 115–120.

Jansen, Lynn A., and Daniel P. Sulmasy. 2002. "Sedation, Alimentation, Hydration, and Equivocation: Careful Conversation about Care at the End of Life." *Annals of Internal Medicine* 136, no. 11: 845–849.

Lo, Bernard, and Gordon Rubenfeld. 2005. "Palliative Sedation in Dying Patients: 'We turn to it when everything else hasn't worked.'" *JAMA* 294, no. 14: 1810–1816.

Lynn, Joanne. 2001. "Perspectives on Care at the Close of Life. Serving Patients Who May Die Soon and Their Families: The Role of Hospice and Other Services." *JAMA* 285, no. 7: 925–932.

McCann, Robert M., William J. Hall, and Ann-Marie Groth-Juncker. 1994. "Comfort Care for Terminally Ill Patients: The Appropriate Use of Nutrition and Hydration." *JAMA* 272, no. 16: 1263–1266.

Miller, David G., Rebecca Dresser, and Scott Y.H. Kim. 2019. "Advance Euthanasia Directives: A Controversial Case and Its Ethical Implications." *Journal of Medical Ethics* 45, no. 2: 84–89.

Quill, Timothy E., Barbara Lee, and Sally Nunn. 2000. "Palliative Treatments of Last Resort: Choosing the Least Harmful Alternative." *Annals of Internal Medicine* 132, no. 6: 499–493.

Quill, Timothy E., Bernard Lo, and Dan W. Brock. 1997. "Palliative Options of Last Resort: A Comparison of Voluntarily Stopping Eating and Drinking, Terminal Sedation, Physician-Assisted Suicide, and Voluntary Active Euthanasia. *JAMA* 278, no.23: 2099–2014.

Quill, Timothy E., Linda Ganzini, Robert D. Troug, and Thaddeus M. Pope. 2018. "Voluntarily Stopping Eating and Drinking: Clinical, Ethical, and Legal Aspects." *JAMA Intern Med* 178, no. 1: 123–127.

Quill, Timothy E., Vyjeyanthi J. Periyakoil, Erin Denney-Koelsch, Patrick White, and Donna Zhurhovsky. 2019. *Primer of Palliative Care, 7th Edition*. Chicago, IL: American Academy of Hospice and Palliative Medicine.

Rietjens, J.A., L. van Zuylen, H. van Veluw, L. van der Wijk, A. van der Heide, and C.C. van der Rijt. 2008. "Palliative Sedation in a Specialized Unit for Acute Palliative Care in a Cancer Hospital: Comparing Patients Dying With and Without Palliative Sedation." *Journal of Pain Symptom Management* 36, no. 3: 228–234.

Stevens, Kenneth R. 2006. "Emotional and Psychological Effects of Physician Assisted Suicide and Euthanasia on Participating Physicians." *Linacre Q* 73, no. 3: 203–216.

PART I

VOLUNTARILY STOPPING EATING AND DRINKING (VSED) BY PEOPLE WITH DECISION-MAKING CAPACITY

Part I of this book explores voluntarily stopping eating and drinking (VSED) by persons who have serious illness, currently unacceptable suffering or fear about such future suffering or deterioration, and who have decision-making capacity to make a major life and death decision. Part I is divided into six chapters:

Chapter 1. Illustrative Cases, each followed by the editors' views of their most notable characteristics and issues raised. The subsequent five chapters will follow up on these cases, exploring some of the challenges of VSED from different professional perspectives.

Chapter 2. Clinical Issues, including evaluation, initiation requirements, advance care planning, symptom management, cultural considerations, and advantages/disadvantages of the practice.

Chapter 3. Ethical Issues, including comparisons with refusing lifesaving treatment, MAID, and other end-of-life possibilities, and whether VSED constitutes "suicide" and palliative support for it "assisting in suicide."

Chapter 4. Legal Issues, including the perception and reality of VSED's legal status, its potential inclusion in right to refuse laws, and potential conscientious objection by health care providers.

Chapter 5. Institutional Issues, including prevalence and acceptability, barriers, residents' rights, role of hospice, and recommendations for practice in these settings.

Chapter 6. Best Practices, Enduring Challenges, and Opportunities for VSED, including a summary of bottom-line points from the previous five chapters and an assessment of VSED's future place in end-of-life care.

1

Illustrative Cases

The editors have assembled four previously unpublished cases that illustrate the advantages and the challenges of VSED for patients who wish to hasten death. The cases have different authors, some of whom are not one of the volume's editors. At the end of each case the editors have added what they view as some of the "notable characteristics" of the case and the "issues raised" by it.

Case 1.1—Al (Amyotrophic Lateral Sclerosis): Looking for Options to Hasten Death

"What [escape] options do I have?"

Timothy E. Quill

Al was an accountant by day and a Harley motorcycle enthusiast who loved traveling and socializing with his motorcycle "brothers and sisters." In his mid-40s, he developed a headache and had some difficulty physically managing his bike, followed by some detectable weakness on his right side. Al reluctantly made a doctor's appointment and was diagnosed with a localized malignant brain tumor. He was treated with surgery and whole brain radiation therapy and temporarily prohibited from riding his bike. Over the next two years, he was deemed to be "cured" and gradually regained nearly full functioning, eventually getting the green light to return to motorcycle riding, albeit on a "three-wheeler."

Life returned to near normal for the ensuing fifteen years, but then Al gradually developed progressive weakness in his arms and legs. His neurologists were initially baffled. There was no evidence of tumor recurrence, but something was definitely wrong. Motorcycling was quickly out of the question, and it was not long before even walking became a risky challenge. He eventually was diagnosed with amyotrophic lateral sclerosis (ALS), probably due to a late complication of his past whole brain radiation treatment. He couldn't believe what was happening to him, but he adapted as best he could, initially riding on the back of his friends' motorcycles, then requiring a wheelchair for getting around, and eventually becoming completely bed-bound over the next nine months.

With the assistance of Medicaid, Al was able to arrange a group of very dedicated nursing aides who cared for him at his own home 24/7. He couldn't get out of bed by himself, and then needed help with toileting, and eventually with eating. And he kept getting weaker. Al's care at home was excellent, but he began to consider whether he wanted to keep living under these circumstances. His nursing aides were completely opposed to his making any decision toward accepting death for multiple reasons: (1) they cared deeply about him; (2) most felt that making any choices toward death was morally wrong; and (3) they worried he might be depressed.

Al asked for a home visit from me, so his concerns and wishes in this regard could be openly explored. In our visit, he grieved the elements of life he had lost. But Al still enjoyed visits from his motorcycle friends and his family, watching TV and reading, and he genuinely appreciated the loving care from his nursing aides, with whom he had become very close. But areas of enjoyment were not enough for him to keep living. He had always been "fiercely independent" and now he had virtually no privacy or independence in his eyes. He had no severe pain, dyspnea, or other debilitating symptoms that were not being adequately palliated, and he was not clinically depressed. If he lived in Oregon, Al would have requested and might have qualified for physician-assisted death (he was an adult with decision-making capacity, though his prognosis may have been too long to qualify). But he lived in Rochester, New York, where such options were (and still are) not legally allowed.

He asked about his options, and I told him about the possibility of voluntarily stopping eating and drinking (VSED). Al could no longer feed himself at this point as his arms were too weak, but his aides had become very skilled at preparing soft foods that he both tolerated and enjoyed. I informed him that he could refuse all food and fluids, and we could palliate any symptoms that occurred as a result. The process would likely take 10–14 days from start to finish, provided he was fully committed to not drinking. His nursing aides were adamantly opposed to this decision, so we also discussed that to pursue this option he would probably need to be admitted to an inpatient facility. Because VSED had not been previously instituted in our hospital and might have been perceived to be ethically controversial, I also suggested two things that would be wise if Al wanted to pursue this in the hospital: a psychiatric consult to ensure full decision-making capacity (though I doubted it was really clinically needed) and, more important, an ethics consult to reassure the hospital administration that this action is permissible. With our hospital never having previously cared for a patient choosing VSED, we were perhaps overly cautious to minimize the degree of potential "second-guessing" of the decision by our administration. In any case, the consultations also lessened the moral distress of the inpatient providers, many of whom had not carefully considered these issues in the past.

Sometimes people who learn they can have an escape through VSED or other potential last-resort options feel less trapped by their illness and choose at least for a while to keep eating and drinking. However, shortly after being informed of this option, Al decided to pursue it as soon as possible. Not surprisingly, his home health aides and their agency decided they could not support him doing VSED at home. After discussing the potential plan with our hospital administration, I admitted Al to our palliative care unit. We also discussed the plan with our staff members and gave them the option of not participating if any felt they could not morally live with their role in his death (none choose this option). Our psychiatry and ethics consultants found Al to have decision-making capacity, and made the analogy between VSED and stopping life-sustaining therapy, which he clearly would have a right to do.

He fully stopped eating and drinking within 24 hours of arrival to our unit. Our staff talked with his home health aides about any tips they had about his physical care, and they were invited to visit as family members as long as they did not try to undermine his decision. Al had a steady stream of visits from his motorcycle friends, who were supportive but deeply saddened by the impending death of their friend. His home health aides also visited and tried to make peace with his decision. Not eating and drinking for him was not difficult, as his now advanced ALS made the eating process a prolonged ordeal every day that he was glad to give up. Our staff also found caring for him very meaningful as they came to grips with his decision and how sometimes common sense can resolve what appears to be a major ethical, medical, and legal dilemma. Al died 12 days after starting VSED, surrounded by several friends and one of his former nursing aides, remaining alert, engaged, and appreciative until the very end.

Notable Characteristics

- VSED was the only feasible, legal way Al could hasten death.
- He asked about potential life-ending options and was then informed of the possibility of VSED.
- VSED was not difficult for Al, given how much of an ordeal eating and drinking had already become. He also received excellent palliative support.
- He preferred to remain at home, but he was unable to otherwise care for himself without the assistance of home health aides (toileting, changing position, manipulating his environment in any way). His home health aides were not comfortable caring for him if they were not allowed to feed him. He then gained admission to a nearby palliative care unit.
- VSED provided time for saying goodbye. His home health aides visited regularly, and eventually most came to understand if not fully accept his decision.

Issues Raised

- Should Al have been able to remain at home (with home hospice) despite his aides' objection to not being allowed to feed him? Should his other providers and his family all have tried harder to replace those aides with others who would support his choice so that he could remain at home? Should his aides have been more strongly encouraged to accept his VSED despite their moral objections to it? Were their moral objections personal, or were they professional?
- How would things have proceeded if Al had not had good palliative care?
- Is VSED analogous to stopping life-sustaining therapy, or is it different because it concerns "basic" care, not "medical" care?
- While Al's care at home was "excellent," how would non-optimal care affect the voluntariness of a decision to VSED?

Case 1.2—Bill (Breast Cancer): Preference for Medical Aid in Dying

"What right do they have to say how I should die?"

Timothy E. Quill

Bill was a 55-year-old man who had metastatic breast cancer. He was a self-employed, "fiercely independent" man who successfully ran his own small business. He was married with no children, and had many hobbies, interests, and strong opinions. His life was very full and satisfying. He had a family history of aggressive breast cancer in many female relatives, but he was the first male to have contracted the disease. He had witnessed several very difficult deaths from cancer in other family members, and he had already joined the Hemlock Society to be sure his own end-of-life options would include controlling the manner and timing of his own death, which was clearly what he wanted when his time came. He was not afraid of death, but he wanted no part of becoming physically dependent on others, much less experiencing severe suffering should it occur in his future.

Bill began hormonal treatment shortly after having a bilateral mastectomy after his initial diagnosis. When his disease progressed, he then tried chemotherapy which he tolerated. It seemed to keep his disease at bay for a time. He specifically asked his primary treating oncologist for a palliative care consultation with me personally because of my past advocacy of open access to a physician-assisted death, part of what he wanted access to in the future should he "need it." By that time in my career, my advocacy in this domain ironically had made it more difficult for me personally to provide access to the medications needed to successfully achieve this end (although he would have qualified by his prognosis if he lived in any of the U.S. states where MAID is currently legal, the practice was and is still illegal in New York State).

Bill was very angry that this option was not openly available to him should he become terminally ill in the future, and he was not at all satisfied or interested in considering the other potential last-resort options such as voluntarily stopping eating and drinking (VSED) which he thought was "immature and barbaric." His contact with the Hemlock Society was also not very satisfying. Access to barbiturates had become increasingly restricted, and other potentially lethal medication combinations that were being advocated seemed less certain to be effective.

His metastatic cancer very slowly progressed with no major crises over the next six months until Bill developed a pathological fracture in his right femur (main long bone in his leg). He was admitted to the hospital and almost immediately developed another fracture in his left humerus (upper arm). He was now bed-bound, dependent on others for toileting or moving around at all, but without any vital organ deterioration that would "naturally" end his life. He was beginning to live out his worst nightmare. He had little or no pain if he was still, but any movement could be excruciating.

He again privately requested a medically assisted death from me with full knowledge that I could probably not provide it, and again he lamented how unfair he found his situation to be: "What right do they have to say how I should die?" While in the hospital Bill participated in teaching conferences where he articulated his wishes and values, hoping to influence how the medical establishment thinks about these options in the future. He even completed a video interview with me on the subject, which was published online as part of a series of articles in the *New York Times.*

Although Bill clearly wanted and was ready to die, he had no life-sustaining therapies (such as a breathing machine or dialysis for kidney failure) that could be legally stopped to achieve that end, and his symptoms, while severe with movement, did not seem severe enough to warrant palliative sedation to unconsciousness. Because his anger was at times very severe and we were concerned that it might possibly be distorting his judgment, we asked psychiatry to help us determine if his thinking was being altered by clinical depression. However, the consulting psychiatrist learned once again that both his passion and this request were consistent with long-standing personality traits and long-held views and values, and there was no distortion in his thinking from any mental illness.

I contemplated whether again to raise the possibility of initiating VSED, which he initially found to be so unacceptable; in my opinion it was his only realistic option in New York State given his clinical circumstances. When I did again raise this possibility, his initial response was a similar burst of anger and lament. But we also discussed that if he was serious about wanting an escape through death, VSED was probably his only non-violent option. (He was well aware that suicide using guns was not 100% effective, and that even if it "worked," his wife would be left devastated by the event.)

Over the next 24 hours, Bill accepted VSED and wanted to start right away. I asked that he undergo consultations with psychiatry and with medical ethics, which he agreed to (more for me than for him in his mind). Both consultations found that he had decision-making capacity and that this choice was consistent with his long-standing views, values, and personality. Bill was clearly a person who valued being in control of his life and his situation, and VSED put him back in the "driver's seat" of his life and his death. Having come to know Bill over the days since his admission to our palliative care unit, our staff was also supportive if he chose this option, and felt it made sense according to what they had learned about him.

Once he started to VSED, Bill did not waver. At his request we offered him nothing to eat or drink, and he assiduously avoided swallowing even the tiny amounts of liquid saliva used to keep his mouth moist. He lamented he could not have the option of a clinician-assisted death that he believed to be more rational, humane, and responsive to his situation. But he also acknowledged that VSED was far better for him than a lingering death filled with unacceptable dependence on others for all aspects of his care, and probably increased lack of control of his own body and mind as his disease inevitably would progress. Bill died quietly and relatively peacefully about twelve days after starting VSED. It was not the death he wanted, but it was the "least worst" solution given the options available (Battin 1996).

Notable Characteristics

- Bill was clear from start that he badly wanted not only to avoid great suffering but also to avoid being physically dependent on others.
- He was angry he could not access Medical Aid In Dying (MAID).
- He initially rejected VSED as "immature and barbaric." When the option was raised again later and he realized it was his only realistic, non-violent way to escape his condition, he pursued VSED decisively and never wavered.
- He agreed to psychiatric exams before pursuing VSED, but he did so probably more in deference to his physician than for his own protection.
- He was well supported by caregivers throughout the process and died peacefully in twelve days.

Issues Raised

- Should the option of VSED be raised with a patient who does not ask about it? Should the subject be raised only for those patients inquiring in some way about methods to hasten death, or should it be discussed with all terminally ill patients?

- In the majority of jurisdictions where informed consent requires physicians to discuss all options that a reasonable patient would deem significant, with which patients must physicians discuss VSED?
- If VSED is raised and the patient initially firmly rejects it, should it be raised again later if and when his conditions worsen?
- Should we respect Bill's decision based on his desire to avoid physical dependence as much as we would if his primary reason were to avoid other forms of physical suffering?
- Should a psychiatric evaluation be required for *all* patients seriously considering VSED, or just those where there is clinical suspicion about lack of decision-making capacity or presence of significant mental illness?

Case 1.3—Mrs. H. (Early Alzheimer's Disease): How Best to Time VSED

"Someday, Robby, someday . . . "

Robert K. Horowitz

My 85-year-old mother ended her life by voluntarily stopping eating and drinking (VSED) to terminate the progression of her dementia. I recorded several of our discussions about VSED, and Mom granted me full permission to share their content, including the quotations below, to humanize our experience.

Mom learned about VSED from an acquaintance whose adult son "L" had a progressive neuromuscular disease. I am a palliative care physician who cared for L during his last years and through his death by VSED. Mom was moved by his autonomy and decisiveness in the face of tragedy, and she came to me to learn more about VSED, which she considered "a much better way to go than going to one of those . . . [nursing] homes. . . . I did not want that in the worst way. . . . So, I did ask you, because who else was I going to ask?" As I spelled out the process and its challenges, Mom smiled, her eyes brightened, and with a shake of her finger and nod of her head she forecast, "Someday, Robby, someday . . . ."

Mom's dementia was exposed a year later when Dad's death ended his compensations for her losses. Ever compulsively dependable and keenly attuned to place, people, and propriety, Mom began receiving notices of unpaid bills, got lost driving familiar roads, and grew more isolated, suspicious, and critical. Her internist established the diagnosis of dementia, soon confirmed by a dementia expert and a geriatric psychiatrist. This revelation devastated Mom, who had described dementia as a "nightmare" into which her own mother disappeared forty years earlier, ultimately dying frail, lost, and alone in a nursing home.

We four children encouraged her to consider assisted living, to which our characteristically proper Mom seethed, "No fucking way!" To accommodate her insistence on remaining in the home she and Dad built to live and die in, we hired 24-hour aides, an intrusion that infuriated her. She begrudgingly tried antidepressant and dementia medications, as well as talk and physical therapies. Over months of continuing decline, we took her car keys, turned off the stove gas, and installed an automated medication dispenser, which became for her a maddening, squawking symbol of her dwindling independence and of our expanding privations.

Mom complained in enduring our protective encroachments until, provoked by one too many humiliations, she revisited "that thing we talked about," VSED. "I cannot go much longer, Honey . . . my memory is getting worse all along . . . little by little, and all too much I am losing the ability to express myself the way I want to. . . . I don't have a car, I can't walk too well . . . . It gets sad, you know?" Her dreaded, promised "someday" had arrived, one year after her dementia was formally diagnosed.

A trusted physician colleague agreed to take us on, starting with a home visit. Mom was delighted, and more light-hearted than she'd been in months, because she now believed it possible to avert the mounting fate she so dreaded. After meeting with our family, the doctor met privately with Mom. When they emerged an hour later, he announced two things. First, despite her real and evolving dementia, Mom retained capacity to make decisions about VSED, something which aligned with her long-held and very public sentiments. Second, she was "serious about VSED, but not ready"; she intended to live some more.

Mom's deferral was both relieving—more time to savor, remember, connect!—and distressing, because before her loomed a window of unknowable but finite duration during which she would remain able to carry out VSED before dementia's progression shut it, forever. There followed three months of joys and tensions, sweet connection, and anguished goodbyes, and two more visits from the doctor, before they emerged from their third private dialogue with his announcement, "She's ready, now." My heart sank and soared. Grief and relief. Mom dutifully reviewed her calendar and selected a date five weeks hence that would not taint any of the family birthdays, anniversaries, or other celebrations she still meticulously recorded.

Mom then mothered us with reassurance about our sorrow and trepidation: "This doesn't frighten me, this doesn't discourage me." In response to a few friends' protests about her decision to die, she reflected about VSED, "I don't think of it as suicide, but darn it all, it is." We came to realize that, applied to our Mom, the tired catchphrase "fiercely independent" was neither cliché nor hyperbole, but a literal description; facing down dementia, she was savage, a ferocious adversary choosing to die in order to not succumb to it.

The Sunday before "day one," three and a half months after her first visit with her physician to discuss VSED, Mom shared her last family supper— take-out burgers, French fries, and ice cream sundaes with the works. Monday, she signed onto home hospice. With her cheerful approval this time, we hired experienced hospice nurses to be as remote as reasonable and as involved as necessary. Mom played host the first four days, dressed neatly in slacks, sweater, and beaded necklace, reminiscing and saying goodbyes to selected friends and family, reading her favorite mysteries, and resting in her recliner. She felt "a touch dry," a symptom quelled by a frozen teething ring sprayed with Biotene, and, as it intensified, eased with modest doses of lorazepam. Low-dose opioids relieved her chronic and escalating musculoskeletal pains. Hunger never troubled her, because, being a lifelong binge dieter, she had plenty of practice and endurance; she giggled with pleasure and pride as her refractory leg edema receded.

From day five onward, the family and professional caregivers tended to Mom, who would be dressed forevermore in flannel pajamas, and mostly in bed. She was ever quieter, slower to respond, feeling "dopey but good," sharing occasional smooches, hugs, and tender words. She denied worry or fear at any point. Day eight was her last conscious one. I held her for our last brief conversation, in which we exchanged "I love you's." She then rubbed her belly, and whispered, "50 pounds lighter," chuckling at her exaggeration, and I think her victory. Day nine her breathing became erratic, her arms cooled, and as her "dears" gathered around her bed at home, watching every breath with dread and desire, grief and relief, remembering and marveling, she slowly exhaled her last one.

Notable Characteristics

- Mrs. H. already knew of VSED, so that caregivers were never faced with dilemmas about whether and when to inform her.

- To a person who strongly desires not to live long into dementia, VSED while still decisionally capable may be a very viable option for escaping impending dementia.
- Just when to initiate VSED is a difficult decision. This patient's readiness and the support of her family were assessed periodically. The long period of delay was nerve-wracking to the family but provided time for sharing and "goodbye."
- Mrs. H. refused to enter a nursing home. Home hospice was employed once VSED began (initiating VSED was what made her illness terminal enough to qualify for hospice). Comfort issues were well managed.

Issues Raised

- In pre-emptive VSED to avoid advanced dementia, when to initiate VSED is a delicate and difficult decision. How can one be confident that one is not acting too early (missing out on precious time with family and friends) or waiting too long (losing the mental capacity to initiate and carry out VSED)?
- Should the patient's "readiness" for VSED as well as his or her capacity to make a major life and death decision be periodically assessed by a professional caregiver?
- If VSED really is "suicide," what consequences does that have for the patient? For the patient's family?
- Can a patient with no terminal illness (one that results in life expectancy of six months or less, if it runs its normal course) qualify for hospice merely by beginning VSED?

Case 1.4—G.W. (Lung Cancer): Family and Staff Conflict

". . . renegade acts of compassion"

Ty Markham and Margaret P. Battin

From Ty Markham:

G.W. Lamb, Jr. (my dad) was a retired corporate accountant and known as a "man's man," which is to say he knew how to take charge of just about any situation, and did. When confronted with his final demise at 76, living on his ranch in rural Texas, he was stoic and decisive. The lobectomy to rid a metastatic small-cell cancer from his lung was ultimately unable to stop its spread to his occipital visual cortex. Dad always looked for the "writing on the wall" and could see it even better as his visual field narrowed and faded. He wasn't surprised when, after one last attempt—a 6-week course of radiation treatment—failed, his oncologist suggested home hospice. He was crestfallen, but took the news "like a man" and signed a "VSED agreement" with only slight noticeable hesitation while I, my mom, and the hospice nurse looked on. For a man nearing his 78th birthday he was still mentally sharp and articulate. He listened daily to the political and financial news right up to the point that he was fading in and out of consciousness. We knew he was getting close when he stopped his nightly ranting over the 6:00 news.

Mom, on the other hand, was already showing early signs of dementia at 75. She was quickly losing the last bit of life she knew, and had long been slowly losing her sense of confidence that she could handle things on her own. In her near-panic, she over-compensated by obsessing on the VSED details. She took quite seriously the one about "resisting" the urge to give in to the patient's pleas for water or food. She understood it correctly I'm sure, as it was meant to avoid prolonging his suffering. We took turns sitting for hours next to Dad's hospital bed in the family room. I saw how, every time she refused him a sip of water, he would roll his eyes and groan. A heartbreaking memory to this very day.

When it was my turn, I couldn't do it. I'd seen a documentary that I couldn't get out of my mind—one in which a man who'd survived many days in the desert explained what it was like to go without water till near death. It was considered the most painful way to die. Dad's suffering was so palpable, and so painful to watch, that I kept dipping the small mouth-sponge in the water so he could suck on it. Even as weak as he was, he would raise his arm to try to hold my arm in place to keep me from taking the sponge away until he finished getting all the water out of it.

At one point, my mother caught a glimpse of this and vigorously chastised me aloud (in front of Dad), for doing "the one thing they told us NOT to do!" I knew she was desperate and afraid. But it broke my heart to see the pain in Dad's expression as he heard that utterance. I whispered in his ear afterwards that I would continue no matter what, and he turned his head toward me and slowly mouthed the words "Thank You." As he weakened over the remaining days, Dad made a few more attempts to show gratitude for the water (he never seemed to want food) before he finally slipped into a coma and died two weeks after starting VSED.

I'll never forget the heated interchanges with my mom over my insubordination to the VSED "rules." She was well-meaning and earnest. But so was I. And I'll never regret my renegade acts of compassion, nor the bits of relief that I was able to render for my father in his last days of suffering.

From Margaret P. Battin:

I didn't know Ty Markham's father, but I do know Ty herself, and when I interviewed her—in my little cabin in southern Utah, late in the evening, by the light mostly of candles, recorded on my cellphone—I could see something deeply authentic here: the anguish of someone for whom a death of a much-loved one by VSED hadn't gone quite so well. This case—written by Ty in her own words, unredacted—leaves many questions open. Where did the VSED "agreement" Ty's father signed "with only slight noticeable hesitation" come from? Did somebody make it up? If offered by the hospice, was VSED presented as an ordinary option in their menu of end-of-life care, despite the fact that neither VSED nor an agreement like this is standard hospice care? Did Ty's father understand himself to have other options, or did he think he was expected to do this—just part of what a "man's man" would have to do? When her father signed the document, Ty was sitting in a chair a few feet away; she never saw the content of the document.

Later, when asked for more details about her father's agreement to embark on VSED, Ty wrote, "I only recall how the form was presented orally to my dad. She [the hospice nurse] explained to him that hospice would try to keep him as comfortable as possible, but he could speed up the process if he chose to not have food or water once the process of dying (organs shutting down) begins. I remember his hesitation at that decision. He looked down, grimaced, and with a slight shake of his head as if to indicate 'I don't like this,' he apparently agreed to this plan and signed the document. I didn't have any immediate reaction to that choice until I saw up close and in the moment his torment while dying."

Further, Ty wrote, "What could've helped is if the hospice nurse had forewarned us of the dilemma beforehand by saying something like: 'There may come a time where he'll start to become agitated by the discomfort of thirst and become demanding of immediate relief. You'll have to weigh whether it is better to give immediate relief even if it means prolonging the experience. This difficult choice can cause conflict among family. Here's a way we can help if that arises . . . ?' (and perhaps suggest we call the nurse to administer a sedative, or whatever)."

What's important about this case is that it didn't go entirely well. There wasn't, apparently, adequate consent. There wasn't mutual understanding between the daughter and the mother about how to proceed, and the conflict between them only got worse as the father's dying process continued. There's no real evidence that the local hospice, in a remote area, however well-meaning, understood optimal dry-mouth care, or that they realized that a very fine water mist that does not provide the volume of liquid that sponges do could still be good for comfort and not prolong life and suffering as much. It does show how powerful popular conceptions of the suffering of dying by thirst can be—formed, for instance, by seeing a documentary about a man barely surviving many days in the desert—but it doesn't show how those perceptions could be effectively addressed.

Was the hospice organization well versed in standard palliative care for a person doing VSED? Would there be any way to address the daughter's and the mother's different responses to the hospice instructions? Would there be any real way to have this family understand what it was getting into, or how to have it go better in these specific circumstances? This case is best seen, perhaps, as a cautionary tale for the casual recommendation of VSED where adequate information, realistic consent, and effective palliative care are not fully available—which may, after all, be the case in many remote and not-so-remote corners of the world where people die.

Notable Characteristics

- This patient and family may not have been adequately informed of the potential difficulties of VSED. Palliative approaches to address these difficulties should be discussed upfront with patient and caregivers.
- Home hospice in the patient's rural area was not experienced in palliative support for VSED.
- Once VSED began, conflict between the patient's wife and himself, and between his wife and his daughter, was often sharp.
- The patient's daughter could not accept his suffering from thirst. The patient, not having realized the potential complications, left no clear instructions or wishes about what was to be done if they occurred.

Issues Raised

- Adequately informing the patient and all involved family members of the possibility of VSED and its potential associated challenges is crucial before the process is initiated.
- If major family conflict arises once VSED is initiated, a family meeting between the hospice team and the family should be immediately scheduled, and consideration should be given to stopping versus re-committing to the VSED process.
- VSED should only rarely be pursued if competent palliative support is not available, and in those circumstances sophisticated, coherent, and knowledgeable family support would be essential.
- Patient and family caregivers should clearly and accurately know in advance what to expect from hospice and from professional caregivers after VSED is initiated. The approach to a patient who has clearly chosen VSED at one point but then subsequently pleads for water to relieve thirst should be discussed in advance with patient and caregivers.
- Is a "written agreement" to VSED necessary or prudent when the patient has capacity? What issues and conditions should be addressed in such an agreement?

The chapters that follow pursue in depth the clinical, ethical, legal, and institutional aspects of VSED, independent of the cases presented above. At many points within each of the chapters, however, reference will be made to specific elements of these cases.

Reference

Battin, Margaret P. 1996. *The Least Worst Death*. New York: Oxford University Press.

2

Clinical Issues

Timothy E. Quill, Judith K. Schwarz, and V. J. Periyakoil

Voluntarily Stopping Eating and Drinking (VSED) is the process whereby a person with current or prospective serious illness chooses to completely stop eating any food and drinking any fluids with the intention of hastening her own death (Quill et al. 2018, Horowitz, Sussman, and Quill 2016). The context is usually the presence of a serious progressive illness that may or may not be terminal but that has become associated with an unacceptable quality of life by the patient's own personal standards. VSED is also sometimes motivated by anticipation of future unacceptable suffering or concern about losing the cognitive capacity to initiate or sustain the process in the future. VSED is the product of a voluntary choice made by a patient with full decision-making capacity, and is therefore different from the "natural" process of losing one's appetite and ability to drink toward the very end of life as death approaches. Death is definitely intended with VSED, and it usually occurs within two weeks provided the person assiduously avoids drinking.

2.1. Background Issues—Palliative Care and Hospice

Palliative care should be part of the standard of care for all seriously ill patients whether or not they are engaged in active, disease-directed treatment or are knowingly approaching the end of their lives. Palliative care involves biological, psychological, social, and spiritual care for patients with serious illness. Patients receiving palliative care may simultaneously have a wide range of disease-directed treatment philosophies: (1) They may want to receive any and all potentially effective disease-directed medical treatments, potentially including aggressive treatments such as chemotherapy, cardiac surgery, organ transplantation, and cardiopulmonary resuscitation. (2) They may set partial limits (do-not-resuscitate, no breathing tubes) but receive all other potentially effective disease-directed treatments available.

(3) They may set more limits, still treating easily reversible problems such as infections or dehydration, and accepting hospitalization if needed, but no intensive care unit, for example. (4) They may prefer to be managed with comfort measures only (as in hospice).

When palliative care is provided by a patient's main treating physicians, it is sometimes called "primary palliative care." More complex palliative problems (e.g., difficult-to-treat symptoms, requests for assistance in dying) might require involvement by a formally trained palliative care specialist. This practice is sometimes called "specialty palliative care" (Quill and Abernethy 2013).

Hospice is a formal program designed to provide palliative care to patients who accept that they are terminally ill and that they are more likely than not to die in the next six months. It is a special subgroup within the larger palliative care umbrella. The transition to hospice is very difficult for many patients and their families, as they have to accept that disease-directed medical treatment is no longer effective and/or no longer meaningful to them, and that all subsequent medical treatment will be directed toward comfort and support (Casarett and Quill 2007). Many of those who make the transition to hospice, however, are subsequently very grateful about the care they subsequently receive and frequently wish in retrospect that they had made the transition earlier.

Whereas palliative care is mainly a medical consultation service like cardiology or oncology, hospice is also a medical insurance benefit provided by Medicaid, Medicare, and many other insurers. Hospice potentially offers and pays for: (1) up to two to four hours per day of home health care aides at the patient's own home as needed, (2) regular weekly visits by an RN and social worker, (3) all palliative medications and assistive devices (e.g., commodes, shower chairs . . .), (4) phone consultation backup systems day and night, and (5) additional bereavement care for the family after the patient dies. The medical aspects of hospice care can be provided and supervised by the patient's primary care clinician or primary treating subspecialist, or by a palliative care consultant or a designated hospice clinician. Usually one main treating clinician serves that role from the time of enrollment in a hospice program until the patient's death.

Although hospice care is generally associated with high levels of patient and family satisfaction, there are also significant limits to hospice services. For example, most hospice at home relies heavily on family members and friends providing physical care (toileting, bathing, assistance with meals, etc.), and not everyone has such a support network. Furthermore, the hospice medical insurance benefit, at least in the United States, requires that the patient be more likely than not to die in the next six months. Hospice therefore may not cover patients such as those with early dementia, who may want a hospice philosophy of care (comfort measures only) but are likely to live several years rather than months if the disease follows its usual course. Nonetheless, hospice is the standard of care for many patients who accept that they are dying, and it can adequately address and relieve most if not all end-of-life suffering.

2.2. Background Issues—Unacceptable Suffering and Deterioration

Despite the potential of palliative care and hospice to address most end-of-life suffering, some patients worry about potential future unacceptable suffering or deterioration as their condition progresses. This is particularly worrisome for those who have witnessed harsh suffering or extreme decline before death in a family member or friend, or those with early dementia who value their ability to be in control of their minds, bodies, and lives, and do not want to endure where their disease is likely taking them in the future.

Some patients are bold enough to raise questions about what "options" they might have to hasten their deaths in the future should this perceived need arise. Others might be more cautious and wait for their clinicians to open the door to such discussions. Taking a family history of how family members have died can be a good entrée into this discussion, as can asking questions about what such patients are "hoping for" and what they are "afraid of" in their future (Quill 2000). Clinicians may be hesitant to ask these questions because they might then be asked to do things that are illegal or that exceed their own personal moral boundaries (Meier, Back, and Morrison 2001). But some patients are already thinking about these issues, some of whom are desperate to find a safe person with whom to talk and to help them learn what is possible if an unacceptable condition develops in their future.

This hypothetical discussion about potential future access to a controlled death was very valuable to each of the patients presented in the opening chapters of this book, including the following three examples:

- Rob's mother (Case 1.3) was reassured that there could be an escape from her slowly progressing cognitive impairment through VSED, but she was uncertain how long to wait. If she initiated the process too early, she might miss out on meaningful time with her family and friends that she was still enjoying. If she waited too long, she might lose the mental discipline needed to sustain the process and override her basic instincts to drink and eat. Nonetheless, she was reassured knowing that a pre-emptive escape was possible.

- Al, the biker with ALS (Case 1.1), appreciated the loving care provided by his caregiving team at his own home, but he eventually decided that the dependency created by his progressive weakness was more than he wanted to bear. If he lived in Oregon or other jurisdictions where it is legal, he might have preferred to receive medical aid in dying (MAID). But even if MAID was legally available, he would likely have been too weak to take the medication himself. So, VSED gave him back a sense of control of his own destiny and being less trapped by his illness.

- Bill, the man with widely metastatic breast cancer (Case 1.2), would have been very reassured by the possibility of future medically assisted death (MAID) at a time of his choosing if he lived in a jurisdiction where it was legally available. But he lived in a state where MAID was illegal. He was angry and tormented by the absence of this option, and he thought that VSED sounded cruel and inhumane when first considered. Not long thereafter he reassessed his options and pursued VSED.

Other patients, especially those who have not had regular access to health care in their pasts because of poverty or other social issues, may not be at all interested in this conversation about "last-resort options" that could hasten their deaths. In fact, they may find the existence of these options frightening, and clinicians opening up an informing conversation may undermine the fragile trust that such patients may have in the health care system. At least in theory, now that they have access to health care, such patients will tend to want "everything" that has any possibility of prolonging their lives, even if it entails considerable suffering (Quill, Arnold, and Back 2009).

Patients who are interested in learning about options for hastening their own deaths may make general inquiries about the possibility of achieving death at a time of their own choosing. Many will be reassured by knowing there are legally available options, although most will never actually need them if they receive adequate palliative care (Ganzini, Goy, and Dobscha 2009; Ganzini et al. 2006; Schwarz 2007). A small number of patients, however, reach a point where they are ready to die "right now" because their current circumstances have become unacceptable to them. Sometimes these real-time requests are triggered by suffering related to difficult-to-treat symptoms. Sometimes they may be driven more by relentless debility and dependence from their progressive illness which they find unacceptable, and other times these requests are driven by fear of losing the cognitive capacity to act in the future.

The vast majority of these patients live in places where MAID is not legally available, and many are in clinical circumstances where they would not qualify based on prognosis even if it were legal. For these patients VSED may be the best, or perhaps, as Bill experienced above, the "least worst" of the available options (Battin 1996). The prevalence of the practice of VSED at the end of life is not well known. Forty percent of a sample of hospice nurses in Oregon have seen a case of VSED (Ganzini et al. 2003), and it reportedly accounts for 2.1% of deaths in the Netherlands (Ivanovic, Buche, and Fringer 2014; see also Appendix C). These estimates are probably conservative given the likelihood that some patients initiate their own version of VSED without the assistance (neither permission nor even awareness) of their physicians, nurses, or other health care professionals for fear they would not support their VSED and might even intervene to prevent the process (Stangle, Schnepp, and Fringer 2019).

2.3. Evaluation of Requests for VSED

Requests for any kind of assisted death, including but not limited to VSED, should be the beginning of a conversation that includes a careful evaluation of "why now" (Quill 1993; Quill and Battin 2020). All aspects of the patient's suffering and quality of life should be explored, including biological, psychological, social, spiritual, and religious dimensions. *Why is this request coming at this particular time? What is making your situation so unacceptable that you would rather die than keep living?*

The patient should be carefully evaluated for any underlying psychiatric problems that may be distorting their perception of their current situation, including anxiety, depressive, cognitive, and eating disorders. If significant past or present uncertainties are present in these domains, the patient should be evaluated by an experienced psychologist or psychiatrist (Ganzini, Goy, and Dobscha 2008; Ganzini et al. 1994). On the other side of the coin, evaluating clinicians should also look for and explore where the patient has experienced hope, love, connection, and meaning in the past, including where it is still present and where it may be surprisingly absent (Byock 2014). Close family members should be interviewed to get their perspective on the meaning and timeliness of the patient's request. If significant family members are unaware of this discussion and exploration, the reason for their exclusion should be carefully explored. The main treating clinician should look for common ground with the patient, but, if there are uncertainties, consultations should be considered from clinicians with special expertise in the patient's underlying disease, palliative care, psychiatry, and/or ethics depending on the situation.

In addition to thoroughly addressing the "why now" of the patient's request, clinicians should have an awareness of the full range of "last resort" options that might address the patient's clinical situation (Quill, Lo, and Brock 1997; Quill, Lee, and Nunn 2000). These potentially death-hastening measures were defined and described in the Introduction, and summarized there in Tables I.2 and I.3 (Section I.2). Voluntarily stopping eating and drinking is one of those options that we now explore in more depth.

2.4. VSED—Key Practical Matters to Consider in Advance

One of the unique and most important aspects of VSED is that it is largely patient initiated and patient controlled (provided the patient knows about it). In theory, VSED could be completed in its entirety without any clinician involvement or assistance. While VSED might have the advantage of requiring that the patient be highly motivated when carried out independently, we argue strongly that entirely eliminating clinicians would be a real loss in terms of (1) ensuring fully informed consent, (2) making sure the patient has access to best possible symptom management before VSED is initiated, (3) providing added support and information to the patient and family as the process unfolds, (4) helping address uncertainty about how to proceed if the patient becomes delirious during the late stages of VSED, and (5) providing bereavement support for the family after the patient dies.

Involving clinicians for the first time when the patient is in a crisis after VSED has been initiated is problematic for all concerned, as there will likely be no common understanding of the contextual issues that led the patient to the decision. For patients with early cognitive impairment like Mrs. H.,

Rob's mother, timing was a critical factor that needed both open discussion and potentially negotiation between clinician, patient, and family. Initiating VSED too early might mean missing out on being alive for a period of time that may be meaningful and valuable to the patient and family. On the other hand, if she waited too long the "window of opportunity" could be lost as she might lose the cognitive ability to remember why she was not eating and drinking, which would then make no sense as she became very thirsty and possibly hungry. For these reasons, if at all possible at least one main treating clinician should be involved from before initiation, and fully aware about what is transpiring in all phases of the VSED process.

In addition, all core family members should be consulted or at least informed to some degree unless the patient explicitly prohibits contacting them. If particular family members are being excluded, this limitation should be fully explored and understood and hopefully mutually resolved in a way that minimizes the risk of a family member being psychologically harmed as a by-product of the process, and also to anticipate and plan for any family conflict that might emerge once the process is initiated. It was clear when one of us (Tim Quill) first met with Mrs. H. that she and her son had discussed VSED and were on the "same page" about it being a reasonable future option, but it was less clear that her daughters were accepting of the process. Their becoming more informed led to eventual acceptance and fuller understanding of their mother's decision, and their risks of bereavement problems diminished as a result of subsequent discussions in advance of Mrs. H. initiating the process.

2.5. Requirements to Initiate VSED for Patients with Decision-Making Capacity

The requirements to initiate VSED ideally should be as follows:

- A main treating clinician who agrees to be the primary "medical quarterback" for the entire VSED process should explore the following questions with the patient, health care proxy, and family:
  - Why has VSED become a question right now?
  - Are there any concerns about the patient's current decision-making capacity?
  - Have they discussed how to proceed if the patient loses capacity during the VSED process?

- Have all four advance care planning documents outlined in the next section been considered and/or completed?
- Are there any other unique individual concerns about the process?
- Do the patient and all caregivers understand what to expect physiologically and psychologically going forward as VSED unfolds?
- Does the patient currently have decision-making capacity for a major life and death decision? Many times patients have been considering these options for a considerable time, and the decision is consistent with long-standing views and values. In these situations it may be sufficient to have the patient evaluated by the main treating clinician, and a palliative care consultant or experienced hospice clinician (MD, NP, PA, RN, or MSW depending on availability and experience) could provide a second opinion. If they all agree that the decision makes sense given the patient's medical condition and personal values, then it should be reasonable to move forward.
- Does the main treating clinician have a clear understanding of the "*why now*" from the patient about her decision to initiate VSED? What are the unacceptable symptoms or future concerns driving the decision? Might the decision change with better symptom management? What is it that makes the future unacceptable *right now* at this point in time as opposed to postponing the decision for a defined or undefined period?
- A formal psychiatric evaluation to ensure adequate capacity to make a decision of this magnitude should be obtained if there is significant uncertainty about the patient's mental capacity to make a major medical decision (see Box 2.1).

Box 2.1 Indications for a Formal Psychiatric Evaluation before Initiating VSED

- Current evidence of delirium, dementia, or major mental illness
- Past psychiatric history of major depression, bipolar disorder, or psychosis
- Apparent inconsistency of VSED with the patient's previous life narrative, values, or religious practices
- Uncertainty about family dynamics influencing decision toward VSED
- Ambivalence about whether and when to proceed

2.6. Formal Advance Care Planning

Because of the risk of developing delirium from dehydration and/or electrolyte abnormalities late in the process, all patients seriously considering VSED should discuss in advance their preferences for how to manage such situations with their families and main treating clinician. Before starting VSED they should consider implementing all four of the following **advance care planning documents** to make their future wishes clear should they lose capacity after initiating VSED. The first three do not take effect until the patient loses decision-making capacity (up until that time, patients should be making their own real-time decisions with their clinicians and family members). The fourth document will guide both current and future treatment from the time it is completed and properly signed.

1. **Health Care Proxy (HCP)** (aka durable power of attorney for health care or health care agent) directive allows the patient to formally designate a person to make decisions on her behalf if she loses decision-making capacity in the future. The job of the HCP is to make decisions as she believes the patient would if she was still capable, using what is known about the patient's views and preferences. This process is called "substituted judgment," so it is critical that the HCP both knows that is her responsibility and that she makes it a point to learn about the patient's views and values under likely future clinical circumstances. Based on that knowledge, the designated HCP may then be asked to make decisions accordingly for the now incapacitated person about providing or continuing to withhold food and fluids if delirium occurs and questions arise about continuing or stopping the VSED process.

2. **Advance Instructional Directive** (also called a **Living Will**, or just **Advance Directive**) is also completed while a person still has decision-making capacity about the kinds of medical treatment he would and would not want if he loses the ability to make medical decisions on his own in the future. Living Wills can provide overarching guidance. One person might want "*comfort measures only*." Another person with very different views and values might want "*all treatments no matter how aggressive including cardiopulmonary resuscitation if they have any chance of helping me live longer.*" A third person might want something in between, "*no resuscitation or breathing machines or intensive care, but I would want relatively easy treatments such as antibiotics, fluids, and*

hospitalization if they might help me live longer without suffering too much." In this particular circumstance where a person is planning to initiate VSED, he should specify in his Living Will how he would want feeding handled if he loses capacity late in the process, and nonverbally or verbally expresses a desire to be fed. For example, "*If late in the process of forgoing oral intake I become confused and verbally or nonverbally express a desire for food or drink, please give me the smallest amount possible to keep me comfortable.*" The patient might also write instructions specifying that requests for liquids made when in a confused or delirious state that are inconsistent with his previous informed choice should be treated aggressively with other comfort measures, such as proportionate sedation, that do not include giving fluids. The idea here is to give the health care team and the proxy decision makers guidance as to patients' wishes should they lose decision-making capacity after VSED is initiated. (See Chapter 8, Section 8.1, and Appendix A for more detailed information about advance care planning in this domain.)

3. **Advance directive videos** are coming into use as a way to literally hear the patient's voice if they lose decision-making capacity in the future. These videos allow the patient's family and future caregivers and clinicians to directly hear and see what the patient has expressed in the past in her own voice if and when the ability to participate in such discussions is lost. These carefully prepared videos are a powerful way to ensure that the patient's own views and values will be seriously integrated into medical care at this phase of life. They can be particularly helpful to guide to family members or privately hired nursing aides who provide a great deal of bedside care (In My Own Words 2020).

The next document covers the patient's *current and future* wishes about cardiopulmonary resuscitation, mechanical ventilation (breathing machines), and other potentially life-prolonging therapies (i.e., antibiotics, intravenous fluids . . .). Unlike the three *advance* directives just outlined, which are only activated when and if a patient loses the ability to make her own decisions, the next directive holds for any and all current and future situations where the life-extending treatments mentioned might be initiated or withheld.

4. **Practitioner Orders for Life Sustaining Therapy (POLST) forms** are documents specifying what kinds of medical treatments a person would and would not want *right now* if the need arose. In a sense,

POLST forms are both current care and advance care directives. They serve as actual medical orders to guide treatments in the patient's current and future circumstances. In addition to addressing cardiopulmonary resuscitation, mechanical ventilation, and intensive care unit treatment, POLST forms can guide whether or not to hospitalize or to treat with antibiotics, intravenous fluids, artificial hydration, and nutrition should the potential need arise, as well as the possibility of providing "comfort measures only" as might occur in hospice. (See https://polst.org/national-form/ for a representative POLST form.) If a patient loses decision-making capacity in the future, his clinician would look to any advance directives that have been completed and see if they provide guidance for the kinds of treatment the patient would and would not want under this new condition, and whether his POLST form needed to be updated. If the patient wishes oral feedings to be limited in the future, that decision must be added to the section regarding comfort measures. If someone was designated by the patient to be his health care proxy, that person would be the main family representative to help make POLST decisions as well as other major medical decisions, though the views and values of other family members or close friends would be considered if they shed light on the patient's views and values.[1]

Hospice referral should also be recommended to all patients contemplating VSED if it is available. If a patient with early dementia initiating VSED did not qualify for hospice based on an uncertain prognosis before VSED is initiated, a palliative care or "pre-hospice" evaluation might be started with a plan to activate hospice home services once VSED is underway. Such patients might need to forgo all fluids for several days before contacting hospice for a formal enrollment evaluation. If the patient seems resolute in his desire and ability to forgo further oral intake, hospice enrollment often proceeds without limitation, as the patient would be expected to die within approximately two weeks. If VSED is being considered for a patient already enrolled in hospice, it would be worthwhile to explore the plan first with the main treating hospice clinician and the hospice medical director and main administrator, and

---

[1] Other states may have similar forms such as Medical Orders for Life-Sustaining Treatment (MOLST), so interested patients or family members should discuss the best form for their state with their health care providers.

then later with the patient's assigned nurses and aides. Some hospices now have position statements regarding how staff is to respond to VSED requests that may or may not parallel facilities' response to MAID requests where the latter practice is legal. The backup services and added support provided by hospice can clearly enhance the quality of care and support available at home once VSED is initiated, but to be successful, the process also requires support from family members and other caregivers.

If hospice services are not available, or if the available programs are not accepting of a patient embarking on VSED, then arrangements should be attempted with other available home care services to provide additional support. The patient, family, and main treating physician should work together to find the best support services available given these limitations, which may sometimes include admission to an inpatient hospice or palliative care unit.

This was the case with Al, the motorcyclist with ALS (Case 1.1 in the previous chapter) who would have preferred to carry out VSED in his own home where he was getting excellent care 24/7 from his home health aides. After thorough exploration of his "why now," the home hospice physician was supportive of his decision, but his home health aides could not accept it. They had become profoundly attached to Al and didn't feel comfortable "helping him to intentionally die" in this way. Al was totally dependent on these home aides for all aspects of his physical care, including toileting, skin and mouth care, and positioning, so he was eventually admitted to an inpatient palliative care unit after checking with its hospital administration and legal team to ensure permissibility from their perspective. He got excellent support and care there while carrying out the VSED process.

2.7. Managing Symptoms and Complications Once VSED Is Initiated

Once VSED starts, very predictable symptom management issues emerge:

Hunger and Thirst: Hunger usually disappears within 24–48 hours as the patient's own metabolic system tries to generate calories by creating ketones (which leads predictably to a "fruity" breath smell). Thirst, or the experience of a very dry mouth, is a much more challenging and ongoing symptom to manage, as this sensation can generate a strong desire to drink that requires considerable will power to overcome.

Strong will power is a common characteristic of those who choose and successfully complete VSED, including the cases in this volume.

Mouth Care: Also critical is the provision of excellent mouth care, which usually includes the repeated application of lip balm, keeping teeth brushed, and rinsing with mouthwash and then spitting out rather than swallowing any remaining liquid. Hospice often provides swabs that can be moistened with small amounts of liquid, or a moistened washcloth that has been frozen can be provided to the patient. Cool water or artificial saliva should be offered frequently as a means to "rinse and spit" to keep the mucus membranes lining the mouth feeling moist. Spraying a small amount of a fine mist of water into the mouth can also relieve feelings of a dry mouth. These interventions are most beneficial during the first week of forgoing oral intake, when the patient can usually cooperate with these comfort measures. By the second week, most patients will be sleeping for longer periods, and they may not remember or realize they are trying not to swallow any fluids offered for moistening purposes. If a patient trying to VSED regularly swallows significant amounts of fluids, the dying process could go on for many weeks or months.

Delirium can occur late in the VSED process and may be accompanied by behavior that suggests the patient wants something to drink, with no memory of her previous desire to hasten death by VSED. This possibility should be discussed in advance with the patient and family, and agreement reached regarding how the family and caregivers should respond. The patient's wishes and preferences in this regard should have been clearly documented in a formal Advance Directive, also discussed in detail with their designated healthcare proxy (see section above on Advance Care Planning). Should this situation arise, the patient should first be gently reminded of his prior decision to forgo fluids, and why that decision was made. If the request for fluids persists, the previously identified comfort measures should be provided, starting with those that do not introduce fluids to the patient who has now, most likely, lost decision-making capacity. If requests for fluid persist, small amounts should be offered to the patient. In addition, medication to relieve any associated anxiety or underlying pain should be provided. Often, the patient is able to settle and falls back to sleep. On rare occasions the patient may rehydrate himself and may even begin to eat, at which point the entire VSED process would need to be re-evaluated. (Strategies for anticipating and responding to these challenging circumstances are explored in Chapter 8, Sections 8.4 and 8.5.) **Severe agitated delirium** if it occurs during VSED is often accompanied by very significant patient and family suffering, and may require proportionate palliative sedation. This possibility of severe delirium late in the process should also be discussed with patient and family during the advance care planning process so it is not unanticipated if it occurs.

Other Symptom Management. The other symptom management issues that emerge as VSED gets fully underway (debility, weakness, dyspnea, and eventually decreased awareness) are very familiar to hospice providers from caring for other dying patients. Even if the patient was previously able to be out of bed, after several days of forgoing all oral intake she will likely become bed-bound due to weakness and low blood pressure. Once bed-bound, round-the-clock caregiving and presence must be provided to prevent falls, address symptoms including confusion, and keep family caregivers from becoming physically and emotionally overwhelmed. Delirium and/or agitation sometimes accompany the final stages of VSED as the major organs and regulatory processes begin to fail. Hospice clinicians should be immediately notified if delirium or agitation occur, as specific medications that can help relieve those distressing symptoms are usually provided in the home hospice–provided "emergency pack."

2.8. Impact of Culture on VSED

Food is a primary way to express aspects of culture. Traditional cuisine is passed down from one generation to the next. Many culturally relevant holidays are marked with preparation of signature food items with associated rituals. Eating is a communal event, and feeding someone is a way of expressing love and concern.

The word "starve" has origins in the Old English word *steorfan*, meaning "to die." The World Health Organization estimates that 821 million people suffered from hunger in the year 2017 (World Health Organization 2018). Twelve percent of the global population is afflicted by chronic and persistent food insecurity, and struggle without reliable access to sufficient quantity of affordable and nutritious food. Food insecurity disproportionately impacts minority populations. Deaths due to starvation are common in patients from developing countries in Asia and the Pacific regions, sub-Saharan Africa, Latin America, and the Caribbean. Food insecurity (Munger et al. 2015; Olsen 1999; Hill et al. 2011; Kaiser et al. 2003; Ahluwalia, Dodds, and Baligh 1998; Alaya, Baquero, and Klinger 2008; Chilton and Booth 2007) disproportionately impacts minority populations who may live in food deserts (Dubowitz et al. 2015a; Dubowitz et al. 2015b; Woodruff et al. 2020; Walker, Keane, and Burke 2010; Dhillon et al. 2019) or may not have the financial resources to buy adequate quantities of healthy food. Minority patients and their families may be particularly sensitized to the role of nutrition in fostering health and longevity and may be opposed to being personally offered the possibility of VSED in their futures, much less initiating it themselves.

To make this matter even more complex, most seriously ill patients eventually lose hunger and thirst as a natural part of the very late stages of their illness. When a patient is not able to eat or drink, family members may ask for artificial ways to provide nourishment to the patient to prevent them from "starving." When a patient stops eating and drinking in the last few days of life, loved ones may unwittingly infer that the lack of food and fluids caused the death and feel that artificial food and fluids would have prevented death.

Faith and religion also deeply impact how patients and families view the role of food and fluids at the end of life. Some religions have ritualistic practices that condone starving to death. Jainism allows and even admires the practice of *sallekhana* (Braun, 2008), the act of facing death voluntarily through fasting. Sallekhana is not considered suicide by Jain religious leaders, as it is a potentially admirable act of letting go of desires, not an act of violence or sin.

In many other traditions, on the other hand, a patient who decides to implement VSED may be seen as committing suicide, an act opposed by most religions. Not providing food and fluids to a patient, even if motivated by the person's explicit request, may be seen by loved ones as committing the sin of starving him to death. VSED may also be seen as the patient "playing God" by determining his fate and time of death.

In some traditions food also has deep cultural value in the afterlife. Buddhist mythology describes six realms of existence: (1) the realm of Gods and heavenly beings, (2) the realm of demons, (3) the realm of hell, (4) the realm of the hungry ghosts, (5) the realm of animals, and (6) the realm of humans. Humans who die on an empty stomach are consigned to become "hungry ghosts"—creatures that wander eternity with huge empty stomachs and great longing for food (Teiser 1996). Hungry Ghost festivals are celebrated in the seventh month of the lunar calendar in Asia, where families leave offerings of food for their ancestors who may have become hungry ghosts (*China Daily* 2004).

Patients and families who believe in hungry ghosts may become very anxious at the thought of dying on an empty stomach. If a patient loses hunger or thirst as a normal part of the dying process, they may request oraxegenic (appetite stimulating) medications to enhance appetite or artificial feeding to enhance caloric intake. On the other hand, a patient may choose to implement VSED after extensive discussion and informed consent even if she is fully capable of eating and drinking. If such a patient later becomes confused and asks for food and fluids, the loved ones may feel deeply constrained to feed her even if all involved, including the patient, may have initially agreed to the full VSED process.

VSED can have a different, more positive role in certain cultural and medical circumstances. The future possibility of VSED could potentially mitigate suffering even if the patient eventually does not choose to implement it. Consider the following case illustration (some details masked to protect the patient and family).

Mr. Z., a Korean-American with End-Stage Pancreatic Cancer

Mr. Z. was a 70-year-old Korean-American with metastatic pancreatic adenocarcinoma. He lived in his own home with his wife who had dementia. He was her primary caregiver. They had three adult children: two sons and one daughter. His older son lived out of state. His daughter lived locally and was very involved in his care. His younger son also lived locally, but he had a chronic mental illness and was completely estranged from the patient.

Mr. Z. had already undergone chemotherapy with gemcitabine after his initial diagnosis. His primary adverse effect from chemotherapy was severe anorexia. The fact that he did not have an appetite was extremely distressing to him, and he did not want to experience it again with more chemotherapy. Even after having been off chemotherapy for a few months, his appetite had not completely returned. When Mr. Z. decided to forgo further chemotherapy, his oncologist referred him to the palliative care clinic. He came to his palliative care visits accompanied by his daughter. He had very little pain or other physical symptoms. At the encouragement of his daughter, he tried various oraxogenic (appetite stimulating) medications, with limited response.

One of his key priorities was attending his Korean-American Christian church on Sundays. He would drive himself and spend almost the entire day there, where he was "the mayor of his church." He loved to socialize and eat there and spend quality time with his "church family."

As Mr. Z.'s illness advanced, his functional status deteriorated. Even with someone else driving him to church, he eventually became too tired to sit in the pew. He could not eat, as he had no appetite. Once he was no longer able to attend church, he stated that he was ready to die and enrolled in home hospice care. He was in great distress due to lack of appetite, lack of taste, and profound weakness. Mr. Z. often said that he was tired of "just sitting around waiting to die." He wanted to hasten his death but was too debilitated to complete the legal process of requesting MAID (which had been legalized in his state). In response to his statements in this domain, his palliative team educated him about the option of VSED. As he was already profoundly anorexic (eating only a few bites each day), he was eager to learn more about VSED and discussed it extensively with his palliative team. He was still holding out hope, however, that he could reconcile with his estranged son. Though he died without achieving that reconciliation, discussing VSED as a viable and accessible option provided him with a sense of control and helped mitigate his deep existential distress.

Mr. Z. illustrates some of the often overlooked positive aspects of having VSED as an end-of-life possibility. Seriously ill patients who may or may not have legal access to physician-assisted death may welcome other potential options for hastening death. Even in states where MAID is legal, the steps required to access this option are quite onerous. Many patients do not qualify for MAID because they are not terminal enough, and others may be too debilitated to complete the legally required documentation and evaluation, as was the case with Mr. Z. Furthermore, MAID may be morally unacceptable to the person even where it is legal, while other last-resort options such as VSED may be more acceptable to them. Most religions, including Mr. Z.'s (Christian), do not condone suicide. (It is not clear whether or not his religion would have considered VSED a form of suicide, and Mr. Z. did not ask his religious leaders about their view about this as he was considering VSED as an option.) Nonetheless, VSED may offer a legally permitted and morally acceptable pathway for some seriously ill patients in profound existential distress to potentially achieve a desired death. Even when patients do not actually stop eating and drinking, discussing VSED as an accessible option within their control, with no associated legal concerns and fewer religious ones, may help alleviate their suffering even if they do not carry it out.

2.9. Advantages of VSED as an Option to Achieve a Desired Death

VSED has a well-defined beginning, middle, and end that lasts from 10 to 14 days providing the patient adheres to the process. To some extent the timeframe can vary by how well hydrated patients are at the outset, as well as how acutely ill they are, but the biggest variable is the need to be very determined about not drinking. If patients adhere to the requirements of the process they tend to be coherent for the majority of the time. However, all patients seriously considering VSED in the near future should anticipate the distinct possibility of developing delirium late in the process, and have an approach clearly spelled out in their formal advance directives and discussed with their healthcare agent and family. Then delirium, if it occurs, is much less likely to undermine the process.

VSED's relatively predictable timeframe once initiated is radically different from the open-ended, sometimes seemingly endless process of others who gradually die without using VSED. Families can often come together and have a meaningful, time-limited period to say good-bye and work on life closure issues.

VSED is more directly patient initiated and controlled in comparison to other last-resort options, and it does not require that the patient experience severe unrelievable or unbearable symptoms in advance of initiating it. In fact, the patient does not have to have what is usually considered to be an imminently "terminal illness," so VSED is potentially available to those (like Mrs. H.) with mild to moderate dementia who still have sufficient decision-making capacity but are very worried about their future because it can be so long with so much debility.

Clinicians tend to be more comfortable with VSED than they are with MAID. They perceive the process of VSED to be both patient initiated and patient controlled, and they see their role in a patient's hastening death in this way to be supportive but not instrumental. VSED could theoretically be completed without any clinician involvement, whereas with MAID, the clinician's role as a prescribing assistant makes her a critical partner in the process.

Most but not all hospice programs will support VSED, especially if the patient has an otherwise qualifying terminal illness or was already enrolled. Other hospices may enroll patients whose prognosis is more uncertain after they have initiated VSED such that they are then "terminal," and their role helping clinicians and family members manage symptoms and make the most of the dying process seems much more familiar and comfortable. Some religiously affiliated hospices might not accept patients who are initiating VSED because they view it as a form of suicide, though again there is considerable variation. The demographics of patients who have initiated and successfully completed VSED in the past suggest that patients tend to be over 80 years old, have a large disease burden, are already dependent on others, and have a poor self-perceived quality of life, a desire to die at home, and a wish for control (Bolt et al. 2015; Ganzini et al. 2003).

2.10. Disadvantages and Challenges of VSED as an Option to Achieve a Desired Death

First, VSED can be too slow a process for the patient if he has acute, extreme, immediate physical suffering. Ten days to two weeks is a lifetime if suffering is severe, and other aggressive symptom management methods, including sedation, may be much preferable. (NB: The usual two-week waiting period generally required for access to lethal medication for MAID makes that practice subject to the same criticism if a patient waits to make a request until symptoms are severe and unmanageable.)

Second, VSED is only a realistic option for resolute, disciplined persons who have the wherewithal to exert control over their basic bodily drives and who are not experiencing overwhelming acute physical suffering. The level of resoluteness, control, and discipline needed will probably require patients with progressing but not yet severe dementia to initiate the process earlier than they would really like to, because of the fear of losing the ability to initiate and sustain this relatively demanding process. The patient's level of commitment to the VSED process may wane if it is not particularly strong at the beginning in the face of progressive weakness, very persistent thirst, and potential delirium late in the process.

Third, VSED also requires significant caregiver buy-in and support. However weak a patient is when VSED is started, she gets progressively weaker over time and rapidly will need 24/7 support and presence. Caregivers must also fully accept the patient's decision to stop eating and drinking, and they must work assiduously not to undermine the patient's decision or to expose her to the sight or smell of food during the process. This task of avoiding food and drink may become much more difficult if the patient becomes delirious and forgets about his decision and now wants to have something to drink and eat.

Fourth, a significant percentage of patients who initiate VSED may lose capacity for decision making sometime after initiation. Ideally they have planned for this possibility, and have completed an AD for SED to guide the process of continuing to withhold food and fluids. This may be hard to implement if the patient's expression of desire for food and drink becomes insistent. In Chapter 8 we will outline strategies for approaching these circumstances in more depth.

Patience, persistence, and flexibility are needed from the caregivers under these circumstances as they may struggle with differences between the patient's wishes at the time of initiation and the requests of a delirious patient who is very thirsty and cannot recall why he is not drinking. At some level and to some degree, ambivalence is likely to be present in this process for all patients, and this can potentially become amplified as the now delirious person tries to deal with a very primitive survival drive to drink. Not only will caregivers have to deal with potentially conflicted feelings from the patient, but mixed feelings and ambivalence are also likely to arise in caregivers themselves if the process becomes more difficult and conflicted around not drinking despite being very thirsty, and around wanting the process to end sooner than it may. Additionally, conflicts of interest around the cost of care as well as the amount of time and psychic energy needed for caregiving are to some degree inevitable, to say nothing about the complexity of human relationships under all circumstances, which will likely become intensified and exaggerated under these circumstances.

2.11. Revisiting the Initial Cases.

Case 1.1. Al, the Motorcyclist with ALS

Al was ready to die and readily accepted the fact that VSED was his only realistic option. He was not severely symptomatic, so intensification of symptom management was not needed and palliative sedation not indicated. He was on no life-sustaining treatments that could be stopped other than his assisted feeding. He would have preferred staying at home to die, but his home health aides were not comfortable caring for him if he was not allowing them to feed him, which they viewed as assisting him in a suicide. He was therefore admitted to an inpatient palliative care unit where, after consultations with an independent palliative care consultant and an ethics team, at his request he stopped being fed and hydrated by his caregivers (he was too weak to self-feed). His symptoms were well managed, and a steady stream of old friends came to visit over his final two weeks for storytelling, reminiscing and saying good-bye. His symptoms were relatively easily managed, and he remained coherent throughout the process that lasted two weeks from beginning to end. His home health aides visited him regularly to provide support, and most eventually accepted his decision to some degree.

Bottom Line Points
- VSED can be an acceptable escape for patients with a wide range of problems who feel they are not dying rapidly enough.
- VSED requires dedicated, committed caregivers who are willing and able to support the process.
- Sometimes initiating and carrying out VSED will require admission to an inpatient facility, where the staff will need to be educated about the process.

Case 1.2. Bill with Widely Metastatic Breast Cancer

Bill wanted access to MAID and remained angry and frustrated that he could not gain legal access because he lived in New York, where the practice was (and is) illegal. Other last-resort options that could be legally accessed, including VSED, were explored. He also looked at the underground options for accessing a more direct form of physician-assisted death, but was unable to make firm plans in this regard. Later in his illness, several long bones spontaneously fractured and he ended up admitted to our inpatient palliative care unit. His pain was controlled as long as he stayed still, so palliative sedation was not indicated. We revisited VSED, arguably his only remaining realistic death-hastening choice, which he then initiated and carried out. His symptoms were well managed, and he did have some meaningful time with his family, but he also remained angry he could not have the control that he wanted. He died 10 days after initiating VSED.

Bottom Line Points
- VSED will sometimes be a disappointing second choice for those who would prefer a more definitive intervention like medical aid in dying or euthanasia.
- On the other hand, VSED may provide a desired escape to death for people with serious illnesses and without better legal options.

Case 1.3. Mrs. H. with Progressive Dementia

A consulting physician had several meetings over six months with Mrs. H. and her family to explore the possibility of VSED as an option. She became increasingly worried about losing decision-making capacity and losing the ability to live and die in her own home, so she eventually picked a date. She and the physician met one additional time to ensure that she was still clear about her decision, and to make sure that her family was still accepting and supportive. She then started VSED after a celebratory meal. Her symptoms of dry mouth and progressive weakness were relatively easy to manage. Her family and she had a meaningful celebration of her life over the following two weeks, at the end of which she died peacefully in her own bed in her own home, as was her wish.

Bottom Line Points
- VSED may provide a meaningful escape for those with mild to moderate dementia who fear a prolonged death from advanced dementia.
- It is hard for patients with mild to moderate dementia who are still enjoying much of their lives to decide when to initiate VSED because of the risks of losing precious time by acting too soon and of losing capacity to initiate and carry out the process.

Case 1.4. G.W. with Lung Cancer

G.W.'s death was filled with family conflict over his final time. His decision-making capacity became much less clear as the VSED process progressed. His "past self" before the brain surgery was relatively clear about wanting VSED, but his "current self" was much less clear about and less committed to the plan. His wife felt she was honoring his previously stated wishes to withhold food and drink, but his daughter felt that his current wishes should be honored, and he should be offered and then given food and drink if desired in the current moment. The struggle between patient, wife, and daughter continued until his death.

Bottom Line Points
- There may be significant differences between what one thinks earlier in an illness that one might want later in terms of an escape, and what one actually wants when the time comes, especially if capacity becomes diminished.
- Significant conflict can arise if the patient loses capacity during the VSED process, and there may be very differing views about how to honor the patient's prior directives and their current requests within and among families and healthcare providers. (In Part II of this book we will be exploring whether and how stopping eating and drinking [SED] might be an option for those who lose capacity for decision making before activating the process.)

The Korean-American Pastor

The final case in this chapter (Section 2.8) was a Korean-American pastor with a progressive terminal illness whose son had a mental illness. The pastor's quality of life was acceptable as long as he could go to church, but once that outlet became impossible he felt his life had lost meaning and his symptoms and debility became unacceptable. He began exploring the full range of last-resort options and even initiated a brief trial of VSED, which he gave up on relatively quickly for uncertain reasons. He eventually died on hospice without using any death-hastening option.

Bottom Line Points
- VSED can sound like a reasonable option in the abstract, but it can be very hard to execute and follow through with unless one is very committed and has thoroughly thought it through in advance.
- Because VSED usually has several phases with different kinds of clinical challenges over a timeframe of up to two weeks or more, it may require a more complex, multi-layered level of meticulous informed consent before initiation than many other major medical decisions.

- Carrying out VSED may encounter significant barriers because of the deep, culturally complex meanings of feeding and eating.

References

Ahluwalia, Indu B., Janice M. Dodds, and Magda Baligh. 1998. "Social Support and Coping Behaviors of Low-Income Families Experiencing Food Insufficiency in North Carolina." *Health Education and Behavior* 25, no. 5: 599–612.

Ayala, Guadalupe X., Barbara Baquero, and Sylvia Klinger. 2008. "A Systematic Review of the Relationship Between Acculturation and Diet Among Latinos in the United States: Implications for Future Research." *Journal of the American Dietetic Association* 108, no. 8: 1330–1344.

Battin, Margaret P. 1996. *The Least Worst Death*. New York: Oxford University Press.

Bolt, Eva E., Martijn Hagens, Dick Willems, and Bregie D. Onwuteaka-Philipsen. 2015. "Primary Care Patients Hastening Death by Voluntarily Stopping Eating and Drinking." 2015. *Annals of Family Medicine* 13, no. 5: 421–428.

Braun, Whitney. 2008. "Sallekhana: the Ethicality and Legality of Religious Suicide by Starvation in the Jain Religious Community." *Medicine and Law* 27, no. 4: 913–924. PMID: 19202863.

Byock, Ira. 2014. *Four Things that Matter Most: A Book About Living*. New York: Simon and Schuster.

Casarett, David J., and Timothy E. Quill. 2007. "'I'm Not Ready for Hospice': Strategies for Timely and Effective Hospice Discussions." *Annals of Internal Medicine* 146, no. 6: 443–449.

Chilton, Mariana, and Sue Booth. 2007. "Hunger of the Body and Hunger of the Mind: African American Women's Perceptions of Food Insecurity, Health, and Violence." *Journal of Nutrition, Education, and Behavior* 39, no. 3: 116–125.

China Daily. 2004. "Zhongyua Festival—Hungry Ghost Festival." *China Daily*, August 30, 2004 (retrieved October 20, 2008).

Dhillon, Jaapna, L. Karina Diaz Rios, Kaitlyn J. Aldaz, Natalie De La Cruz, Emily Vu, Syed Asad Asghar, Quintin Kuse, and Rudy M. Ortiz. 2019. "We Don't Have a Lot of Healthy Options: Food Environment Perceptions of First-Year, Minority College Students Attending a Food Desert Campus." *Nutrients* 11, no. 4: 816–830.

Dubowitz, Tamara, Madhumita Ghosh-Dastidar, Deborah A. Cohen, Robin Beckman, Elizabeth D. Steiner, Gerald P. Hunter, Karen R. Flórez, Christina Huang, Christine A. Vaughan, Jennifer C. Sloan, Shannon N. Zenk, Steven Cummins, and Rebecca L. Collins. 2015a. "Diet And Perceptions Change With Supermarket Introduction In A Food Desert, But Not Because Of Supermarket Use." *Health Affairs* 34, no. 11: 1858–1868.

Dubowitz, Tamara, Shannon N. Zenk, Bonnie Ghosh-Dastidar, Deborah A. Cohen, Robin Beckman, Gerald Hunter, Elizabeth D. Steiner, and Rebacca L. Collins. 2015b. "Healthy Food Access for Urban Food Desert Residents: Examination of the Food Environment, Food Purchasing Practices, Diet and BMI." *Public Health Nutrition* 18, no. 12:2220–2230.

Ganzini, Linda, Tomasz M. Beer, Matthew Brouns, Motomi Mori, and Yi-Ching Hsieh. 2006. "Interest in Physician-Assisted Suicide Among Oregon Cancer Patients." *Journal of Clinical Ethics* 17, no. 1: 27–38.

Ganzini, Linda, Elizabeth R. Goy, and Steven K. Dobscha. 2008. "Prevalence of Depression and Anxiety in Patients Requesting Physicians' Aid in Dying: Cross Sectional Survey." *British Medical Journal* 337: 1682.

Ganzini, Linda, Elizabeth R. Goy, and Steven K. Dobscha. 2009. "Oregonians' Reasons for Requesting Physician Aid in Dying." *Archives of Internal Medicine* 169, no. 5: 489–492.

Ganzini, Linda, Elizabeth R. Goy, Lois L. Miller, Theresa A. Harvath, Ann Jackson, and Molly A. Delorit. 2003. "Nurses' Experiences With Hospice Patients Who Refuse Food and Fluids to Hasten Death." *New England Journal of Medicine* 349, no. 4: 359–365.

Ganzini, Linda, Melinda A. Lee, Ronald T. Heintz, Joseph D. Bloom, and Daren S. Fenn. 1994. "The Effect of Depression Treatment on Elderly Patients' Preferences for Life-Sustaining Medical Therapy." *American Journal of Psychiatry* 151, no. 11: 1631–1636.

Hill, Brittany G., Ashely G. Maloney, Terry Mize, Tom Himelick, and Jodie L. Guest. 2011. "Prevalence and Predictors of Food Insecurity in Migrant Farmworkers in Georgia." *American Journal of Public Health* 101: 831–833.

Horowitz, Robert, Bernard Sussman, and Timothy Quill. 2016. "VSED Narratives: Exploring Complexity." *Narrative Inquiry in Bioethics* 6, no. 2: 115–120.

In My Own Words. 2020. Video Advance Recording Service, Oakland, CA. http://inmyownwords.com (accessed June 5, 2020).

Ivanovic, Natasa, Daniel Buche, and Andre Fringer. 2014. "Voluntary Stopping of Eating and Drinking at the End of Life—a "Systematic Search and Review" Giving Insight Into an Option of Hastening Death in Capacitated Adults at the End of Life." *BMC Palliative Care* 13, no. 1: 1.

Kaiser, Lucia L., Hugo Melgar-Quiñonez, Marilyn S. Townsend, Yvonne Nicholson, Mary Lavender Fujii, Anna C. Martin, and Cathi L. Lamp. 2003. "Food Insecurity and Food Supplies in Latino Households with Young Children." *Journal of Nutrition, Education, and Behavior* 35: 148–53.

Meier, Diane E., Anthony L. Back, and Robert S. Morrison. 2001. "The Inner Life of Physicians and Care of the Seriously Ill." *JAMA* 286, no. 23: 3007–3014.

Munger, Ashley L, Tiffani D.S. Lloyd, Katherine E. Speirs, Kate C. Riera, and Stephanie K. Grutzmacher. 2015. "More Than Just Not Enough: Experiences of Food Insecurity for Latino Immigrants." *Journal of Immigrant and Minority Health* 17, no. 5: 1548–1556.

Olson, Christine M. 1999. "Nutrition and Health Outcomes Associated with Food Insecurity and Hunger." *Journal of Nutrition* 129, no. 2: 521S–524S.

Quill, Timothy E. 1993. "Doctor, I Want to Die. Will You Help Me?" *JAMA* 270, no. 7: 870–873.

Quill, Timothy E. 2000. "Initiating End-of-Life Discussions with Seriously Ill Patients: Addressing the 'Elephant in the Room.'" *JAMA* 284, no. 19: 2502–2507.

Quill, Timothy E., and Amy P. Abernethy. 2013. "Generalist Plus Specialist Palliative Care—Creating a More Sustainable Model." *New England Journal of Medicine* 368, no. 13: 1173–1175.

Quill, Timothy E., and Margaret P. Battin. 2020. "Physician Assisted Death: Understanding, Evaluating and Responding to Requests for Medical Aid In Dying." UpToDate (website), Robert M. Arnold, section editor: https://www.uptodate.com/contents/physician-assisted-dying-understanding-evaluating-and-responding-to-requests-for-medical-aid-in-dying.

Quill, Timothy E., Robert Arnold, and Anthony L. Back. 2009. "Discussing Treatment Preferences with Patients Who Want 'Everything.'" *Annals of Internal Medicine* 151, no. 5: 345–349.

Quill, Timothy E., Rebecca Dresser, and Dan W. Brock. 1997. "The Rule of Double Effect—a Critique of its Role in End-of-Life Decision Making." *New England Journal of Medicine* 337, no. 24: 1768–1771.

Quill, Timothy E., Linda Ganzini, Robert D. Truog, and Thaddeus M. Pope. 2018. "Voluntarily Stopping Eating and Drinking Among Patients With Serious Advanced Illness-Clinical, Ethical, and Legal Aspects." *JAMA Internal Medicine* 178, no. 1: 123–127.

Quill, Timothy E., Bernard Lo, and Dan W. Brock. 1997. "Palliative Options of Last Resort: a Comparison of Voluntarily Stopping Eating and Drinking, Terminal Sedation, Physician-Assisted Suicide, and Voluntary Active Euthanasia." *JAMA* 278, no. 23: 2099–2104.

Schwarz, Judith K. 2007. "Exploring the Option of Voluntarily Stopping Eating and Drinking Within the Context of a Suffering Patient's Request For a Hastened Death." *Journal of Palliative Medicine* 10, no. 6: 1288–1297.

Stangle, Sabrina, Wukfried Schnepp, and Andre Fringer. 2019. "The Need to Distinguish between Different Forms of Oral Nutrition Refusal and Different Forms of Voluntary Stopping of Eating and Drinking." *Palliative Care & Social Practice* 13:1–7.

Teiser, Stephen F. 1996. *The Ghost Festival in Medieval China*. Princeton, NJ: Princeton University Press.

Walker, Renee E., Christopher R. Keane, and Jessica G. Burke. 2010. "Disparities and Access to Healthy Food in the United States: A Review of Food Deserts Literature." *Health and Place* 16, no. 5: 876–884.

Woodruff, Rebecca C., Regine Haardörfer, Ilana G. Raskind, April Hermstad, and Michelle C. Kegler. 2020. "Comparing Food Desert Residents With Non-Food Desert Residents on Grocery Shopping Behaviours, Diet and BMI: Results From a Propensity Score Analysis." *Public Health Nutrition* 23, no. 5: 806–811.

World Health Organization. 2018. "Global Hunger Continues to Rise, New UN Report Says" (September 11, 2018). https://www.who.int/news-room/detail/11-09-2018-global-hunger-continues-to-rise---new-un-report-says (accessed June 5, 2020).

3

Ethical Issues

Paul T. Menzel

3.1. Introduction

Legal and ethical assessments of VSED raise two kinds of questions: What behavior is permissible for patients, providers, and/or family? What are they obligated to do, or not do? The legal version of these questions is comparatively factual: what does the law *actually* permit? The ethical version, by contrast, is directly normative: what *ought* a patient, family member, or a medical provider be permitted to do? To be sure, ethical and legal considerations are often closely related. Legal permissions and requirements can greatly influence our moral judgments. In this chapter the ethical questions are usually pursued directly, without looking for answers that might depend on the facts of the law. Quite often, though, ethical and legal principles come together.

The ethical questions themselves divide into at least two basic sorts:

1. *What is the right thing to do?* We ask this sort of question when we ask whether for Al (the biker with ALS), for example, VSED would be a morally defensible step for him to take, or a morally wrong one.
2. *What are people permitted to do?* This is the sort of question we ask when assessing VSED as an overall practice: Is it an ethically permissible way for patients to hasten death? Is it permissible for providers and family to support it? Ethical permission still involves a judgment of right and wrong about behavior, but the focus is not only the patient's act, but others' action in response to it: would it be morally wrong for them to interfere and attempt to stop the act? To say that VSED is an ethically permissible choice is to say that such interference would be wrong, that others should respect the choice. This naturally slides into the language of rights: if VSED is permissible, the patient has a moral right to pursue it—a right in the sense of a "moral liberty," moral protection against interference or condemnation.

The questions pursued in this chapter are usually of the second sort: Is VSED a morally permissible way to hasten death? Actions by different parties come within the scope of such assessment: (a) the patient's act of VSED, (b) the support for that action that might come from health care providers and family, and (c) caregivers' choice to inform, or not to inform, them of their option to use VSED. All three are examined.

Throughout, three assumptions will be made: that (1) the patient who would pursue VSED has decision-making capacity; (2) the patient is adequately informed about VSED, its alternatives, and its typical progression and possible complications; (3) the patient understands her diagnosis and her prognosis with and without further treatment; and (4) any decision to pursue VSED is made voluntarily and without coercion, pressure, or manipulation. The focus in the chapter is thus on whether "clean" VSED, uncorrupted by any deficiencies in these respects, is ethically permissible.

Ethically assessing VSED will inevitably involve comparison with other end-of-life options and our beliefs about them, especially refusing lifesaving treatment (RLST). The moral right of patients with decision-making capacity to refuse treatment, even lifesaving treatment, is so firmly embedded in our beliefs that it can serve as the "anchoring" right in this discussion. The more similar we see RLST and VSED to be, the more likely we are to regard VSED as permissible. If providers are ethically permitted (even obligated) to provide palliative care when patients RLST, providers will be permitted (or even obligated) to provide palliative care for those who VSED.

A different comparison, with medical aid in dying (MAID), is also important. Since the ethical case for MAID is much more contested than it is for RLST, critics of VSED are likely to see VSED as more comparable with MAID than with RLST. Insofar as VSED is similar to MAID, the ethical case for VSED becomes more questionable.

In addition to the pursuit of moral consistency among VSED, RLST, and MAID, a central role will be played in the analysis by the principle of *patient autonomy*. In one of its standard formulations, the principle bids us to "respect the capacity of individuals to choose their own vision of the good life and act accordingly" and to engage "the patient's own powers of deliberation, choice, and agency" (Steinbock, London, and Arras 2013, 36 and 45). Reflecting *self-determination*, moral autonomy requires others to respect patients' decisions about their own lives.

Why should autonomy have such moral weight? It is hard to see why if we understand it primarily in terms of preferences, for even a competent person's preferences and desires may be volatile, fragile, and superficial, a function of serendipitous and questionable factors in people and their environments. Indeed, "preferences," as if they were a consumer's, are a misleading veneer of autonomy (O'Neill 2002, 47–48). A better understanding focuses more on *respect for persons*. Two of the first things such respect requires is to avoid deception and minimize coercion. If deception were routinely legitimate, how could individuals relate to each other as reflective, decision-making beings (the paradigm of persons) rather than objects to be manipulated? And if coercion were routinely justified, what would be the point of being a person, with capacity to reflect, form values, have convictions, and make decisions?

Autonomy gains yet additional force from our conceptions of *ownership*. "It's my life, not yours," said by patient to provider, is obviously true. Consciousness itself demands this use of possessive pronouns—self-consciousness does, at least. "My life" is life with *my* body, with *my* mind. I therefore have privileged use of my body and mind. When I use them to labor, work, and create, for example, the products are rightfully at least partly mine—thus the right not to be enslaved is fundamental. Others inevitably influence my mind and body, but they may not control them without my consent unless I am adversely affecting others. The title of the film "Whose Life Is It Anyway?" captures this self-ownership aspect (Badham 1981). It is utterly basic to persons, beings with the kind of consciousness in which they can think of their bodies *as their own*. The kind of ownership involved here is all the more powerful because it is so close to our very identity—we "own" our minds and bodies because we *are* our minds and bodies.

3.2. Refusing Lifesaving Treatment

One of the most powerful manifestations of these points about self-determination, respect for persons, and self-ownership is a patient's right to refuse medical treatment—a right secure enough to serve as an "anchoring right" in ethical comparisons with VSED.[1]

The terms with which the law categorizes this right are instructive. Administering medical treatment to competent persons without their informed consent is "battery"—the unauthorized harmful *or* offensive invasion of the body or contact with it. Why should the protection against

---

[1] Significant elements of the substance of this section were articulated in Menzel 2017, 636–639.

imposing treatment hold even against invasions that are merely "offensive," not harmful, and even when there is good reason to think treatment would be helpful? Two reasons stand out (Cantor 2006, 106).

First, bodily integrity: treatment is typically an invasion of the body, and if anything should be within persons' province of control, their own bodies should be.[2] Here the self-ownership element behind autonomy is clearly at work. Second, patient decision-making capacity: if patients can be asked and are capable of responding if they are asked, they should be asked. An extremely basic moral judgment is present here: when people have the capacity to consent, they should be asked, and their voluntary choices should be respected. If we do not ask, we do not treat or respect them as persons— the beings with agency and capacity that they are. And asking is not genuine if the person's response does not matter—the right of informed consent must include the right to refuse.

The right to refuse medical treatment thus has a strong moral foundation and is more than just a legal right. In the United States in the late 1970s and 1980s, moreover, the right came to include the refusal of *lifesaving* (or life-sustaining) treatment, at least in situations of terminal illness and suffering.[3] Even if lifesaving treatment is firmly included within its scope, though, the right encounters other questions whose answers have important implications for the scope of VSED. Among the most important is whether the right should extend to refusing lifesaving treatment when a person's illness is not "terminal."

Non-Terminal Illness

In situations of terminal illness and continued suffering, the basis of the right to RLST is relatively obvious: who is better positioned to discern the value of the remaining life with suffering than the person experiencing that time? How much of the power of this question changes when the person is not terminally ill?

[2] Justice Cardozo in *Schloendorff* 1914, 129: "Every human being of adult years and sound mind has a right to determine what shall be done with his own body."

[3] Pope 2013; Meisel, Cerminara, and Pope 2020, para. 7.06[A-3] and 6.03[F]. See also *Satz* 1978, discussed in Meisel, Cerminara, and Pope 2020, para. 12.02[C-4], and *In re Browning* 1990, discussed in Meisel, Cerminara, and Pope 2020, para. 5.01[A].

On the one hand, very little.[4] If anything, suffering in non-terminal illness may last longer and therefore be all the worse. Moreover, while an illness may not be "terminal" in the sense of death being likely within six months, life may still be on a steady downhill slide in which the patient is losing the things she most associates with being alive (in progressive dementia, for example). On the other hand, what if the refusal occurs in a situation where the illness or injury is not terminal at all—a 25-year-old accident victim, for example, who, after initial stabilization, refuses the limb amputation still needed to save her life. May we impose treatment there?

Two factors affect how likely we are to stick to a right of refusal in non-terminal situations: degree of bodily invasion and potential for later retrospective consent. A tasteless pill or food additive are different than surgery or tube-feeding. Most lifesaving treatments are invasive, however, and thus especially objectionable to impose in the face of refusal. It is, after all, the patient's own body that would be invaded.

The prospect of retrospective consent can matter, too. If providers have very good reason to think that a burn patient, for example, will end up saying, after recovery, that it was right to give him lifesaving treatment even though he refused that treatment at the time because of his horrendous pain, we may think treating him despite his current refusal is justified.[5] This justification does not simply override autonomy to achieve patient benefit. The appeal is to the patient's eventual consent, still reflecting a kind of respect for autonomy. Moreover, such an appeal has a natural check: whether the patient will later validate her choice having been overridden.

While patients' decisions to RLST are more open to challenge in non-terminal illness situations when a low degree of bodily invasion and high likelihood of retrospective consent can sometimes justify imposing treatment, the default rule remains the right to refuse. The burden of proof falls on the person who wants to treat to show that the degree of bodily invasion is minor or the likelihood of retrospective consent high. Generally the moral

---

[4] *In re Browning* 568 So. 2d 4.10 (Fla. 1990): the patient's right to refuse treatment holds "regardless of his or her medical condition." This and many of the other legal developments in the last half of the 20th century concerning the right to refuse medical treatment, including most of those mentioned in the previous paragraphs, are admirably summarized by Norman Cantor in his engaging memoir (2020, 101–123).

[5] The contention of several physicians attending Dax Cowart (Burton 1989; Cowart and Burt 1998). Dax never did subsequently consent (Pope 2005, 694–695).

right to refuse lifesaving treatment applies in non-terminal as well as terminal illness situations.[6]

The Comparison with VSED

We are now in a position to compare RLST with VSED. Both are sometimes pursued by patients in non-terminal as well as terminal illness situations. In both, people reject something vital to life that directly involves their bodies. To be sure, there are some factual differences between RLST and VSED, but the moral relevance of these differences is questionable.

In RLST a patient decides what other people will do to her body; in VSED she refuses to do something to herself. What difference, though, should this make? Why would self-ownership and bodily integrity be any less important in what you may do to yourself than in what others may do to you? If others are wrong when they invade your body by imposing treatment, why would they be justified in forcing food into you? *The reasoning in this rhetorical question is not that food and water are medical treatment, but that forced feeding is similarly an intrusion into the patient's body.* One should note, too, that for a patient determined not to eat, forced feeding can only be accomplished by imposing a feeding tube or intravenous line. Imposing medical treatment without consent is thus implicit in any effective denial of a patient's right to VSED.[7]

A second, more widely cited descriptive difference is that while RLST may not assuredly hasten death—the patient may live without treatment

---

[6] The right may have other exceptions as well. They might include, for example, the young anorexic who needs additional nutrition, patients with treatment-resistant depression, and those who wish to hasten death because they are circumstantially "tired of life." These may involve incapacitated individuals, in which case they are not truly exceptions, or they may be justified exceptions to the right to RLST. Perhaps there are even more exceptions to any right to VSED. In any case, acknowledging cases that may constitute limits to the right is no reason to deny the right in its typical, non-exceptional situations.

[7] This needs qualification. There are ways short of imposing treatment in which the right, though not strictly blocked, can be undermined: by not providing requested palliative support for a VSED patient who needs that to proceed, or by not informing a patient of the VSED option. See the "Providing Assistance" and "Information" sub-sections below. There are also more unusual ways: tempting the patient to eat once she has begun VSED (holding food close to her, accompanied by "don't you want some of this ___ that you love so much?"), verbally badgering the patient, or threatening to withhold something cherished (seeing her grandchildren one more time, for example).

anyhow—VSED carried through assiduously will always result in death. In exercising the right to RLST a person is said to *allow death to come*, not to *cause* it; the underlying disease is the cause of death. In VSED, the patient's action causes the death.

Yet the moral relevance of this difference, too, is doubtful. In a refusal of LST, the causes of the specific death, occurring when it does, are multiple: the underlying condition or disease that sets the stage for a decision to refuse LST *and* the decision to refuse. To say that the only cause was the underlying disease would not explain why this death occurred as soon as it did and in the way it did. In the typical case of VSED, too, there are multiple causes: the refusal to eat and drink, as well as the underlying condition that motivates the person to embark on VSED.

As to intention, even in a permissible refusal of treatment a patient's intention may be to hasten death. An antibiotic for pneumonia, for example, may be refused with just that intention and that hope. There can even be definitive evidence of this—if the patient were to express distinct disappointment, for example, when she failed to die despite refusing treatment.

It might be argued that a somewhat different distinction, active/passive, distinguishes VSED from RLST. Not treating is passive inaction, and treating is active. VSED, though, is hardly passive. It's an active steeling of oneself against the desire to eat. Yet this view of how the action/inaction distinction applies to VSED compared to RLST is simplistic, too. Refusing, even in RLST, is an active element; it's deciding *not* to do something, true, but deciding to refuse is often experienced as very much a decisive act of the patient. Moreover, refusing treatment can often require various other active steps to accomplish, especially when treatment is being discontinued. In VSED we see the same mix of both active and passive elements. VSED is not-eating as well as an assertive act of refusing to eat. Even if the active/passive difference were morally relevant,[8] it does not readily distinguish RLST from VSED.

Might terminal illness limit the right to VSED more than the modest limitations that terminal illness allows on the right to refuse treatment? Again, it would be hard to justify treating VSED differently. Bodily integrity and self-ownership are as much at stake in VSED as in RLST. If they are the moral

---

[8] The moral relevance of the difference, often stated as the distinction between doing and allowing harm, has elicited a huge critical literature in contemporary philosophy; see Woollard and Howard-Snyder 2016 for a high-level survey. A useful collection of articles on the distinction as used and contested in bioethics is Steinbock and Norcross 1999.

underpinnings of the general protection accorded refusing treatment even when one is not terminally ill, why would they not also protect VSED in that situation? A clinician's refusal to inform about the VSED option or provide support for it may dissuade a person from VSED, but ultimately the only way to prevent a determined person from hastening death by VSED is by imposing medically delivered nutrition and hydration, violating the patient's right to refuse treatment.

We have seen that in unusual situations, a high probability of retrospective consent may justify rejecting a patient's decision to RLST, at least in situations absent terminal illness. Theoretically, such retrospective consent could also justify overriding a patient's choice of VSED. In the actual circumstance and process of VSED, however, this reasoning is likely to be even more problematic than it is already with RLST. VSED demands fortitude and persistence from patients, and inherently it allows them time to reverse their decision.[9] Thus, so many cases of VSED are free of the prospect of a patient retrospectively consenting to not having been allowed to stop eating and drinking that retrospective consent does not normally need to be considered.

Take Mrs. H., the patient with clear signs of Alzheimer disease (Case 1.3, Chapter 1). She was not terminally ill in the conventional sense of a six-month prognosis, but many other factors virtually eliminated any prospect that she would later thank family or providers were they to have stopped her from completing VSED: (1) her direct experience with her own mother's advanced Alzheimer's, (2) her steadfast refusal to consider a nursing home, (3) her expressions that she would know when it was time to pull the VSED trigger, and (4) her decisive admission to a home hospice program when she began VSED.

In a comparison with the right to refuse lifesaving treatment, VSED thus stands up reasonably well. The moral grounds for respecting it as a patient's choice are so similar to those for respecting a refusal of LST that the legitimate scope of VSED, too, is not limited to terminal illness.

---

[9] Moreover, lifesaving treatment may look frightening and burdensome to a patient, leading the person to focus too much on the difficulty of enduring it, losing sight of its positive potential; that's one reason we may on occasion be confident that patients will later agree with rejecting their choice. By contrast, what the prospective VSED patient faces if she continues to accept food—normal eating and drinking—is usually not burdensome or frightening. The prospect of eating and drinking does not mislead. Precisely the opposite—sometimes it is the difficulty of not eating and drinking that may mislead.

3.3. Suicide

We have yet to deal with arguably the most important ethical objection to VSED: that it is a form of suicide and fundamentally different in this respect from RLST.[10] In suicide a person *intentionally aims* at her own death and *directly causes* it; in a typical VSED, too, a person intends to die and directly causes the death. As a matter of descriptive fact, then, VSED is a form of suicide. (Keep in mind the working definition of VSED from the Preface and Chapter 1: it does not include failure to eat and drink when eating and drinking are painful or medically burdensome, or when appetite is naturally suppressed.)

In the moral framework in which this is raised as an objection, intentionally and directly causing the death of any innocent person (oneself or others) is never ethically permitted. In the Natural Law version of the framework dominant in traditional Roman Catholic moral theology, one is not permitted to destroy intentionally any fundamental natural good of human existence, one of which is bodily life itself (Boyle 2017, 256 and 260).

The focus of the objection is not on the contrast between active killing and death from omission; it is on *intentionally causing* death. In refusing treatment the purpose is typically "to relieve the patient of a . . . procedure that was of limited usefulness . . . or unreasonably burdensome," and omitting treatment, even medically delivered food and fluid, is then not a decision to kill and should not be equated with suicide (U.S. Bishops' Pro-Life Committee 1992, 393). At other times, however,

> the harsh reality is that . . . withdrawal of nutrition and hydration . . . directly intend[s] to bring about a patient's death . . . . Whether orally administered or medically assisted . . ., [food and fluids] are sometimes withdrawn not because a patient is dying, but precisely because a patient is not dying (or not dying quickly) . . . . (U.S. Bishops' Pro-Life Committee 1992, 393, emphasis added).

The view is clear: when, as in VSED, people intentionally cause their death and cause it with certainty, they impermissibly commit suicide.[11]

---

[10] Significant elements of the substance of this section were articulated in Menzel 2017, 638.

[11] Some argue that the doctrinal Roman Catholic position should not reach this conclusion. John Paris has articulated the various grounds in classic Catholic sources for frequently not regarding the refusal or withholding of food and water, including by mouth, as prohibited suicide. The elements in Catholic moral theology that provide grounds for such a relatively liberal position on VSED include

Can the Principle of Double Effect (PDE) be used to support VSED? Is VSED analogous to the classic medical case that employs this principle, the use of morphine? In the traditional Catholic view administering morphine is licit because the act itself is pain-relieving and not inherently wrong, and the death it might eventually cause, though foreseen, is not intended. The intention is to relieve pain. Moreover, the relief of pain is accomplished by the morphine and not by causing the patient's death. This is precisely where administering a possibly lethal dose of morphine differs from VSED. The person who pursues VSED does it precisely in order to hasten death, with certainty death will follow, and only the death, not the stopping eating and drinking itself, accomplishes the patient's goal.[12] The PDE does not rescue VSED.

Some may try to defend VSED against this view by claiming that only actions, not omissions, can cause death and constitute suicide; therefore, since VSED is the omission of food and water, it cannot be the cause of death and thus cannot be suicide. But that response on behalf of VSED does not work. Omissions, especially intentional ones, can be causes (O'Rourke 2005, 540). Even if it is an omission, VSED still causes death. It may be "suicide by omission," "passive suicide," or a "singular form" of suicide, but it is suicide nonetheless (Birnbacher 2015; Jox et al. 2017, 187).

Once we move outside an ethical framework where all intentional killing of innocent persons is inherently and always wrong, however, the descriptive and conceptual fact that VSED is a form of suicide does not have to make it objectionable. Why should hastening death *intentionally*, ensuring it *with certainty*, and being its *primary cause*, make the act that hastens death morally wrong if what the action brings about, death sooner rather than later, is a good thing compared to living with great suffering or in a condition of severe deterioration like advanced dementia? The characteristics of VSED's relationship to death—intention, certainty, causation—may make VSED

---

a fuller understanding of non-obligatory "extraordinary" care as care with "disproportionate" or "excessive" burdens, an emphasis on "hope of benefit" and "friendship with God" as the ultimate goods that extended life can sometimes threaten, and wariness about a too exclusive focus on the slippery notion of intention. On these important elements in Catholic moral tradition, see Paris 1992 and O'Rourke 2005.

[12] For a somewhat more extended discussion of Double Effect and VSED, see Menzel 2017, ftn 26. For a detailed application of Double Effect and the prohibition of suicide to VSED, see Jansen and Sulmasy 2002, especially 846, 848. The intricate relationship between Double Effect and the prohibition of intentional, directly caused death is pursued by Boyle 2017, especially 262, 272. An extensive critical analysis of PDE is provided by Sumner 2011, 56–71.

different than either "letting death come" or the pain-relief focused, Double Effect cases like morphine, but why do they make it *wrong*? Intentionally ensuring and causing a good result would, if anything, seem to be better than merely letting the same result come about with no action. *Moreover, as long as SED is voluntary and not foisted on patients by others, it is within their moral prerogative as much as is RLST.* Either can be foolish or wrong in a specific situation, but liberty-rights include the freedom to make foolish choices.

Providing Assistance

These are powerful arguments against the view that VSED is inherently wrong because it is a form of suicide, yet one of the strongest threats to VSED's legal and moral acceptability still pivots off its descriptive status as suicide. In U.S. law, while neither completed nor attempted suicide is a crime in the sense of something for which the person may be punished, others may stop the attempt, and in most jurisdictions no one is legally permitted to assist it. The resulting complication for VSED is clear. To be a comfortable path to death, VSED is best medically managed and accompanied by palliative care. But if VSED is suicide, VSED may then involve caregivers in assistance in suicide. This poses no moral difficulty for those who see nothing wrong with assisting a justified suicide, but it threatens to greatly complicate the normal legal and moral picture.

Assume for the moment that VSED is suicide. Under what circumstances would palliative care for VSED patients qualify as *assistance* in the suicide? Jox and colleagues argue that it sometimes does, as determined by two requirements: (1) when the assistance or its promise is "instrumental for the death to occur," and (2) when the assisting person "knows and at least partially shares the patient's intention to induce death" (Jox et al. 2017, 188). The first is a kind of causal condition—a "but for . . .," necessary but not sufficient cause: were it not for the palliative care or its promise, the patient would not have initiated, or would not have completed, her VSED. This condition is arguably satisfied, for example, when a patient who has been distinctly hesitant about VSED decides to pursue it once palliative care is explained and arranged by attending caregivers, or when a patient proceeding with VSED repeatedly asks for reassurance of such support. In other cases it could be clear that palliative support does not constitute causal assistance: when the clinician support comes along later in the process without having been promised earlier, or when the patient seems determined to continue VSED in any case (Jox et al. 2017). The point of Jox and colleagues is not that to say that when the supportive care qualifies as assistance in a suicide it is necessarily wrong, but that it is in fact assistance in suicide and thus needs to be justified as such.

Once the limited real alternatives for caregivers are clearly seen, however, pragmatic considerations provide the justification. Review the ethical picture from the start. To block a determined person from hastening death by VSED, a caregiver would need to do one of three things: (1) suppress her "revulsion at the prospect of physically overcoming and restraining people" and feed them against their will (Cantor 2006, 112); (2) engage in the seeming hypocrisy of letting patients embark on VSED but then pull them back from the final phase of dying from VSED once they are no longer able to resist the imposition of food and fluid; or (3) continuously badger them from the start to have food and fluid while not palliating weakness and dry-mouth. None of these is morally defensible, for the patient is acting within her moral rights. In such a context, it would be callous, indeed, for providers to deny appropriate palliative care. Thus, in practice, the assistance involved in supportive care is ethically permissible *even if* (a) VSED is suicide, (b) the care supporting it qualifies as real assistance, and (c) assisting in a suicide is generally not permissible.[13]

The ethical justification of palliative care for VSED is thus strong, a function finally of three convincing points. First, the competent act of VSED is itself a morally protected liberty. Second, caregivers should respect that liberty even when they might think a particular patient should not exercise it. Third, when a patient does exercise it, caregivers should serve their patient's best interest—that is, with palliative support.

The conclusion is important, for supportive care is crucial if VSED is to be a realistic option. At the same time, however, such strong ethical justification does not necessarily forbid all efforts of a provider to discourage VSED (see Section IV below). The conclusion may also tolerate exempting providers as conscientious objectors to the whole process of VSED, provided they can refer to alternative accepting providers.

---

[13] Reasoning very similar to this, though not exactly the same, was used by the Supreme Court of South Australia in *H Ltd v J* 2010 to avoid the conclusion that assisting with VSED is the criminal offense of assisting a suicide. The judge had previously concluded that VSED was not suicide, but stated that even if it was suicide, "merely respecting a competent refusal falls short of the required encouragement to constitute aiding and abetting." See White et al. 2014, at 382–384. The quotation is White and colleagues' description of the judge's position, not the judge's own words.

Terminal Illness and "Suicide"

Despite the fact that VSED literally is suicide, in many of its settings people may just not regard it that way. "Suicide" can be a highly elastic term even when the technically necessary and sufficient elements of intention, certainty, and causation are present. Alan Alberts, for example, employed VSED to ensure that he would not live years into his relentlessly advancing dementia. With that goal sharply focused in his mind, his wife Phyllis Shacter writes that "it never occurred to either of us" that Alan's refusal to eat and drink could be suicide; it was making the best of what would otherwise be a much worse road to death (Shacter 2016, 95; Shacter 2017).

If we do not regard a patient's refusal of even the most clearly lifesaving and non-invasive medical treatment as suicide (for example, a basic antibiotic for pneumonia), why should we see the refusal to eat and drink as suicide? The patient's intention in some refusals of LST is to hasten death, not merely to draw a line on burdensome or insufficiently beneficial medical treatment to see what happens. Many people, of course, may just see the refusal of lifesaving treatment differently in regard to "suicide" than they see a refusal to eat and drink merely because RLST concerns treatment. But that does not engage the crucial question of why that difference should matter if intention and causation are the same in both, and if the death that both accomplish is better than living longer.

The variable use of the "suicide" label is starkly visible not only in the common perception of RLST but in efforts to legalize medical aid in dying (MAID). Advocates of MAID legalization often insist that it is not "assisted suicide." The view that as a matter of terminology it is not "suicide" is shared by the American Association of Suicidology (American Association of Suicidology 2017). The chances of legislative and voter approval of legalization appear to be influenced by the label used. Referring to MAID as "aid in dying" instead of "physician-assisted suicide" need not be sleight-of-hand labeling. When the assistance in hastening death is restricted to persons with a "terminal" condition, as it has been in many jurisdictions where MAID has been legalized, it is descriptively correct to refer to it as "aid in dying"—the patient already *is* dying. And yet at the same time, with its characteristics of intended death, assured death, and directly caused death, a patient's act in using MAID is also suicide. Descriptively, the act is both.

Perhaps perceptions of "suicide" in regard to VSED reflect similar observations. Even when VSED hastens a death that would otherwise be further off than six months—to avoid the imminent progression of dementia past the point of retaining decision-making capacity, for example—the situation can still be legitimately seen as "terminal." Progressive dementia that relentlessly deepens, even if slowly, is likely to be experienced personally as a "terminal" condition. It is utterly different than normal old age, for one is literally progressively losing one's mind. It, too, is a terminal condition in the terms that matter to people (Menzel 2013, 342–343).

Outside morally absolutist frameworks about suicide, context is likely to matter. What people generally see suicide to be when they regard it as tragic or wrong is intentionally causing one's death *when one is not already dying*. Thus, VSED in contexts that people see as terminal will often not be seen as suicide. Literally VSED is suicide, but many will not see it that way when it is neither tragic nor impermissible. "Suicide" will have become a normative term; it's "suicide" when it's wrong and "aid in dying" when it's not.[14]

In summary, justification for a moral right to VSED may not be provided by exactly the same reasons that undergird the right to RLST, but those reasons come close. The additional considerations that will suffice are readily available: (a) if truly competent and voluntary suicide is not inherently wrong, (b) if VSED is not suicide, or (c) if, though VSED literally is suicide, assisting it is still permissible. As long as refusing food and water by mouth is voluntary and not foisted on patients—the same limitations we put on RLST—VSED is a patient's moral prerogative. Both reflect self-determination, respect for persons, and bodily self-ownership.

3.4. A Different Comparison: Medical Aid in Dying

While many of the elements that underlie the moral right to RLST also apply to VSED, fewer of them apply to MAID, making MAID's justification more

---

[14] Some authors approach the question of whether VSED is suicide in a normative vein that seems even more pragmatic: because VSED and its assistance are, for all practical purposes, legally permissible, they do not warrant the "suicide" label. See Schwarz 2011. We should keep in mind, however, the dangers that can attend denying the label "suicide" to MAID and VSED and reserving it for the tragic, allegedly pathological and often violent acts we without hesitation regard as "suicide." Phoebe Friesen argues with considerable nuance and detailed evidence that drawing such a strong distinction stigmatizes those who attempt suicide as mentally ill when not all are, fails to respect them in their individual situations, and hampers optimal treatment. Drawing the distinction is thus a two-edged sword: it has benefits for MAID and VSED, but it unjustifiably stigmatizes those who commit "suicide" with a morally pejorative label (Friesen 2020, especially 34–35).

difficult than VSED's. VSED does, however, share some descriptive characteristics with MAID that morally challenge VSED.

Like refusing treatment, VSED is ultimately a refusal to let others do
things to one's body (force-feeding, tube-feeding). MAID is different: a patient asks others to do something to her body (or at least *for* her, so she can
in turn do something to her body). MAID, unlike VSED, does not bar others
from doing what they might want to do (force-feed). Consequently, the arguably most fundamental aspect of any right to hasten death—control of the
patient's body by the patient—protects VSED nearly as clearly as it protects
RLST, but the same claim cannot be readily made for MAID.

To be sure, the ultimate moral relevance of this difference between
rejecting what others may want to do and asking them to act to accomplish
the same end can be doubted. Those who focus on the beneficial effect for
the patient may find the difference irrelevant and conclude that MAID,
RLST, and VSED are morally equivalent options for avoiding suffering and
living too long. Others who focus less on effect and more on the primary
prerogatives of patients are likely to see the difference as important, leading
them to regard RLST as the most firmly protected, VSED as a close second,
and MAID as more questionable.

These differences, debatable as they are, may explain some of the varying
scope we accord to the legitimate use of RLST and VSED compared to MAID.
Permissible VSED, like RLST, is not limited to terminal illness, whereas we
find such a limitation on MAID in many of the jurisdictions where it is legally permitted. The strong bodily integrity and self-ownership elements
at the heart of our respect for a patient's refusal of treatment and choice to
stop eating and drinking are not as clearly available to MAID. Consider the
worries we have about MAID creating a culture where people are expected to
die when they get to be "burdens," or are readily allowed to end things when
they are only "tired of life." Perhaps we should, and do, have similar worries
about the use of RLST and VSED, but in those cases the concerns tend to get
pushed aside by the strength of the underlying right to control what is done
to one's body. In the case of MAID, that strongest moral ground is not as
available. Thus, restrictions on MAID such as terminal illness or an underlying serious medical condition are not as difficult to justify as they would be
on RLST or VSED.

In one outstanding respect, however, VSED does resemble MAID more
than it does RLST—suicide. In both VSED and MAID, the patient intends
death and can cause it with assurance. If suicide carries a burden of absolute

(or nearly absolute) wrongdoing, then VSED will be as difficult to justify as MAID, and for the same reasons. But that's a big "if." As has been noted previously, one does not clinch the ethical case against VSED simply by pointing out that it can be accurately described as "suicide." Hastening death with explicit intention and assured causal effect may not be any worse than hastening death without such intention or assured effect.

In the final analysis, VSED's substantial similarity with RLST lends it considerable moral protection. Yet it shares some significant similarities with MAID, too, that expose it to some of the ethical challenge faced by MAID.

3.5. Information, Encouragement, Persuasion

If the previous analysis is correct, a competent patient's voluntary choice to stop eating and drinking is morally permissible: the choice is ethically protected and should be respected by others. Also permissible is provider support of VSED patients with effective palliative care even if that support is regarded as assisting in a suicide; providers may even have a duty to provide such care. These conclusions, though, do not settle all questions around the practice of VSED. Should a patient who does not ask about a VSED option be informed of it? May a patient ever be positively encouraged to pursue VSED, not just accurately informed of it? May a patient ever be discouraged from pursuing it?

Information

Some may claim it is permissible for providers not to inform any of their patients about VSED (Jansen and Sulmasy 2002; Quill et al. 2018, 125). A stronger version would claim that not including VSED in information is permissible even if the patient has asked what their options are for hastening death. A stronger version yet would add that not only is failing to inform ethically permitted, but that a provider should not inform. Jansen and Sulmasy take such a position. First, they argue that "the option to engage in VSED is not . . . part of standard care offered to patients at the end of life," and thus one is not obligated to inform patients of it (Jansen 2004, 72). Moreover, a physician "should not even mention this practice to the patient because, by doing so, the patient may be tempted or influenced to choose it," in which case the physician would be "advising, assisting, or tempting others [the patient] to engage in wrongdoing" (Jansen and Sulmasy 2002, 848). On certain further assumptions about complicity, it might even be claimed that a physician who does not inform has no obligation to refer the patient to someone else.

Even for a provider firmly opposed to VSED because of her personal views or her ethical tradition, however, such a position is difficult to defend. If morally and legally it is permissible for patients to refuse food and water (though in a particular case it may not be the right thing for them to do), how can it be proper to deprive them of the information needed to exercise that choice? Professional caregivers are usually in the best position to provide accurate information about VSED and what is in store for patients who pursue it.

The opposite extreme may be no more defensible: inform all patients about the option of VSED, including those who neither ask about it (specifically or generally) nor give any hint they might be interested. Patients are often vulnerable to seeing themselves as a burden to others, not only to themselves, and no one, especially not providers imbued by their patients with special authority, should contribute to a culture of pressure to die sooner than a person truly wants. Providers should exercise discretion and perceptive contextual judgment in threading the needle between two risks—not telling the patient of a viable option they might well end up wanting to pursue (and have every right to pursue), and telling the patient so much, or so abruptly, or in such a tone, that the patient feels nudged or pressured to choose it. Both risks should be minimized. In the abstract, neither is so much worse than the other that we should always err on the side of avoiding one and not the other. Effectively confining people to a life they reasonably want not to continue by not informing them of certain things they have every right to do to hasten death throws up more than a minor obstacle.

Between these extremes, a moderate position emerges as ethically sensible: Recognize that people generally have a right to know their permissible options *and* that no one should do anything that would pressure them to hasten death. Then, attempt to discern the particular balance of words and information that will best respect individual patients. Such discernment is a difficult responsibility, but that is what professional ethical judgment sometimes calls for. Bill, the patient with indolent breast cancer, may be a good example. He desperately sought options to escape an unacceptable medical situation, and VSED was his only legal option. When first informed of it he was not interested, thinking it undignified and too hard. His condition continued to worsen. Faced with the dilemma of whether to raise the VSED option with him again, his providers decided they would, and Bill decisively pursued it. Their judgment may have been hazardous, but it turned out wise.

An ensuing question is inevitable: to carry out their responsibilities regarding information, should caregivers who work in contexts where patients are most likely to have an interest in hastening death have a basic clinical knowledge of VSED? Hospice staff and palliative care physicians and nurses, at least, may reasonably be expected to have such knowledge. Just as palliative care should be made available to any patient who considers refusing lifesaving treatment, we may well want to say that basic information about VSED should be readily available. All clinicians who care for dying patients should at least be aware of VSED as a potential last-resort option, even if they do not approve of it personally.

Encouragement, Discouragement, Persuasion

Is it ever defensible not only to inform a patient about VSED but also to encourage it? Is it ever defensible to discourage it?[15]

It is tempting to say "No" for both. That may be the ethically safe position, for discouragement can constitute a real barrier to a choice that is permissible for the patient to make, and encouragement beyond adequate and unbiased information risks pressuring the patient on the delicate matter of hastening death. Nonetheless, exceptional situations can call for advice beyond information.

A nurse or physician may sense, for example, that a patient who has been repeatedly asking about (even pleading for) a way to hasten death, is unable to absorb what he was told in being informed about VSED—particularly the fact that when supported with good palliative care, dying from VSED is typically not an uncomfortable death. "I just couldn't do that," he says more than once. Would it be permissible for the provider patiently to explain once again the typical course of VSED, adding mildly encouraging words such as "if you really want not to live further in your condition . . . , I suspect you could do this. We would do our best to make you as comfortable as possible." Would that be intrusive pressure, or a wise and discerning boost for a

---

[15] Beauchamp and Childress (2001, 93–98) lay out a spectrum of influence on a patient, from information to persuasion to manipulation and coercion.

patient who would ultimately, in terms of his own values, benefit from such encouragement?

Similarly, in the opposite direction, a provider may sense that a patient who is about to embark on VSED is not going to have the persistence to follow through with it, or she might be missing out on opportunities for recovery or improved quality of life. Having informed the patient of the relevant facts about choosing to die in this way, the provider may wonder out loud with the patient how committed she is to it. Perhaps the proper description of this is not "discouraging" the patient but frankly sharing thoughts about whether it is in fact a wise course given the patient's character and medical condition. But even if it is mild discouragement, why say it is never permissible?

Very different from this, and not acceptable, would be a presumptuous kind of discouragement: a firm "oh you don't want to do that" in response to the patient having said she's considering VSED, for example. Or "that would be suicide, you know," said in a tone that was unmistakably condemning. In some ethical frameworks, of course, VSED might indeed be wrong because it is suicide, but that is not the only plausible framework from which to judge VSED. Certain kinds of encouragement, too, as well-meant as they might be, can be improper: "you know there are a lot of people in your situation who have done this [VSED] . . . " to a patient who has not shown any interest in VSED after caregivers shared that it was a legal and potentially viable option. Improper nudging in either direction takes its worst form when it is an outright attempt to persuade the patient to adopt the provider's own moral point of view. That said, conscientious objection may still allow a clinician to exit upon referral to a more receptive practitioner if she is morally opposed to the practice which her informed patient now wants to pursue. Because the patient has the moral right to pursue VSED, however, the objecting clinician, even if it on the basis of moral conscience, should refer (see Chapter 4, Section 4.9).

3.6. Conclusions

1. Though VSED can reasonably be seen as morally objectionable by particular individuals and within certain ethical traditions, it is not reasonable to deny patients the liberty to hasten death by VSED. Others should not interfere with such a choice, and they ought not to condemn a patient for initiating it. The permissibility of VSED is built on the

same elements that underlie the moral right to refuse lifesaving treatment: bodily integrity and self-ownership, self-determination, and respect for persons. Any society that views RLST as morally protected should extend the same protection to VSED.

2. Clinician support for VSED—hospice and palliative care in particular—is at least permissible, if not obligatory. Such care is not forbidden assistance in a suicide, even if VSED is suicide and even if the care is indispensable assistance. Since patients are within their moral rights in choosing to stop eating and drinking, providers are permitted to provide all care that is in the patient's subsequent best interest. On normal principles of professional fidelity to patients, caregivers may even be obligated to provide such care unless they refer.

3. Neither a practice of refusing to inform any of one's patients of their permissible VSED option, nor a practice of informing all of one's patients of this option, is ethically defensible. Patients generally have a right to know their permissible options that fit their clinical situation; information should not be withheld that a particular patient might find to be critically important. No one, however, should do what could easily be interpreted as pressuring a patient to hasten death. Caregivers cannot escape the responsibility to use discerning and artful judgment in choosing what should be conveyed to different patients.

4. Beyond providing accurate information, providers should seldom offer explicit encouragement or discouragement of VSED. In occasional circumstances of patients' questionable perceptions of VSED's difficulty or ease, however, providers may sensitively encourage or discourage a patient's impending choice, though that should never slide into attempting to persuade the patient of the provider's own moral viewpoint.

3.7. Ethical Issues Review of Initial Cases

Case 1.1. Al, the Biker with ALS

Diagnosed with ALS after years of struggling with a malignant brain tumor, Al quickly progressed to being completely bed-bound and not able to self-feed, assisted 24/7 by dedicated nursing aides. During a requested physician home visit, he explained how strongly he felt about his independence and privacy and asked directly about his options for not prolonging life. He was informed of VSED in considerable detail and quickly decided to pursue it. When and if he was ready to initiate VSED, he had the option of admission to an in-patient palliative care unit.

Al strongly preferred to remain at home, but his aides and their agency decided they could not support him in VSED. He was subsequently admitted to hospital palliative care. Within 24 hours of admission he completely stopped eating and drinking. A steady stream of motorcycle friends visited, as did many of his home health aides, graciously trying to make peace with his decision. Given the depth of his previous medical ordeals, he did not find VSED difficult. His common-sense view was that it was simply the best of his options. Twelve days later, peacefully, he died.

Bottom Line Points
- Al directly asked about his options for hastening his death before being informed of VSED. Providers faced no dilemma about whether or when to inform him.
- Physicians deemed him to have capacity, and he was clear and decisive in his decision. Such a "clean" decision avoided ethical dilemmas that sometimes confront other cases.
- Al's home aides strongly objected to withholding oral feeding; several thought their collaboration would be "assisting a suicide." He disagreed but accepted their decision and was admitted to in-patient care, where many of his home health aides visited him. Personal and ethical tension was greatly reduced by the gracious attitudes of both.

Case 1.2. Bill with Indolent Cancer

Bill was angry that MAID was not legally available. Upon first learning of VSED, he thought it "immature and barbaric." His metastatic cancer progressed to pathological fractures of leg and arm, he was confined to bed, and any independent movement became excruciating. He thought it so unfair that MAID was not an option.

He considered suicide with a gun but knew that even if it worked, it would leave his wife devastated. His physician chose to again raise the possibility of VSED as the only non-violent option. Within a day, Bill opted for it. Already hospitalized in a palliative care unit, the staff had gotten to know him and his strong "right to die" attitudes; they firmly supported him in his choice. He started immediately, never wavered, and died relatively peacefully twelve days later.

Bottom Line Points
- Bill's VSED decision, in a situation where he had no other viable option, was consistent with his long-standing views about independence and the "right to die."
- After he had angrily dismissed VSED as "barbaric" when first discussed, Bill's physicians courageously raised it again, reasoning that within the framework of his values, it was his only viable option. Their decision was validated by the fact that Bill rather quickly chose it and never wavered in carrying it out.

Case 1.3. Mrs. H. with Early Alzheimer's

Mrs. H. had known about VSED from its successful use by an acquaintance and had been moved by that person's autonomy and decisiveness. When her diagnosis with progressive dementia solidified, she was adamant about remaining at home. Several years later she raised the possibility of VSED. Lengthy conversation with a physician led him to tell the family that she's "serious about VSED, but not ready." Months of joy and tension followed. From a subsequent conversation came a different report: "She's ready now." Both grief and relief followed. She would face down the future ravages of dementia by acting now.

Soon thereafter she signed on to home hospice and began VSED. For several days she was gracious host to friends and family. Her mouth comfort issues were competently managed. She lapsed into unconsciousness after eight days and died a day later, surrounded by loved ones.

Bottom Line Points
- Mrs. H's private consultations with a trusted physician about dementia, VSED, and her desired timing created delay, with consequent anguish and stress, but they also established that the VSED she eventually pursued was truly her desire.
- In a preemptive pursuit of VSED to avoid future advanced dementia, there is no way to avoid the difficult question of when to initiate VSED.

- Patient and family confronted the dual reality of grief at hastening death when valuable time is still left, but deep satisfaction in defeating what they saw as the nightmare of future severe dementia.
- Mrs. H. acknowledged the reality of VSED as "suicide" even though she did not think of her final path that way herself.

Case 1.4. G.W. with Lung Cancer

When at the age of 78 all treatments for G.W.'s metastatic cancer failed, he took the news like the decisive, take-charge, stoic person he'd been all his life. He arranged for the home hospice his oncologist had suggested and, still mentally acute, soon signed a "VSED agreement" with them. His wife, with signs of early dementia, obsessed about the hospice details, including the advice to resist the urge to give in to any of her husband's potential later pleas for water or food. His wife and his daughter Ty were almost always with him as VSED proceeded.

G.W. would often roll his eyes and moan when his wife would refuse his requests for water. Ty could not resist providing him some sips, to which he would slowly say "thank you." His wife chastised G.W. for his request and Ty for acceding to it. Daughter and wife had heated exchanges over this. His daughter never shared the alleged agreement between patient and hospice. Apparently the hospice nurse did not forewarn them of the difficulties that might emerge.

Bottom Line Points
- Patients considering VSED should be adequately informed about its process, including difficulties and what can be done to address them. Providers should be prepared to offer competent palliative support.
- Providers should come to a clear agreement with patients, orally or in writing, about what will be done for them during VSED. The agreement should be available to proxies and close family members, and preferably discussed with them.
- What constitutes compassion can be complex. The daughter insightfully acknowledged that providing her father his requested water was not the only compassionate action; it might be equally compassionate to refuse the request and not prolong a difficult process.
- To address such dilemmas that often emerge after the patient loses decision-making capacity, serious consideration should be given, before starting VSED, to writing an advance directive for stopping eating and drinking (AD for SED) later in the process.

References

American Association of Suicidology. 2017. "Statement of the American Association of Suicidology: 'Suicide' Is Not the Same as 'Physician Aid in Dying,'" approved October 30, 2017. https://suicidology.org/wp-content/uploads/2019/07/AAS-PAD-Statement-Approved-10.30.17-ed-10-30-17.pdf.

Badham, John (director). 1981. "Whose Life Is It Anyway?" (film). Beverly Hills: Metro-Goldwyn-Mayer.

Beauchamp, Tom L., and James F. Childress. 2001. *Principles of Biomedical Ethics, 5th ed.* New York: Oxford University Press.

Birnbacher, Dieter. 2015. "Ist Sterbefasten eine Form von Suizid?" *Ethik in der Medizin* 27, no. 4 (December). Unpublished English version from the author: "Is Voluntarily Stopping Eating and Drinking a Form of Suicide?"

Boyle, Joseph. 2017. "Intention, Permissibility, and the Consistency of Traditional End-of-Life Care." In *Euthanasia and Assisted Suicide: Global Views on Choosing to End Life*, edited by Michael J. Cholbi, 255–275. Santa Barbara, CA: Praeger/ABC-CLIO.

Burton, Keith. 1989. "A Chronicle: Dax's Case as It Happened." In *Dax's Case: Essays in Medical Ethics and Human Meaning*, edited by Lonnie D. Kliever, 1–12. Dallas: Southern Methodist University Press. Reprinted in Steinbock et al. 2013, 343–347.

Cantor, Norman L. 2006. "On Hastening Death Without Violating Legal and Moral Prohibitions." *Loyola University Chicago Law Journal* 37: 101–125.

Cantor, Norman L. 2020. *My Eccentric Family: Memories from a Communist, Mafioso, Zionist Past.* Tel Aviv-Yafo, Israel: eBookPro Publishing.

Cowart, Dax, and Robert Burt. 1998. "Confronting Death: Who Chooses, Who Controls?" *Hastings Center Report* 28, no. 1 (January–February): 14–24. Reprinted in Steinbock et al. 2013, 348–353.

Friesen, Phoebe. 2020. "Medically Assisted Dying and Suicide: How Are They Different, and How Are they Similar?" *Hastings Center Report* 50, no. 1 (January–February): 32–43.

H Ltd v J (2010, 107 SASR 352).

In re Browning 568 So. 2d (Fla. 1990).

Jansen, Lynn A. 2004. "No Safe Harbor: The Principle of Complicity and the Practice of Voluntary Stopping of Eating and Drinking." *Journal of Medicine and Philosophy* 29, no. 1: 61–74.

Jansen, Lynn A., and Daniel P. Sulmasy. 2002. "Sedation, Alimentation, Hydration, and Equivocation: Careful Conversation about Care at the End of Life." *Annals of Internal Medicine* 136, no. 11 (June): 845–849.

Jox, Ralf J., Isra Black, Gian Domenico Borasio, and Johanna Anneser. 2017. "Voluntary Stopping of Eating and Drinking: Is Medical Support Ethically Justified?" *BMC Medicine* 15: 186–190.

Meisel, Alan, Kenneth Cerminara, and Thaddeus M. Pope. 2020. *The Right to Die: The Law of End-of-Life Decisionmaking, 3rd ed.* New York: Wolters Kluwer Law & Business. Loose-leaf publication from 2004, with annual supplements.

Menzel, Paul T. 2013. "Advance Directives, Dementia, and Eligibility for Physician-Assisted Death." *New York Law School Law Review* 58, no. 2: 321–345.

Menzel, Paul T. 2017. "Voluntarily Stopping Eating and Drinking: A Normative Comparison with Refusing Lifesaving Treatment and Advance Directives." *Journal of Law, Medicine & Ethics* 45, no. 4 (Winter): 634–646.

O'Neill, Onora. 2002. *Autonomy and Trust in Bioethics.* Cambridge, UK: Cambridge University Press.

O'Rourke, Kevin D. 2005. "The Catholic Tradition on Forgoing Life Support." *The National Catholic Bioethics Quarterly* 5, no. 3 (Autumn): 537–553.

Paris, John. 1992. "The Catholic Tradition on the Use of Nutrition and Fluids." In *Birth, Suffering, and Death: Catholic Perspectives at the Edges of Life*, edited by Kevin W. Wildes, Frances Abel, and John C. Harvey, 189–208. Dordrecht, Netherlands: Springer.

Pope, Thaddeus M. 2005. "Monstrous Impersonation: A Critique of Consent-Based Justifications for Hard Paternalism." *University of Missouri-Kansas City Law Review* 73, no. 3: 681–713.

Pope, Thaddeus M. 2013. "Clinicians May Not Administer Life-Sustaining Treatment Without Consent: Civil, Criminal, and Disciplinary Sanctions." *Journal of Health and Biomedical Law* 9: 213–196.

Quill, Timothy E., Linda Ganzini, Robert D. Truog, and Thaddeus M. Pope. 2018. "Voluntarily Stopping Eating and Drinking Among Patients with Serious Advanced Illness—Clinical, Ethical, and Legal Aspects." *JAMA Internal Medicine* 178, no. 1: 123–127.

Satz v. Permutter 362 So. 2d 160 (Fla. Ct. App. 1978), affirmed 379 So. 2d 359 (Fla. 1980).

Schloendorff v. New York Hospital 211 NY 125 (1914).

Schwarz, Judith K. 2011. "Death by Voluntary Dehydration: Suicide or the Right to Refuse a Life-Prolonging Measure?" *Widener Law Review* 17, no. 2: 351–361.

Shacter, Phyllis R. 2016. "Not Here by Choice: My Husband's Choice about How and When to Die." *Narrative Inquiry in Bioethics* 6, no. 2 (Summer): 94–96.

Shacter, Phyllis R. 2017. *Choosing to Die, a Personal Story: Elective Death by VSED in the Face of Degenerative Disease.* Self-published, information at info@PhyllisShacter.com.

Steinbock, Bonnie, and Alastair Norcross, eds. 1999. *Killing and Letting Die, 2nd edition.* New York: Fordham University Press.

Steinbock, Bonnie, Alex J. London, and John D. Arras, eds. 2013. *Ethical Issues in Modern Medicine, 8th ed.* New York: McGraw Hill.

Sumner, L.W. 2011. *Assisted Death: A Study in Ethics and Law.* New York: Oxford University Press.

U.S. Bishops' Pro-Life Committee. 1992. *Nutrition and Hydration: Moral and Pastoral Reflections.* Washington, DC: U.S. Catholic Conference. Reprinted in Steinbock et al. 2013, 391–397.

White, Benjamin P., Lindy Willmott, and Julian Savulescu. 2014. "Voluntary Palliated Starvation: A Lawful and Ethical Way to Die?" *Journal of Law and Medicine* 22: 375–386.

Woollard, Fiona, and Frances Howard-Snyder. 2016. "Doing vs. Allowing Harm." In *The Stanford Encyclopedia of Philosophy* (Winter 2016 edition), edited by Edward N. Zalta. https://plato.stanford.edu/archives/win2016/entries/doing-allowing/.

4

Legal Issues

Thaddeus M. Pope

4.1 Introduction

In Chapters 2 and 3, we saw that VSED may be an "exit option" that is both medically and ethically reasonable for some patients who want to hasten their death to avoid living under present or future conditions that they judge intolerable. Nevertheless, patients, families, and clinicians will be reluctant to participate in VSED if they fear adverse legal consequences such as criminal charges, civil liability, or disciplinary investigations. Therefore, in this chapter we aim to reduce this uncertainty and fear by clarifying the legality of VSED.

We begin by establishing that clinicians and medical societies widely perceive VSED to be legal. While there continues to be variability, particularly in long-term care settings, as we will see in Chapter 5, legal uncertainty is generally not a significant barrier. Indeed, a patient's right to VSED has been well recognized and widely accepted. This is arguably true even in jurisdictions where courts or legislatures have not addressed VSED. This is because VSED falls squarely within broader (and even more clearly settled) patient rights to refuse treatment and care.

After establishing both the legal right to VSED and clinician acceptance of this right, we move to address more specific legal concerns. First, caregiver support for VSED probably does not constitute the crime of assisted suicide. Second, VSED probably does not constitute abuse or neglect of a vulnerable adult. Third, VSED generally has no impact on life insurance. Fourth, clinicians may have duties to discuss VSED. Fifth, clinicians have rights to conscientiously object to participating.

Finally, note that while the clinical and ethical discussions in Chapters 2 and 3 have broad application, legal analysis is jurisdictionally specific. Accordingly, the following discussion is primarily focused on the major common law jurisdictions: Australia, Canada, New Zealand, United

Kingdom, and United States (Atiyah and Summers 1987). Furthermore, in federal systems like Canada, Australia, and the United States, health care is regulated primarily at the state or provincial level. Consequently, there are material variations among states and provinces even within these countries (Meisel, Cerminara, and Pope 2020; Trowse 2020).

4.2. VSED Is Widely Perceived to Be Legal

Establishing the legality of VSED is necessary, but insufficient, to induce participation by interested patients, families, and clinicians. Equally important is how these parties perceive the legality of VSED. After all, clinicians and patients sometimes believe that end-of-life medical interventions are (or might be) prohibited even when they are not (Goldstein 2012; Meisel 1995; Sherazi 2008). While erroneous, these perceptions matter. Clinicians are unlikely (or less likely) to offer interventions when they think they are illegal (Johnson 2009; Johnson 2012). Therefore, it is important to address not only VSED's actual legality but also its perceived legality or general acceptance within professional health care (Pope and Anderson 2011).

Over the past decade, VSED has become increasingly recognized as a legitimate and appropriate end-of-life option (Pope and Anderson 2011). For example, in the preamble to its 2018 statute legalizing medical aid in dying, the Hawaii legislature observed that "VSED . . . is an option currently available to terminally ill persons in Hawaii" (Hawaii 2018).[1] Similarly, a parliamentary report in Western Australia concluded that a "competent person's absolute right to refuse to eat and drink is clear at law" (Western Australia 2018). Still, such explicit recognition remains uncommon. More often, end-of-life law reform silently assumes the legality of VSED. Consequently, it is almost never itself the subject of legislation or regulation.

Despite the dearth of affirmative legislative or regulatory authorization, VSED is recognized "as legal" by major professional health care associations. For example, in the United States, official statements supporting VSED as a clinically and ethically appropriate option have been published by the American Medical Women's Association, the American Nurses Association, and the Society for Post-Acute and Long-Term Care (ANA 2017; AMWA

---

[1] A California bill similarly recognized the legitimacy of VSED by proposing to mandate that physicians discuss it with terminally ill patients (California 2009).

2007; Wright et al. 2019). In Europe, official supportive guidance has been released by the Austrian Palliative Society, Dutch Medical Association, European Society for Clinical Nutrition and Metabolism, German Society of Palliative Medicine, International Association for Hospice and Palliative Care, Swiss Medical Association, and World Medical Association (De Lima et al. 2017; Druml et al. 2016; Feichtner, Weixler, and Birklbauer 2018; KNMG 2011; Nauk, Ostgathe, and Radbruch 2014; Swiss Academy of Medical Sciences 2018; World Medical Association 2016).

Notably, VSED is recognized "as legal" not only by these professional societies but also by foremost hospice and palliative care clinicians. For example, thought leaders like Ira Byock, Diane Meier, and Timothy Quill have all recognized the legitimacy of VSED (Byock 1995; Quill and Byock 2000; Miller and Meier 1998). So have leading medical ethicists like James Bernat, Julian Savulescu, and Robert Truog (Baumgartner 2006; Cochrane and Truog 2005; Bernat, Gert, and Mogielnicki 1993; Savulescu 2014). An even broader look at decades of peer-reviewed medical literature shows that this is a near consensus position (Eddy 1994; Eddy 2005; Harvath et al. 2004; Montgomery 1996; Sullivan 1993).[2] One study found that 90% of health care professionals classified VSED as natural death or as refusal of life-sustaining treatment (RLST) (Stangle et al. 2021).

Perhaps the best evidence of VSED's recognition and acceptance is not only policy statements and journal articles but actual widespread practice. VSED has a significant prevalence in many countries. The cases in Chapter 1 are only an illustrative subset of many more (albeit an unknown number of) cases in the United States (Ganzini et al. 2003).[3] Elsewhere, studies show that VSED constitutes nearly two in 100 deaths in the Netherlands and nearly one in 100 deaths in Swiss long-term care facilities (Chabot 2007; Ivanović, Büche, and Fringer 2014; Onwuteaka-Philipsen et al. 2012; Stangle et al. 2020; Stangle et al. 2021; Van der Heide et al. 2012). Peer-reviewed medical literature shows that VSED is also widely practiced in Japan and Germany (Hoekstra, Strack, and Simonet 2015; Shinjo et al. 2017).

Finally, perception, practice, and legality are not independent. They are interrelated and interdependent. That VSED is openly and widely practiced

---

[2] Admittedly, some distinguished clinicians and bioethicists argue that VSED is not a legitimate end-of-life option (Jansen and Sulmasy 2002). Others support VSED but urge additional research (Bolt 2020; Ivanović et al. 2014). In one study 12% of respondents felt that people should not have the right to refuse food or fluids, and an additional 17% were unsure (Alzheimer's Australia 2014).

[3] We collect dozens of additional personal narratives in Appendix E at the end of this book.

is relevant not only to its practical availability but also to its legality. The law is very deferential to the medical profession and allows it significant discretion to self-regulate (Dobbs et al. 2020). Consequently, if the medical profession deems a process (like VSED) legitimate, then the law is likely to find it legitimate (Larriviere and Beresford 2008).

4.3. A Patient's Right to VSED Is Settled Law

A patient's right to refuse treatment has been well established in common law jurisprudence since the 1970s (Meisel, Cerminara, and Pope 2020). Capacitated patients may exercise this right even when the refusal will result in their death. Logically and conceptually, this principle has always embraced VSED. After all, if an individual may refuse "any" intervention, then they may refuse "this" intervention. Therefore, it is no surprise that courts have explicitly extended the "right to refuse" principle to VSED.

In the following court cases, the patient wanted to VSED, but a caregiver either thought that was not allowed or wanted clarity and guidance. In every case, the court ruled that the patient could VSED and that clinicians should respect that choice. These cases have been adjudicated by courts in Australia, Canada, the United Kingdom, and United States.

Australia. One of the clearest and most thoroughly reasoned cases is from South Australia (*H Ltd v J 2010*). J, a 74-year-old woman in a long-term care facility, was suffering from muscular wasting disease, such that moving was painful. After long reflection, J announced her plan to end her life by VSED. While the facility was not opposed to J's plan, administrators were uncertain whether they were permitted or obligated to respect J's decision. So, the facility brought the matter to court to get a declaration clarifying the extent to which it could and should lawfully comply.

In 2010, the Supreme Court of South Australia held that the facility not only may, but must, honor J's decision to VSED. In light of J's refusal, the facility had neither a duty nor a lawful justification to hydrate her. The court offered four justifications. First, there is no general common-law duty to provide food and fluid to a resident who refuses it (*H Ltd v. J 2010*, ¶ 36). Second, VSED is not suicide, because there is no duty to feed oneself. "It is doubtful that self-starvation is suicide" (*H Ltd v. J 2010*, ¶¶ 56–65). Third, the facility does not assist suicide by respecting J's decision, because there is no duty to prevent it (*H Ltd v. J 2010*, ¶¶ 67–68). Fourth, while the facility might normally have a duty to provide sustenance to its patients, there is no such duty when the capacitated patient refuses. Any duty to offer care is negated or excused when the person withdraws their cooperation (*H Ltd v. J 2010*, ¶¶ 73–74).

In reaching these conclusions, the South Australia court recognized that most (if not all) of the previous case law on refusing food and water concerned "artificial" nutrition and hydration (e.g., PEG tube, NG tube, or TPN). The court noted that J's case was different, because food is not medicine, and hand feeding is not "medically administered." Nevertheless, the court held that these differences were irrelevant and insufficient to sustain a distinction between suicide and self-determination (*H Ltd v. J 2010*, ¶ 64).[4] Individuals have the right to make choices affecting their personal lives, and clinicians have no responsibility to provide food and fluid when the resident has voluntarily and rationally refused such services (*H Ltd v. J 2010*, ¶¶ 86–88).

Canada. A British Columbia court undertook a similar analysis in 2014, distinguishing artificial and oral feeding. The court held that oral nutrition and hydration (by prompting with a spoon or glass) is "personal" care, not "health" care (*Bentley 2014*, ¶ 84). But like the South Australian court, the Canadian court held that this distinction does not matter. Clinicians may not administer any service (health care or personal care) without consent (*Bentley 2014*, ¶ 46).

Adults have a common-law right to consent or to refuse consent not only to health care but also to personal care services (*Bentley*, ¶ 84). While almost all right-to-refuse cases have been decided in the medical treatment context, that is not the only context in which the right applies. The right to refuse is based on a broader general right to personal autonomy and bodily integrity. In short, capacitated adults have a common-law right to refuse personal care or basic care (*Bentley 2014*, ¶¶ 46, 121).

Unlike the South Australia court, the British Columbia court did not announce a new rule or policy extending the scope of the legal right to refuse from artificial hydration to also include oral hydration. Instead, the British Columbia court observed that a right to VSED had already been established. Other Canadian courts had already found that an adult may refuse to eat or drink and die by dehydration, if he is mentally capable of making

---

[4] The court noted that the negation of provider duties depends upon the continuing operation of the patient's refusal. If the patient revokes her instruction, then the provider's duties are again enlivened (*H v J 2010*, ¶¶ 62, 91). A recent parliamentary report concluded that the same rules would apply in other Australian states (Western Australia 2018).

the decision" (*Bentley 2014*, ¶ 140). Among other authorities, the British Columbia court cited a Quebec case involving Robert Corbeil, a 33-year-old man left quadriplegic after an off-road vehicle accident.

Corbeil requested that clinicians respect his decision to stop eating (Manoir de la Pointe Bleue 1992). The Superior Court of Quebec agreed, concluding that it could counter the will of a VSED patient no more than it could direct a patient to undergo chemotherapy or dialysis. Unlike the South Australia and British Columbia courts discussed above, the Quebec court held that "feeding was a form of medical treatment, and Mr. Corbeil was within his rights to refuse it." But that was not essential to the decision. The Quebec court also noted that the Canadian Law Reform Commission had articulated a right to refuse not only "treatment" but also "care." Therefore, the result would be the same whether (or not) food and fluid is considered health care or personal/basic care.

The British Columbia and Quebec courts are not alone. Other Canadian cases have also confirmed a patient's right to VSED (Astraforoff 1983; Truchon 2019). Indeed, the acceptability of VSED is so well established in Canada that a provincial medical board recently approved using VSED to make a patient's death "reasonably foreseeable," so that she would qualify for medical aid in dying (College 2018).[5]

In sum, there is significant and consistent Canadian precedent holding that adults have a right to VSED. Furthermore, reviewing these cases and their underlying principles, several recent legal academic studies provide further confirmation. They uniformly conclude that VSED is legal across Canada (Downie and Bowes 2019; Mader and Apold 2020).

United Kingdom. Australia and Canada are not the only jurisdictions where courts have announced a right to VSED. In 2012, 74-year-old Englishwoman Monica Cooke was suffering from multiple sclerosis. The disease had robbed her of the ability to move, taste, and smell. Cooke decided to VSED and died eight days later (Evans 2012). The West Somerset coroner held an inquest, concluding that while he normally would record a verdict of suicide, in these exceptional circumstances he was adopting a narrative verdict that records the circumstances surrounding the death without attributing the cause to an individual (Chief Coroner 2016).

---

[5] A court later struck down the statutory requirement that the patient's death be "reasonably foreseeable," because it was more restrictive than the Charter rights recognized by the Supreme Court of Canada (Truchon 2019).

The same year, a 32-year-old Englishwoman suffering from anorexia nervosa sought the right to stop eating and drinking from the Court of Protection. While the court rejected her request, the case is readily distinguishable from typical VSED cases for two reasons. First, the court concluded that the woman lacked capacity. The court stated that if she had capacity, it would have respected her decision. "People with capacity are entitled to make decisions for themselves, including about what they will and will not eat, even if their decision brings about their death" (*A v. E* 2012).

Second, when employing the applicable decision-making test for incapacitated patients, the court held that VSED was not in her "best interest." (We grapple with the legality of SED for incapacitated patients in Chapter 10.) She had a good chance to recover and lead a relatively normal life. In contrast, a typical VSED patient (like the Chapter 1 cases with irreversible, incurable, and progressive ALS, cancer, or dementia) does not have such a chance for recovery. Therefore, the same rules and reasoning that led the court to override the anorexia patient's decision would support a typical VSED patient's decision.

More recently, the General Medical Council (GMC) offered guidance on VSED. The GMC is the licensing authority for more than 300,000 doctors in the United Kingdom. In a 2015 guidance document, the GMC advises that no prohibition prevents a doctor from "agreeing in advance to palliate the pain and discomfort involved for such a patient should the need arise for such symptom management" (General Medical Council 2015). The GMC subsequently confirmed that symptom management includes the symptoms which arise from VSED which progresses to that individual's death. "Doctors may agree with their patients in advance to provide medicines or treatment to alleviate pain or other distressing symptoms, should the need arise" (General Medical Council 2018). Notably, there have been many high-profile VSED deaths in the UK, yet no liability or sanctions (Culzac 2014; Savulescu 2014).[6]

United States. As a substantially larger country, it is no surprise that there is even more case law in the United States than in Australia, Canada, and the United Kingdom. There are two notable cases from California, two from New York, and one each from Delaware, Georgia, and Florida.

---

[6] Two of the most influential right-to-die campaigners in the United Kingdom, Debbie Purdy and Tony Nicklinson, both died from VSED after losing their high-profile court cases for access to MAID (Richards 2014).

The California case of Elizabeth Bouvia is one of the most famous and widely discussed in bioethics and medical jurisprudence (Bouvia 1986). Bouvia was a quadriplegic patient with cerebral palsy and severe degenerative arthritis. She was capable (with assistance) of eating by mouth. But since Bouvia wanted to hasten her death, she refused spoon feeding. When the public hospital to which Bouvia had been admitted refused to honor this decision, Bouvia sued. In 1986, the California Court of Appeal held that Bouvia had a right to refuse spoon feeding even though she had no terminal diagnosis. The court grounded this right in both the state and federal constitutions. The court further held that Bouvia's refusal was not equivalent to committing suicide.

A few years later, in 1993, the Supreme Court of California confirmed a patient's right to VSED. Howard Andrews was a quadriplegic prison inmate. While he was capable of eating by mouth, he refused to do so (Thor 1993). A prison doctor sought a court order allowing him to force-feed Andrews. But the court denied the request, holding that Andrews' refusal discharged any duty to treat. Furthermore, the court held that "judicial authority uniformly rejects the contention that acquiescing in the decision to forgo a life-sustaining procedure subjects the physician to liability for aiding and abetting a suicide."[7]

While an individual's right to VSED has been established by the highest court in California, it has only been recognized by non-precedential trial courts in New York (Brooks 1987; Cantor and Thomas 2000). Two are worth describing here. In the first case, the court ruled that a facility was neither obligated nor empowered to feed a resident who refused (Gallagher 1984; Goodman 1984; Margolick 1984). G. Ross Henninger was an 85-year-old retired college president. After a stroke, he decided that he was unable to participate in the things that made his life meaningful. So, he stopped eating. Henninger's nursing home went to court, presenting the question: "whether the patient may elect to end his life by starvation" (Plaza Health 1984).

The court first determined that Henninger had capacity at the time he elected to discontinue eating, and that he made that decision knowingly and

---

[7] The court notes that "a necessary distinction exists between a person suffering from a serious life-threatening disease or debilitating injury who rejects medical intervention that only prolongs but never cures the affliction and an individual who deliberately sets in motion a course of events aimed at his or her own demise and attempts to enlist the assistance of others" (Thor 1993). The court explained that the attitude or motive of the individual in the former situation "may be presumed not to be suicidal." Therefore, those who assist such an individual "would not be aiding and abetting a suicide" and have "no duty to intervene on this basis" (Thor 1993).

willingly. While the facility had a prima facie duty to provide nutrition to its residents, that duty was discharged when Henninger refused. The court held that the facility was "not obligated or responsible" to feed him under such circumstances. In summarizing its ruling, the court stated, "I will not, against his wishes, in fact order this . . . person to be . . . force-fed in any manner, or to be restrained for the rest of his natural life" (Plaza Health 1984).

In the second New York case, a quadriplegic patient sought an order requiring a hospital to respect his decision refusing nourishment. The court ruled the action was premature. Since the patient was not yet in the hospital, there was no real dispute. Nevertheless, the court stated that it would honor the same request, if (and when) it arose within the context of a live case or controversy (A.B. 1984).

Outside California and New York, courts in other US states have also recognized a right to VSED.[8] For example, Anna Gordy was a 96-year-old patient in a Delaware hospital. In the early 1990s, she was diagnosed with Alzheimer's (Gordy 1994). While she did not completely stop eating and drinking, she decided "I don't want to eat" and "I eat what I want." Gordy's clinicians determined that unless her nutritional deficiencies were addressed (with a feeding tube), she would die within a few weeks. The Delaware court determined that Gordy made a "rational decision . . . that deserves to be respected." Furthermore, in justifying its conclusion, the court noted that death from dehydration is not cruel and painful.

Outside the health care context, there are cases involving hunger-striking prisoners. For example, Ted Anthony Prevatte was a Georgia inmate who engaged in a hunger strike to get the attention of prison officials. The prison sought judicial permission to feed Prevatte. But the Georgia Supreme Court held that the prison had "no right . . . to feed him to prevent his death from starvation if that is his wish." By virtue of his right to privacy, Prevatte "can refuse to allow intrusions on his person, even though calculated to preserve his life" (Silver 2005; Zant 1982). Prevatte later ended his hunger strike (Atlanta Constitution 1983).

Like Prevatte, Michael Costello was also a prison inmate who was able, but refused, to eat. He sought a declaratory judgment permitting him to "continue his fast devoid of non-consensual medical intervention." In other words, Costello sought to enjoin and restrain the prison from "imposing

---

[8] There are likely more court cases on VSED. But there is no systematic way to locate state court decisions at the trial court level (Pope 2008).

non-consensual medical intervention . . . or hindering or interfering with [his] fast" (*Singletary* 1996). The court held that "state interests did not overcome Costello's privacy right to refuse medical intervention."[9]

Summary. In sum, there is substantial court authority supporting (1) an individual's right to VSED, (2) the clinician's corollary "duty" to not intervene, and (3) the relief of any duty to intervene (Pope 2018). While these cases come from various jurisdictions, they are mutually reinforcing, since they were decided under shared principles of common law (*Clarkson* 1976; *Pictaroia* 2000). Furthermore, the cases are uniform and consistent. There is no negative precedent.[10] No capacitated patient who sought the right to VSED has been denied. Moreover, despite the growing prevalence of VSED, no clinician or family member who participated in VSED has been disciplined, sued, or prosecuted.

4.4. Right to Refuse Includes the Right to VSED

So far, we have established that medical societies and medical literature recognize the legitimacy of VSED. We have shown that nearly a dozen court decisions recognize the legitimacy of VSED. But this may be insufficient to allay all legal uncertainty, particularly in light of some of the opposing moral arguments reviewed in Chapter 3.

First, not all jurisdictions have such decisions (although most have decisions on artificial or clinically assisted nutrition and hydration). For example, despite the clarity of the South Australia judgment, there is no analogous precedent in other Australian states or territories. Similarly, despite precedent in California, Delaware, New York, Georgia, and Florida, there are no analogous precedents in other US states and territories.

Second, uncertainty may remain even in those jurisdictions with VSED court decisions. Judge-made law is always decided in the context of specific factual cases. While the court may resolve the situation facing the parties to

---

[9] While cases from the prison context seem inapposite to most patients, they are telling. Legally, it is difficult to involuntarily treat prison inmates (Winnebago County 2020). It is even more difficult to involuntarily treat non-inmates who enjoy a greater scope of liberty.

[10] There are some cases in which courts authorized the force-feeding of hunger-striking prisoners (Caulk 1984; Kallinger 1990; Von Holden 1982). But these cases are distinguishable. First, these inmates were not seeking to hasten their deaths. They were protesting prison conditions. Second, with respect to inmates, the state sometimes has an interest in security that outweighs individual rights (Meisel, Cerminara, and Pope 2020 § 5.04[F]).

the case, there is often uncertainty over the scope of application to other non-identical cases (Hart 1961). For example, some may think that just because a court determined that a terminally ill cancer patient may VSED does not necessarily mean that an early dementia patient (in the same jurisdiction) may VSED.

Fortunately, while some clinicians, facilities, and families might like the bright line clarity of on-point precedent, that level of specificity is unnecessary. The right to VSED falls squarely within broader established rights. Since the 1970s, patients have had not only a common-law right but also statutory and constitutional rights to refuse health care interventions even when they are life-saving or life-prolonging. "Doctors cannot owe the patient any duty to maintain his life where that life can only be sustained by intrusive medical care to which the patient will not consent" (Airedale 1993).

This right to refuse has been most saliently and most frequently articulated in the context of paradigmatic medical interventions like mechanical ventilation, blood transfusions, and dialysis. While VSED does not fit as squarely and neatly into the "health care" category, it still fits within a patient's right to refuse. First, oral food and fluid probably is health care. Second, patients have a right to refuse not only health care but also basic or personal care.

VSED Is Included in the Right to Refuse Health Care. The legal definition of "health care" is usually quite broad. In many US states the term includes "any care, treatment, service, or procedure to maintain, diagnose, or otherwise affect a person's physical or mental condition" (Minnesota § 145C.01(4)). Water surely fits, because it affects a person's physical condition.

The fit is even tighter upon a closer inspection of VSED. First, as described in Chapter 2, it is almost always overseen and supervised by licensed health care professionals (Cantor 2020; Pope and Anderson 2011). Many of these patients are already dependent upon specialized personnel, training, and equipment. Second, many patients VSED in health care facilities, as in several of the Chapter 1 cases. Third, VSED is treated as health care by the health care professions which have developed guidelines and policy statements. We have collected many of these as additional resources in Appendix D at the end of this book.

Finally, the published court cases discussed above suggest that VSED is properly framed as a refusal of "health care." Many of these cases did not focus on the individual's refusal of food and water itself. Instead, they focused on the patient's right to refuse interventions (such as force-feeding or administering a feeding tube) directed at overriding such a refusal. In other words, a right to VSED is derivative from the right to refuse health care.

VSED Is Included in the Right to Refuse Basic Care. Some legal commentators get distracted by an overly narrow focus on whether oral nutrition and hydration is "health care" or whether it is "personal" or "basic" care (Jotkowitz 2009). But an obsession with this definitional question is misplaced. It does not matter whether oral food and nutrition is "health care" or "treatment."

Patients have the right to refuse any intervention (Pope and Anderson 2011). They may refuse not only health care but also personal care or basic care. Nothing turns on the artificiality or ordinariness of the intervention (Cochrane and Truog 2005; Cochrane and Truog 2006). The courts have long rejected the relevance and coherence of a distinction between "ordinary" and "extraordinary" treatment (Meisel 2016). Former US Chief Justice Rehnquist colorfully captured the point, observing that one's bodily integrity is violated just as much by "sticking a spoon in your mouth" as by "sticking a needle in your arm" (Oyez 1997).

Chief Justice Rehnquist is right. All individuals have the right to be free from unwanted touching. To undermine a capacitated patient's VSED by forcibly administering water by mouth or tube would be a "battery" (Pope and Anderson 2011; Pope 2013). The right to refuse any intervention, even when well-intended and physiologically beneficial, has been established since the early 1900s. Feeding a patient contrary to a patient's instructions is a battery (Morton 2007). As Justice O'Connor observed in the same U.S. Supreme Court case: "Whether or not the techniques used to pass food and water into the patient's alimentary tract are termed 'medical treatment,' it is clear they all involve some degree of intrusion and restraint" (Cruzan 1990).

4.5. Assisted Suicide Laws Generally Do Not Apply

Until now, this chapter has focused on establishing a right to VSED. But even if the patient has a right to VSED, some are concerned that other duties or constraints may conflict with that right. Most notably, clinicians and families worry that VSED may fall within the criminal prohibition of "assisted suicide." Assisted suicide remains a crime in every US jurisdiction (Pope 2018).[11] And family members are regularly prosecuted and convicted for

---

[11] A legal prohibition on assisted suicide does not prevent MAID, because the statutes that legalize MAID define it as not constituting assisted suicide. "Actions taken in accordance with this part shall

helping other family members hasten their death (often through violent means like guns). Therefore, if participating in VSED is assisting a suicide, then participating in VSED is a crime.

But the concern is largely misplaced. As we saw earlier in this chapter, court cases from multiple jurisdictions hold that VSED is not suicide (Trowse 2020).[12] Jurisprudence more broadly holds that passively refusing interventions to prevent or delay death is materially different from actively introducing interventions to hasten death. Only the latter have been associated with suicide. If the seriously ill individual who refuses food and fluid is not (legally) committing suicide, then clinicians and family members who support this individual are not committing assisted suicide.

Furthermore, even if participating in VSED might otherwise constitute assisted suicide, it is usually exempted from the scope of prohibition. While VSED does not have a separate, specific statutory exemption like medical aid in dying, both criminal and health care decisions statutes carve out exceptions that usually apply to VSED.[13]

Withholding or Withdrawing Treatment Is Not Suicide. First, a clinician does not commit felony assisted suicide when she withholds or withdraws treatment in accordance with reasonable medical practice. Most jurisdictions have a health care decisions statute that specifically defines care refusals as not constituting suicide. For example, the California law states: "Death resulting from withholding or withdrawing health care . . . does not for any purpose constitute a suicide" (California § 4656).

In addition to this definitional approach in health care decisions statutes, most states also take an exemption approach in their assisted suicide statutes. These laws typically carve out withholding and withdrawing health care from the scope of prohibition (Minnesota § 609.215(3)(b)).[14] In sum, if VSED is withholding "health care," then it is not suicide. If VSED is not suicide,

---

not, for any purposes, constitute suicide, assisted suicide, homicide, or elder abuse under the law" (California § 443.18).

[12] This is especially true when the patient is already dying. But a case from India suggests that VSED is suicide (Joychen 2015).

[13] In Montana, the exception is even more obvious. VSED is exempted from criminal prohibition for the same reason MAID is exempted: the patient's consent (Baxter 2009).

[14] Other state statutes similarly provide that nothing in the prohibition shall: (1) "Prohibit or affect the use or continuation, or the withholding or withdrawal, of life-sustaining treatment, CPR, or comfort care"; (2) "Prohibit or affect the provision or withholding of health care, life-sustaining treatment, or comfort care"; (3) "Affect or limit the authority of a person to refuse to give informed consent to health care" (Ohio § 3795.03).

then supporting it is not assisted suicide. Unfortunately, we cannot be sure whether VSED is the withholding of "health care." Therefore, we cannot be sure whether there is a categorical exception for any type of participation with VSED.

Offering Only Palliative Care Is Not Assisted Suicide. In addition to the withholding and withdrawing exemption, most assisted suicide laws exempt palliative care from the scope of prohibition. Clinician conduct that is solely palliative in nature falls into a safe harbor. For example, the Minnesota statute provides that a health care provider "who administers, prescribes, or dispenses medications or procedures to relieve another person's pain or discomfort . . . does not violate [the prohibition on assisted suicide] unless the medications or procedures are knowingly administered, prescribed, or dispensed to cause death." The exception further provides that nothing in the prohibition shall "prohibit or preclude a physician, certified nurse practitioner, certified nurse-midwife, or clinical nurse specialist who carries out the responsibility to provide comfort care to a patient in good faith." (Minnesota § 609.215(3)(b)).

The clinician's role fundamentally differs between MAID and VSED. With MAID the clinician provides the means through which the patient causes their death. In contrast, with VSED the means are already in the patient's control. Nothing the clinician "administers, prescribes, or dispenses" causes (or is intended to cause) death. As described in Chapter 2, the clinician's primary role (and intent) is palliative.

Of course, the clinician may play roles other than supporting the patient after VSED has already begun. The clinician may counsel the patient about VSED when she is still considering death-hastening options. But this conduct is even less likely to constitute assisted suicide because pure speech is protected under the First Amendment. While material assistance (like writing a lethal prescription) constitutes "assistance," spoken and written communication does not (and cannot) constitute assistance (Melchert-Dinkel 2014).

4.6. Abuse and Neglect Laws Generally Do Not Apply

Clinicians and families are concerned not only that VSED constitutes assisted suicide but also that VSED may fall within criminal and regulatory prohibitions on abuse, neglect, and mistreatment. These laws (often explicitly and specifically) prohibit allowing an older or vulnerable adult to dehydrate (Arizona; Colorado). Moreover, enforcement of these laws is salient given epidemic mistreatment of the disabled and elderly.

But these abuse and neglect laws do not apply when the patient consents. For example, the Utah definition of "neglect" is a "pattern of conduct by a caretaker, without the disabled or elder adult's informed consent, resulting in deprivation of food, water" (Utah). The definition itself excludes consensual deprivation of food and water from constituting neglect. As we saw in the dozen cases discussed at the beginning of this chapter, one can be liable for an omission to provide the necessaries of life only if there were a preexisting duty to act. When the patient refuses food and fluid, there is no such duty (*Taktak* 1988).

Notably, VSED is specifically permitted even by federal health care laws that were promulgated specifically to protect the most vulnerable in society. These regulations tell hospitals, nursing facilities, hospices, and other providers that whatever other care they are obligated to provide, they "are not required to provide care that conflicts with" the patient's own directions (Centers for Medicare and Medicaid Services 2020). In guidelines interpreting these regulations, the US Centers for Medicare and Medicaid Services notes "failure to provide adequate nutrition and hydration to support and maintain health" can place a patient in jeopardy. But when done with the patient's consent, this is not even a "trigger" meriting further investigation (Butler 2009; Centers for Medicare and Medicaid Services 2019; Pope and Anderson 2011; Windsor House 2003).

Nevertheless, even if VSED is not abuse or neglect, it "looks" like abuse or neglect. This is important because families want more than to avoid sanctions. They also want to avoid even investigations and inquiries from adult protective services (APS) and other authorities. Not only are such proceedings stressful, time-consuming, and expensive, but they can also interrupt the patient's VSED (Shacter 2017).

Therefore, as discussed throughout this book (and particularly in Part II and Appendix A), patients should carefully document their VSED wishes. After a patient begins to VSED, they may seem to show an interest in drinking when they have become delirious or lose capacity. With clear documentation in hand, their family can show APS or others that the patient's dehydration is consensual, therefore not abuse or neglect in any jurisdiction.

4.7. Other Issues for Patients and Families—Life Insurance

Patients and families are concerned not only with criminal or civil liability. They are also concerned with other potential adverse consequences. One of the most frequently mentioned concerns is the impact on life insurance. If a patient dies from VSED, will the life insurance company deny the claim? This question arises because most insurance policies have exclusions for suicide.

But a closer look at the policy language shows that the exclusion is not categorical and comprehensive. The exclusion is limited to a two-year period. This means that if the patient undertakes VSED more than two years after purchasing the life insurance policy, then the suicide exclusion does not apply (Goodman 2021). Specifically, life insurance policies typically state: "If the insured, whether sane or insane, dies by suicide within two years from the Policy Date, our liability is limited to an amount equal to the total premiums paid" (Arena 2019). These "suicide clauses" are designed to mitigate adverse selection by discouraging people from buying life insurance when contemplating suicide.

The analysis is more complicated if the patient undertakes VSED within two years of purchasing the policy. But even here, the exclusion applies only if VSED is suicide. While the discussion in Chapter 3 (Section 3.3) indicates the conceptual answer is uncertain, the legal answer is clearer. Most jurisdictions have explicitly declared that withholding and withdrawing health care is not suicide. Without such statutes, any patient that stops dialysis, turns off a ventilator, or deactivates an implanted cardioverter-defibrillator would be committing suicide.

A typical statute states: "Death resulting from withholding or withdrawing health care in accordance with this division does not for any purpose constitute a suicide or homicide or legally impair or invalidate a policy of insurance or an annuity providing a death benefit, notwithstanding any term of the policy or annuity to the contrary" (California § 4656). If VSED is withdrawing "health care," then it falls outside the scope of any life insurance suicide exclusion clause. Moreover, even if VSED is not withdrawing "health care," court cases at the beginning of this chapter held that VSED is not suicide.

4.8. Other Issues for Clinicians—Informed Consent

So far, we have established (1) that VSED is a legal exit option, (2) that it does not constitute abuse or neglect, (3) that it probably does not constitute assisted suicide, and (4) that it probably does not impact life insurance. We turn now to address clinician-specific issues. We move from a discussion of what clinicians *may* do to what they *must* do. Specifically, do clinicians have a duty to disclose this option to seriously ill patients?

Yes, sometimes clinicians must discuss VSED with their patients. First, clinicians have an ethical and legal duty to truthfully respond to patient questions. If the patient specifically asks about VSED or about methods to hasten her death, then the clinician should first determine whether this is really a plea for something else like better symptom management. If the clinician determines that the patient really wants to discuss potentially death-hastening options (or VSED specifically), and the patient has decision-making capacity, then the clinician should either have that discussion or refer the patient to an appropriate resource. The discussion should cover (1) the nature and process of VSED, (2) its likely duration, (3) its benefits, (4) its risks and burdens, and (5) alternatives (Rozovsky 2020).

If the patient does not raise the issue, then the analysis varies from jurisdiction to jurisdiction. Some states (including California, New York, and Vermont) have special end-of-life right-to-know laws. Legislatures enacted these laws because mounting evidence demonstrated that patients were unaware of their options (Meisel, Cerminara, and Pope 2020; Pope 2017). The New York law states: "If a patient is diagnosed with a terminal illness or condition, the patient's attending health care practitioner shall offer to provide the patient with . . . information and counseling regarding . . . end-of-life options appropriate to the patient" (New York). Since VSED may often be an end-of-life option appropriate to the patient, the physician has a duty to at least "offer" to provide information and counseling regarding VSED.

Most of the remaining jurisdictions follow one of two informed consent disclosure standards: the malpractice standard or the material-risk standard (Pope 2017). For example, in the United States about 25 states follow the malpractice standard. The other 25 states follow the material-risk standard. The malpractice standard requires physicians to provide patients with only that information that a hypothetical reasonably prudent physician would disclose in the same circumstances. Since physicians do not customarily discuss VSED with their patients, there is no duty to discuss VSED in these states.

Although the malpractice standard is physician-defined, the material-risk standard is patient-defined. It requires physicians to provide all the information that a hypothetical reasonable patient would consider important or significant in making a treatment decision (Pope 2017). This disclosure duty is broader than the malpractice standard. After all, a reasonable patient may deem information important, even if medical professionals do not customarily discuss that information. Because a seriously ill patient may deem information about VSED to be material (even if they ultimately elect not to use it), physicians in these states have a prima facie duty to discuss it.

But physicians may not have a duty to discuss VSED in every situation. Several exceptions to the duty may apply. First, patients may waive their right to informed consent. Some patients do not want to discuss certain options. Second, if extremely well documented, physicians might avoid discussing VSED by invoking the "therapeutic privilege." Traditionally this exception allows physicians to paternalistically withhold disclosure of information otherwise required when full disclosure would be "detrimental to the patient's total care and best interest" (Nishi 1970; Canterbury 1972). While commentators caution against non-exceptional use of the therapeutic privilege, it may be appropriate in this context. Because some patients may be frightened by VSED, merely bringing it up can be harmful unless the patient gave some indication of interest as a "door opener."

4.9. Other Issues for Clinicians—Conscience-Based Objections

Just because VSED is a legal and accepted option does not mean that any specific clinician or health care facility must participate. Many clinicians will refuse to participate with VSED. So will many hospitals, hospices, and other facilities, especially those affiliated with the Catholic Church (Cavanagh 2014).

This is their right. Laws in most jurisdictions allow both individual and institutional providers to refuse participation in services to which they have a moral or conscience-based objection (Pope 2010; Wolfe and Pope 2020). Indeed, there are often separate conscience clauses for end-of-life treatment. For example, California law provides: "A health care provider may decline to comply with a . . . health care decision for reasons of conscience" (California § 4734).

Nevertheless, a health care provider's right to assert a conscience-based objection is not unfettered. To balance provider rights to act consistent with their personal values and beliefs against patient rights to access legal health care options, the law typically requires both individual and institutional providers to take several steps when asserting a conscience-based objection to either discussing or supervising VSED (Pope 2010; Wolfe and Pope 2020). First, the objecting provider must promptly inform the patient. Second, the objecting provider must make reasonable efforts to assist in transferring the patient to another health care provider that is willing to comply. Third, the objecting provider must provide continuing care to the patient until a transfer can be accomplished.

4.10. Revisiting the Initial Cases

Case 1.1. Al, the Motorcyclist with ALS

Al would have preferred to VSED at home rather than in the hospital. But his home health aides were not personally comfortable with VSED. Al directly asked about his options to hasten death and was informed about VSED.

Bottom Line Points
- Under both state and federal law, clinicians may assert conscience-based objections and refuse to participate in care that violates their religious or personal values. But they must refer the patient to another clinician.
- Patients planning to VSED should screen hospice programs and other providers to make sure that they are willing to participate in VSED.
- There is variability from jurisdiction to jurisdiction regarding exactly when a physician should discuss VSED with a seriously ill patient in the absence of a direct request.
- When the patient makes a direct request for information about her last-resort options, legal and ethical duties require the physician to discuss VSED or refer the patient to another clinician who will discuss this option.
- While hospital administration may be worried about legality and public perception, they have a duty to honor patient refusals unless they have a conscience-based objection.
- If the home hospice were unable to get the proper coverage, they could decline to participate. But duties of non-abandonment require facilitating transfer to a suitable setting.

Case 1.2. Bill, the Man with Metastatic Breast Cancer

Bill would have preferred MAID to VSED. But that option was not available because MAID is illegal in New York.

Bottom Line Points
- Legally, VSED is far more widely available than MAID.
- While MAID is legal in only eleven US jurisdictions and eight other countries, VSED is legally available in all US jurisdictions and most Western countries.
- While MAID is sometimes available as an "underground option" in states where it is clearly prohibited by explicit law, using MAID in these states poses serious legal risks to both the clinician and family.
- Patients have a right to refuse both medical and non-medical intrusions into their bodies, and clinicians have a correlative duty to respect that choice.

Case 1.3. Mrs. H., the Mother with Dementia

Mrs. H was worried about losing decision-making capacity and thus the ability to VSED.

Bottom Line Points
- VSED is only for patients who have decision-making capacity when they begin VSED.
- Patients are presumed to have decision-making capacity until proven otherwise. If there is uncertainty about a requesting patient's capacity, a consultation from a specialist in psychiatry, geriatrics and/or palliative care should be considered for clinical, ethical and legal reasons.
- Because it is difficult to prognosticate precisely when one will lose decision-making capacity, patients who VSED to avoid advancing dementia often die sooner than they would have preferred.
- Patients with fragile cognitive capacity like Mrs. H. should complete an AD for SED to help guide and legally cover family members if they lose capacity once the process is started.
- Even patients with normal cognitive capacity initiating VSED should complete an AD for SED before starting, because they may lose that capacity in later stages of the process.

Case 1.4. G.W., the Father with Lung Cancer

There was family conflict over how to manage G.W.'s VSED, particularly in how to respond to apparent requests for water. G.W. signed a VSED "agreement" with his hospice. But it is unclear what guidance that provided to his family.

Bottom Line Points
- While patients begin VSED with decision-making capacity, they often lose it during the late stages of the process.
- Patients should complete careful advance directives to guide caregivers when they cannot speak for themselves.
- While advance directives are relevant for all adult individuals, they are particularly important for those initiating VSED. These individuals should also complete an AD for SED for when and if they lose capacity late in the process.
- We explore SED by AD in the second half of this book, and legal approaches specifically in Chapter 10.
- We collect tools for completing ADs for SED in Appendices A and B at the end of this book.

References

A v. E, [2012] EWHC 1639 (COP).

A.B. v. C., 477 N.Y.S.2d 281 (Sup. Ct. 1984).

Airedale National Health Service Trust v. Bland, [1993] AC 789.

Alzheimer's Australia. 2014. *End of Life Care for People with Dementia*, https://www.dementia.org.au/files/EOI_ExecSummary_Web_Version.pdf.

American Medical Women's Association. 2018. "Position Statement on Medical Aid in Dying." https://www.amwa-doc.org/wp-content/uploads/2018/09/Medical-Aid-in-Dying-Position-Paper.pdf.

ANA Center for Ethics and Human Rights. 2017. "Revised Position Statement: Nutrition and Hydration at the End of Life." https://www.nursingworld.org/~4af0ed/globalassets/docs/ana/ethics/ps_nutrition-and-hydration-at-the-end-of-life_2017june7.pdf.

Arena v. Riversource Life Ins. No. 19-01043 (3d Cir. Sept. 10, 2019).

Arizona Revised Statutes § 13-3623.

Astraforoff (British Columbia (Attorney General) v.), 1983 BCCA 718.

Atiyah, P.S., and Robert S. Summers. 1987. *Form and Substance in Anglo-American Law: A Comparative Study of Legal Reasoning, Legal Theory, and Legal Institutions.* London: Clarendon.

Atlanta Constitution. 1983. "Obituaries." *Atlanta Constitution*, December 21.

Baumgartner, Fritz. "The Ethical Requirement to Provide Hydration and Nutrition." *Archives of Internal Medicine* 166, no. 12: 1324.

Baxter v. State, 224 P.3d 1211 (Mont. 2009).

Bentley v. Maplewood Seniors Care Society, 2014 BCSC 165.

Bernat, James L., Bernard Gert, and Peter Mogielnicki. 1993. "Patient Refusal of Hydration and Nutrition. An Alternative to Physician-Assisted Suicide or Voluntary Active Euthanasia." *Archives of Internal Medicine* 153, no. 24: 2723–2728.

Bolt, Eva. 2020. "Stop Eating and Drinking." *Pallium*, Nov. 20, https://www.palliumtotaal. nl/magazine-artikelen/stoppen-met-eten-en-drinken/.

Bouvia v. Superior Court, 179 Cal. App. 3d 1128 (Cal. App. 1986).

Brooks (In re), 258 N.Y.S. 2d 621 (Sup. Ct. 1987).

Butler v. United States, No. 4:07CV00519-JMM, 2009 WL 1607912 & 24 (E.D. Ark. June 9, 2009).

Byock, Ira. 1995. "Patient Refusal of Nutrition and Hydration: Walking the Ever-Finer Line." *American Journal of Hospice and Palliative Care* 12, no. 2: 8–13.

California A.B. 2747 (2009).

California Health and Safety Code § 443.18.

California Probate Code § 4656.

California Probate Code § 4734.

Canterbury v. Spence, 464 F. 2d 772 (D.C. Cir. 1972).

Cantor, Norman L. 2020. "Dispelling Medico-Legal Misconceptions Impeding Use of Advance Instructions to Shorten Immersion in Deep Dementia." *SSRN*, https://papers. ssrn.com/sol3/papers.cfm?abstract_id=3712186.

Cantor, Norman L., and George C. Thomas. 2000. "The Legal Bounds of Physician Conduct in Hastening Death." *Buffalo Law Review* 48, no. 1: 83–173.

Caulk (In re), 125 N.H. 226, 480 A.2d 93 (1984).

Cavanagh, Maureen. 2014. "How Should a Catholic Hospice Respond to Patients Who Choose to Voluntarily Stop Eating and Drinking in Order to Hasten Death?" *Linacre Quarterly* 81, no. 3 (August): 279–285.

Chabot, Boudewin E. 2007. *Auto-Euthanasie. Verborgen Stervenswegen In Gesprek Met Naasten*. Amsterdam: Uitgeverij Bert Bakker.

Chabot, Boudewin E., and A. Goedhart. 2009. "A Survey of Self-Directed Dying Attended by Proxies in the Dutch Population." *Social Science & Medicine* 68, no. 10: 1745–1751.

Chief Coroner. 2016. "Guidance No.17 Conclusions: Short-Form and Narrative." https:// www.judiciary.uk/wp-content/uploads/2013/09/guidance-no-17-conclusions.pdf.

Clarkson Co. Ltd. v. Shaheen, 544 F.2d 624 (2d Cir. 1976).

Centers for Medicare and Medicaid Services (CMS). 2020. "Requirements for Providers." 42 C.F.R. § 489.102(c)(1).

Centers for Medicare and Medicaid Services (CMS). 2019. "State Operations Manual, Appendix Q—Core Guidelines for Determining Immediate Jeopardy." https://www. cms.gov/Regulations-and-Guidance/Guidance/Manuals/downloads/som107ap_q_ immedjeopardy.pdf.

Colorado Revised Statutes § 26-3.1-101.

Cochrane, Thomas I., and Robert D. Truog. 2005. "Refusal of Hydration and Nutrition: Irrelevance of the 'Artificial' vs 'Natural' Distinction." *Archives of Internal Medicine* 165, no. 22: 2574–2576.

Cochrane, Thomas I., and Robert D. Truog. 2006. "The Ethical Requirement to Provide Hydration and Nutrition." *Archives of Internal Medicine* 166, no. 12: 1324–1325.

College of Physicians and Surgeons of British Columbia, CPS No. IC-2017-0836 (February 13, 2018).

Cruzan v. Director, Missouri Dept. of Health, 497 U.S. 261 (1990).

Culzac, Natasha. 2014. "Grandmother Starves Herself to Death After UK's Assisted Suicide Laws Left Her with No Alternative." *Guardian*, October 19.

De Lima, Liliana, Roger Woodruff, Katherine Pettus, Julia Downing, Rosa Buitrago, Esther Munyoro, Chitra Venkateswaran, Sushma Bhatnagar, and Lukas Radbruch.

2017. "International Association for Hospice and Palliative Care Position Statement: Euthanasia and Physician-Assisted Suicide." *Journal of Palliative Medicine* 20: 8–14.

Dobbs, Dan, Paul T. Hayden, and Ellen M. Bublick. 2020. *Dobbs' Law of Torts, 2d (Practitioner Treatise Series).* Eagan, MN: Thomson Reuters.

Downie, Jocelyn, and Matthew J. Bowes. 2019. "Refusing Care as a Legal Pathway to Medical Assistance in Dying." *Canadian Journal of Bioethics* 2, no. 2: 73–82.

Druml, Christiane, Peter E. Ballmer, Wilfred Druml, Frank Oehmichen, Alan Shenkin, Pierre Singer, Peter Soeters, Arved Weimann, and Stephan C. Bischoff. 2016. "ESPEN Guideline on Ethical Aspects of Artificial Nutrition and Hydration." *Clinical Nutrition* 35, no. 3: 545–556.

Eddy, David M. 1994. "A Conversation with My Mother." *JAMA* 272: 179–181.

Eddy, David. 2005. "I'm Still Telling Others How Well This Worked for My Mother." In *The Best Way to Say Goodbye: A Legal Peaceful Choice at the End of Life,* edited by Stanley A. Terman, 82–84. Carlsbad, CA: Life Transitions.

Evans, Alex. 2012. "Former Magistrate Starved Herself to Death Supporting Right-to-Die." *Weston Mercury,* October 26.

Feichtner, Angelika, Dietmar Weixler, and Alois Birklbauer. 2018. "Voluntary Refraining from Food and Fluids to Accelerate Death: A Statement from the Austrian Palliative Society (OPG) [Freiwilliger Verzicht auf Nahrung und Flüssigkeit umdas Sterben zu beschleunigen: Eine Stellungnahme der österreichischen Palliativgesellschaft (OPG)]." *Vienna Medical Weekly [Wiener Medizinische Wochenschrift]* 168: 168–176.

Gallagher J. 1984. "Health Facilities' Obligations when a Patient Refuses Treatment." *Health Progress* 65, no. 8: 40–43.

Ganzini, Linda, Elizabeth R. Goy, Lois L. Miller, Theresa A. Harvath, Ann Jackson, and Molly A. Delorit. 2003. "Nurses' Experiences with Hospice Patients Who Refuse Food and Fluids to Hasten Death." *New England Journal of Medicine* 349: 359–365.

General Medical Council (GMC). 2015. "Patients Seeking Advice or Information about Assistance to Die." https://www.gmc-uk.org/-/media/documents/gmc-guidance---when-a-patient-seeks-advice-or-information-about-assistance-to-die_pdf-61449907.pdf.

General Medical Council (GMC). 2018. "Email to Leigh Day, SR1-2099006949," October 30.

Goldstein, Nathan E. 2012. "Prevalence of Formal Accusations of Murder and Euthanasia against Physicians." *Journal of Palliative Medicine* 15, no. 3: 334–339.

Goodman, Ellen. 1984. "Judging the Right to Die." *Washington Post,* February 11.

Goodman, Lee Hugh. 2021. "Litigating the Suicide Exclusion in Life Insurance Policies." *American Jurisprudence Proof of Facts* 3d 20: 227

Gordy (In re), 658 A.2d 613 (Del. Chancery 1994).

H Ltd v. J, [2010] SASC 176 ¶ 1-2 (Austl.).

Hawaii. "Our Care, Our Choice Act." Laws 2018, chapter 2.

Hart, H.L.A. 1961. *The Concept of Law.* London: Clarendon Press.

Harvath, Theresa A., Lois L Miller, Elizabeth Goy, Ann Jackson, Molly Delorit, and Linda Ganzini. 2004. "Voluntary Refusal of Food and Fluids: Attitudes of Oregon Hospice Nurses and Social Workers." *International Journal of Palliative Nursing* 10: 236–241.

Hoekstra, Nina Luisa, M. Strack, and A. Simonet. 2015. "Physicians Attitudes on Voluntary Refusal of Food and Fluids to Hasten Death—Results of an Empirical Study Among 255 Physicians." *Zeitschrift für Palliativmedizin* 16 no 2: 68–73.

Ivanović, Natasa, Daniel Büche, and André Fringer. 2014. "Voluntary Stopping of Eating and Drinking at the End of Life—A 'Systematic Search and Review' Giving Insight into an Option of Hastening Death in Capacitated Adults at the End of Life." *BMC Palliative Care* 13, no. 1. https://bmcpalliatcare.biomedcentral.com/track/pdf/10.1186/1472-684X-13-1.pdf

KNMG, (Koninklijke Nederlandsche Maatschappij tot bevordering der Geneeskunst) [Royal Dutch Medical Association]. 2011. "The Role of the Physician in the Voluntary Termination of Life." https://www.knmg.nl/actualiteit-opinie/nieuws/nieuwsbericht/euthanasia-in-the-netherlands.htm.

Jansen, Lynn A., and Daniel P. Sulmasy. 2002. "Sedation, Alimentation, Hydration, and Equivocation: Careful Conversation about Care at the End of Life." *Annals of Internal Medicine* 136: 845–849.

Johnson, Sandra H. 2009. "Regulating Physician Behavior: Taking Doctors' 'Bad Law' Claims Seriously." *Saint Louis University Law Journal* 53: 973–1032.

Johnson, Sandra H. 2012. "What Law Really Requires." *Hastings Center Report* 42, no. 1 (Jan./Feb.): 11–12.

Jotkowitz, Alan. 2009. "End-of-Life Treatment Decisions: The Opportunity to Care." *American Journal of Bioethics* 9, no. 4: 59–60.

Joychen, P.J. 2015. "Jain Practice of Santhara Illegal: Rajasthan HC." *Times of India*, August 11. https://timesofindia.indiatimes.com/toireporter/author-PJ-Joychen-479195188.cms.

Kallinger (Commonwealth v.), 134 Pa. Commw. 415, 580 A.2d 887 (1990).

Larriviere, Dan, and H. Richard Beresford. 2008. "Professionalism in Neurology: The Role of Law." *Neurology* 71: 1283–1288.

Mader, Sarah, and Victoria Apold. 2020. "VSED as an Alternative to MAiD: A Pan-Canadian Legal Analysis." https://papers.ssrn.com/sol3/papers.cfm?abstract_id=3500173.

Manoir de la Pointe Bleue Inc. v. Corbeil, [1992] Carswell Quebec 1623 (Quebec Superior Court, Canada).

Margolick, David. 1994. "Judge Says Ailing Man, 85, May Fast to Death." *New York Times*, February 3.

Meisel, Alan. 1995. "Barriers to Forgoing Nutrition and Hydration in Nursing Homes." *American Journal of Law and Medicine* 21: 335–382.

Meisel, Alan. 2016. "Legal Issues in Death and Dying: How Rights and Autonomy Have Shaped Legal Practice." In *Oxford Handbook of Ethics at the End of Life*, edited by Stuart J. Youngner and Robert M. Arnold, 7–26. New York: Oxford University Press.

Meisel, Alan, Kathy L. Cerminara, and Thaddeus M. Pope. 2020. *The Right to Die: The Law of End-of-Life Decisionmaking.* New York: Wolters Kluwer.

Melchert-Dinkel (State v.), 844 N.W.2d 13 (Minn. 2014).

Miller, Franklin G., and Diane E. Meier. 1998. "Voluntary Death: A Comparison of Terminal Dehydration and Physician-Assisted Suicide." *Annals of Internal Medicine* 128: 559–562.

Minnesota Statutes § 145C.01(4).

Minnesota Statutes § 609.215(3)(b).

Montgomery, Lori. 1996. "Starving is Legal Suicide Method." *Detroit Free Press*, November 20.

Morton v. Wellstar, 653 S.E.2d 756 (Ga. App. 2007).

Nauk, Friedemann, Christoph Ostgathe, and Lukas Radbruch. 2014. "Physically Assisted Suicide: Help with Dying—No Help with Dying." *German Medical Journal* [*Dtsch Arztebl*] 111, no. 3: A67–A71.

Nishi v. Hartwell, 473 P. 2d 116 (Haw. 1970).

New York Public Health Law § 2997-c.

Ohio Revised Code § 3795.03.

Oyez. 1997. "Vacco v. Quill Oral Argument." *Oyez*, January 8. https://www.oyez.org/cases/1996/95-1858.

Onwuteaka-Philipsen, Bregje D., Arianne Brinkman-Stoppelenburg, Corine Penning, Gwen J.F. de Jong-Krul, Johannes J.M. van Delden, and Agnes van der Heide. 2012. "Trends in End-of-Life Practices Before and after the Enactment of the Euthanasia Law in The Netherlands from 1990 to 2010: A Repeated Cross-Sectional Survey." *Lancet* 380, no. 9845: 908–915.

Pictaroia v. N.E. Utilities, 756 A.2d 845 (Conn. 2000).

Plaza Health & Rehabilitation Center (In re), (Onondaga County, NY Feb 2, 1984) (Miller, J).

Pope, Thaddeus M. 2008. "Involuntary Passive Euthanasia in U.S. Courts: Reassessing the Judicial Treatment of Medical Futility Cases." *Marquette Elder's Advisor* 9: 229–268.

Pope, Thaddeus M. 2010. "Legal Briefing: Conscience Clauses and Conscientious Refusal." *Journal of Clinical Ethics* 21, no. 2: 163–180.

Pope, Thaddeus M., and Lindsey Anderson. 2011. "Voluntarily Stopping Eating and Drinking: A Legal Treatment Option at the End of Life." *Widener Law Review* 17, no. 2: 363–428.

Pope, Thaddeus M. 2013. "Clinicians May Not Administer Life-Sustaining Treatment without Consent: Civil, Criminal, and Disciplinary Sanctions." *Journal of Health & Biomedical Law* 9: 213–296.

Pope, Thaddeus M. 2017. "Certified Patient Decision Aids: Solving Persistent Problems with Informed Consent Law." *Journal of Law, Medicine, and Ethics* 45: 12–40.

Pope, Thaddeus M. 2018. "Law and Ethics in Oncology: Voluntarily Stopping Eating and Drinking Is a Legal and Ethical Exit Option." *ASCO Post*, June 25.

Pope, Thaddeus M. 2018. "Legal History of Medical Aid in Dying: Physician Assisted Death in U.S. Courts and Legislatures." *New Mexico Law Review* 48: 267–301.

Quill, Timothy E., and Ira R. Byock. 2000. "Responding to Intractable Terminal Suffering: The Role of Terminal Sedation and Voluntary Refusal of Food and Fluids." *Annals of Internal Medicine* 132: 408–414.

Richards, Naomi. 2014. "The Death of the Right-to-Die Campaigners." *Anthropology Today* 30, no. 3: 14–17.

Rozovsky, Fay A. 2020. *Consent to Treatment: A Practical Guide, Fifth Edition.* New York: Wolters Kluwer.

Swiss Academy of Medical Sciences. 2018. "Management of Dying and Death." https://www.sams.ch/en/Publications/Medical-ethical-Guidelines.html.

Savulescu, Julian. 2014. "A Simple Solution to the Puzzles of End of Life? Voluntary Palliated Starvation." *Journal of Medical Ethics* 40: 110–113.

Shacter, Phyllis. 2017. Choosing to Die: A Personal Story: Elective Death by Voluntarily Stopping Eating and Drinking (VSED) in the Face of Degenerative Disease. Self-published, information at https://www.phyllisshacter.com/.

Sherazi, Saadia. 2008. "Physicians' Preferences and Attitudes about End-of-Life Care in Patients with an Implantable Cardioverter-Defibrillator." *Mayo Clinic Proceedings* 83, no. 10: 1139–1141.

Shinjo, Takuya, Tatsuya Morita, Daisuke Kiuchi, Masayuki Ikenaga, Hirofumi Abo, Sayaka Maeda, Satoru Tsuneto, and Yoshiyuki Kizawa. 2019. "Japanese Physicians' Experiences of Terminally Ill Patients Voluntarily Stopping Eating and Drinking: A National Survey." *BMJ Supportive Palliative Care* 9, no. 2: 143–145.

Silver, Mara. 2005. "Testing Cruzan: Prisoners and the Constitutional Question of Self-Starvation." *Stanford Law Review* 58: 631–662.

Singletary v. Costello, 665 So. 2d 1099 (Fla. Dist. Ct. App. 1996).

Stangle, Sabrina, Wilfried Schnepp, Daniel Büche, Christian Häuptle, and André Fringer. 2020. "Family Physicians' Perspective on Voluntary Stopping of Eating and Drinking: A Cross-Sectional Study." *Journal of International Medical Research* 48, no. 8; 1–15.

Stangle, Sabrina, Daniel Büche, Christian Häuptle, and André Fringer. 2021. "Attitudes and Professional Stance of Swiss Health Care Professionals towards Voluntary Stopping of Eating and Drinking to Hasten Death: A Cross-Sectional Study." *Journal of Pain and Symptom Management* 61, no. 2; 27–278.

Sullivan, Robert J. 1993. "Accepting Death without Artificial Nutrition or Hydration." *Journal of General Internal Medicine* 8: 220–223.

Thor v. Superior Court, 5 Cal.4th 725 (Cal. 1993).

Taktak v. R, 14 NSWLR 226 (1988).

Trowse, Phillippa. 2020. "Voluntary Stopping of Eating and Drinking in Advance Directives for Adults with Late-Stage Dementia." *Australasian Journal on Aging*, 39, no. 22: 142–147.

Truchon v. Procureur Général du Canada, 2019 QCCS 3792.

Utah Code Annotated § 62A-3-30.

Van der Heide, Agnes, A. Brinkman-Stoppelenburg, J.J.M. Delden, and B.D. Onwuteaka-Philipsen. 2012. *Sterfgevallenonderzoek 2010: Euthanasie en Andere Medische Beslissingen Rond het Levenseinde*. Den Haag: ZenMw.

Von Holden (In re), 87 A.D.2d 66, 450 N.Y.S.2d 623 (1982).

Western Australia Joint Select Committee on End of Life Choices. 2018. *My Life, My Choice: The Report of the Joint Select Committee on End of Life Choices*. https://www.parliament.wa.gov.au/Parliament/commit.nsf.

Windsor House v. Centers for Medicare & Medicaid, DAB No. CR1039 (U.S. Dept. Health & Human Services 2013), dhhs.gov/dab/decisions/CR1039.html.

Winnebago County v. C.S., No. 2016-AP-1982, 2020 WI 33.

Wolfe, Ian D., and Thaddeus M. Pope. 2020. "Hospital Mergers and Conscience-Based Objections—Growing Threats to Access and Quality of Care." *New England Journal of Medicine* 382, no. 15: 1388–1389.

World Medical Association. 2016. "Declaration of Tokyo." https://www.wma.net/policies-post/wma-declaration-of-tokyo-guidelines-for-physicians-concerning-torture-and-other-cruel-inhuman-or-degrading-treatment-or-punishment-in-relation-to-detention-and-imprisonment/.

Wright, James L., Peter M Jaggard, Timothy Holahan, and Ethics Subcommittee of AMDA. 2019. "Stopping Eating and Drinking by Advance Directives (SED by AD) in Assisted Living and Nursing Homes." *JAMDA* 29: 1362–1366.

Zant v. Prevatte 286 S.E.2d 715, 248 Ga. 832 (1982).

5

Institutional Issues

David A. Gruenewald

5.1. Introduction

VSED occurring in an institutional long-term care (LTC) setting merits a separate discussion from VSED in other settings, not only because it is subject to substantially more regulatory scrutiny but also because it entails relatively distinct and unique clinical and ethical challenges. In this chapter, I describe what is known about the experience of VSED in LTC facilities by patients who have decision-making capacity at the time they are making this decision, including the barriers that residents wishing to VSED may encounter. I discuss the important role of hospice in managing conflicts between LTC facilities and residents wishing to VSED. I consider variations in state laws affecting resident rights relative to VSED in the United States. I conclude by offering recommendations for the approach to care of residents wishing to VSED in LTC facilities, and by considering specific care issues that may be encountered in these settings.

5.2. Published Data on Patient Experience of VSED
in Institutional Settings

Little information is available in the published literature on the experience of patients wishing to VSED in institutional LTC settings. Two VSED case series from the Netherlands included a substantial proportion (41%–47%) of residents of LTC facilities (Bolt et al. 2015; Chabot and Goedhart 2009). In one of these studies, common motivations for wishing to hasten death by VSED as reported by their family physicians included somatic symptoms such as fatigue, weakness, and physical deterioration; existential suffering and loss of purpose; and physical dependency (Bolt et al. 2015). However, this study did not report whether motivations to VSED were different in residents of LTC facilities and those living in non-institutional settings. A study of skilled nursing facilities in Switzerland estimated the incidence of death by VSED to be 1.7% (Stängle et al. 2020).

Apart from these studies, to the author's knowledge, no other published work to date has reported how commonly community-dwelling people are admitted to inpatient hospice units or skilled nursing facilities to undergo VSED, the underlying reasons for these admissions, or the quality of the experience of dying by VSED in a LTC facility.

5.3. Institutional Barriers to VSED

Although detailed in many respects, the Royal Dutch Medical Association guideline on caring for people who VSED did not comment on the experience of people who opted to VSED in institutional care settings compared to home settings (KNMG and V&VN 2014). In North America, residents of institutions have at times been blocked from attempting to VSED by the institutions in which they reside, even when the resident has intact decision-making capacity (Pope and Anderson 2011, 373).

As a case in point, in 2011 Armond and Dorothy Rudolph were expelled from the assisted living facility in New Mexico where they resided with only one day's notice after informing facility administrators of their intention to VSED. They subsequently died in a rented home under the care of family members and hospice workers (Pope and West 2014). Taken together with the large number of care facility residents undergoing VSED in the two published series from the Netherlands, it is tempting to speculate that there may be greater cultural resistance to VSED in institutional settings in North America than in the Netherlands (Bolt et al. 2015; Chabot and Goedhart 2009).

Some people with intractable suffering related to serious degenerative and terminal illnesses lack the resources and support from family and friends to pursue VSED at home, while others with similar illnesses and experiences of suffering already reside in institutional care settings. In either situation, the only option for these individuals may be to receive care in a facility, either with facility support during VSED or with "usual" comfort-oriented feeding as part of standard hospice or comfort-focused care (see Chapter 8, Section 8.1).

To the author's knowledge, no studies have examined whether an ill person's desire to VSED is more likely to be enacted in a home setting than in an institutional residential setting (although this likelihood may appear self-evident). As noted elsewhere in this volume, for ill people who don't reside in an institution, VSED is self-initiated usually with some support from family and friends, but doesn't require the mandatory participation of health care providers and staff (although such support is highly advisable).

By contrast, involvement of health care providers and staff is unavoidable for residents of care facilities. Residents wishing to VSED must negotiate the permissibility of VSED with a gauntlet of administrators, providers, and staff. Unless stopped by a persuasive and persistent advocate or health care agent, some facilities may expel residents wishing to VSED once their intention is known, as happened in the case of the Rudolphs in New Mexico (Pope and West 2014). As a way to circumvent limitations on the freedom to VSED in LTC settings, some residents may leave LTC facilities preemptively and de-camp to short-term rental housing where they may pursue VSED with support from family and/or professional home caregivers (Pope and West 2014, 71).

Even if not expelled, residents of care facilities may find their requests to VSED thwarted by the facility's administrative and/or clinical staff (e.g., by badgering them to eat and drink, or by continuing to offer food and drink regularly after beginning a VSED attempt) for a variety of reasons (Box 5.1). Conflicts may arise between the resident's right of self-determination and institutional mandates.

Administrative and clinical leaders in residential care settings are appropriately and understandably concerned about maintaining the safety of residents, and they may fear that allowing a resident to VSED will potentially place the facility at risk for survey citations, loss of licensure, fines, or accusations of abuse or neglect. For example, the occurrence of weight loss, functional deterioration, and labeling resident behavior as "suicidal" may raise concerns of regulators. The mere risk of being investigated, with the time and stress involved, may deter some facility administrators from supporting VSED, even if the facility is ultimately found blameless. Concerns about bad publicity or arousing the attention of activists who object to allowing VSED may be additional deterrents.

Box 5.1 Institutional Barriers to Voluntarily Stopping Eating and Drinking (VSED)

- Some LTC institutions including those with religious affiliation may bar participation.
- LTC administrators and staff may be unfamiliar with responding to requests for hastened death including VSED.
- Specific administrative and clinical concerns regarding VSED include the risk of:
  - Survey citations or accusations of abuse or neglect
  - Quality of care concerns related to weight loss, functional decline, and death (particularly in absence of terminal prognosis)
  - Making the facility complicit in suicide
  - Triggering mandatory reporting of suicidal intent
- Staff may experience moral distress or conscientious objection.
- State laws in a few states indicate that oral nutrition and hydration shall be provided even if life-sustaining treatment or artificial administration of nutrition and hydration are withheld or withdrawn.

Abbreviations: LTC—long-term care; VSED—voluntarily stopping eating and drinking.

5.4. Variations in State Laws around Resident Rights

States vary considerably in how their laws balance resident autonomy and institutional requirements to provide oral nutrition and hydration, and the extent to which state laws regulate these considerations. Some states explicitly prohibit withholding or withdrawing oral nutrition and hydration. For example, state laws in Delaware and Oklahoma indicate that "[e]ven if life-sustaining treatment or artificial administration of nutrition and hydration are withheld or withdrawn, the patient shall be provided with medication or other medical treatment to alleviate pain *and will be provided with oral consumption of food and water*" (American Bar Association 2017; Oklahoma Statutes 2018). However, these laws should not be interpreted to mandate forcible oral feeding and hydration against a resident's wishes.[1]

---

[1] In support of this proposition, New York attorney David Hoffman cites 42 C.F.R. § 489.102(c)(1), 10 NYCRR § 415.44, and 18 NYCRR §§ 487.8 & 488.8. These laws require providing and offering food and fluid unless that care conflicts with the patient's instructions.

By contrast, other states grant "enhanced rights" to vulnerable adults living in institutional settings, including the right to make decisions about their plan of treatment and how to conduct their personal lives. For example, in Washington State, vulnerable adults have enhanced rights in all LTC settings, including skilled nursing facilities, assisted living facilities, and "adult family homes" (group homes). These rights include the right "to direct his or her own service plan and changes in the service plan, and to refuse any particular service so long as such refusal is documented in the record of the resident." Residents also have the right to "receive services in the facility with reasonable accommodation of individual needs and preferences, except when the health or safety of the individual or other residents would be endangered" (Washington 2008; Centers for Medicare and Medicaid Services 2019).

The Washington State LTC Ombudsman Program advocates for resident rights in LTC facilities, including the right to refuse any treatment. The Ombudsman program has an interest in ensuring that LTC facilities respond to and make reasonable accommodation to honor resident rights. Program staff is potentially available to advocate on behalf of residents who request VSED and are encountering barriers or resistance from facility staff to honoring these requests (Washington State Long-Term Care Ombudsman Program 2020).

Advocacy programs such as the Washington State LTC Ombudsman may be especially important for low-income citizens who often lack the social support, health care access, and other resources available to more economically privileged citizens. These individuals may have no alternative to LTC facilities if they wish to pursue VSED. Accordingly, there is a social justice aspect to ensuring the availability of VSED in LTC facilities, especially for people who lack the support and resources to carry out VSED at home.

Based on the foregoing, all stakeholders, including LTC facility administrators and clinical staff, persons considering VSED who reside in or are contemplating entry into a care facility, and their families, should be aware of the policies and attitudes regarding VSED within the facility. Ill older people who are considering VSED may wish to determine whether VSED will be permitted by a care facility before agreeing to facility placement.

5.5. Role of Hospice in Buffering Conflicts Between Interests of Resident and LTC Facility

Hospice agencies may play an important role in buffering conflicts between the right of self-determination of ill people and the concerns of LTC facilities.

When a person wishing to VSED enters hospice care, the focus of health care becomes helping the person who is deteriorating from serious and terminal illness to live as well as possible for whatever time remains, rather than pursuing life-prolonging treatments. In hospice care, an interdisciplinary team of health care professionals addresses the physical, psychosocial, and spiritual needs of the person and his or her family (Hospice Foundation of America n.d.). Enrollment in hospice care may reassure all parties that the resident's care needs and potential sources of suffering are being comprehensively addressed (Gruenewald 2018; Quill et al. 2018; Wax et al. 2018). Furthermore, some hospices may have policies and procedures in place that give voice to the care wishes of residents wishing to VSED and offer guidance to facility personnel on responding to these requests (Post and Blustein 2015, Chapter 17).

However, issues and conflicts may still arise even when hospice is involved in the care of residents who choose VSED (Quill et al. 2018). Some hospice staff may perceive participation in VSED as contrary to their mission to promote comfort and "neither to hasten nor prolong the dying process" (Hospicare.org 2020). Hospices may be unwilling to enroll people seriously considering VSED with a prognosis of more than six months. Or they may refuse to enroll them until several days after VSED has been initiated, especially if they would not otherwise qualify with the requirement of a six-month or less prognosis. Furthermore, patients not otherwise terminally ill who change their minds about VSED after initiation and resume oral fluids will likely be disenrolled from hospice.

Patients who are unable to enroll in hospice may still benefit from palliative care. Indeed, palliative care may be invaluable at any stage of the process, including early on, to clarify goals of care, optimize symptom management, develop a treatment plan aligned with values and goals, and identify resources and supports as needed. Palliative care services for people who are not hospitalized are becoming more widely available, but they are not yet as accessible as hospice care in many communities. When available, palliative care is often accessed by referral from a primary care provider or team.

5.6. Approach to Care of Persons Requesting VSED in Institutional Settings

Recommendations for the care of LTC facility residents who request VSED are shown in Box 5.2 (Gruenewald 2018). Just as for people requesting

Box 5.2 Recommendations for Practice When a LTC Facility Resident Requests VSED

Providers and Interdisciplinary Professional Staff:

- Listen carefully to understand resident's suffering and reasons for the request.
- Ensure resident/family have a clear understanding of disease and prognosis.
- Ensure resident/family and interdisciplinary professional staff have an accurate understanding of the VSED process and know what to expect as VSED unfolds.
- Obtain formal palliative care and/or hospice consultation. This second opinion is especially important if the resident is unlikely to die soon without VSED, or there is lack of consensus.
- Assess decision-making capacity and voluntariness. Consult psychiatry and/or palliative care if uncertain.
- Ensure completion of advance directive. Identify health care proxies and specifically address the resident's desire and reasons to VSED, and their desire to continue VSED if capacity is lost in the process. Video recording of the resident's care preferences regarding VSED is highly recommended.
- Ensure that the DNAR/DNI order is in place. A POLST, MOLST, or equivalent document is strongly advised.
- Consider values of facility staff and legal limits.
- Assess impact of regulations in your state regarding care facility support for withholding and withdrawing oral nutrition and hydration.
- Inform residents requesting hastened death who have decision-making capacity and intractable suffering near end of life about all legally available treatment options, including VSED.
- Clinicians are not required to act against their moral principles, but they must not make moral judgments for residents based on their personal beliefs.
- If clinician has moral/ethical qualms about VSED, refer the inquiring resident to a clinician who doesn't have moral objections to supporting the practice (if possible).
- Identify family, friends, others available for emotional and physical support.
- Ensure availability of front-line caregivers for physical, psychosocial, and spiritual care.

LTC Facility Administrators and Leaders
- Know regulations in your state regarding withholding and with-drawing oral nutrition and hydration.
- Include front-line staff in care planning discussions of resident's request to VSED.
- Educate front-line caregivers regarding clinical scenarios that may arise during VSED, including dry mouth, delirium, and resident requests to resume fluids and food.
- If possible, allow objecting front-line staff to opt out of caring for residents choosing VSED, while ensuring that rigorous attempts have been made to address their concerns.
- Consider facility's ability to ensure around-the-clock staffing.
- Ensure appropriately private setting within facility.
- Ensure rigorous care planning around potential/expected outcomes, e.g., weight loss, dry mouth, skin care, delirium, declining function, requests to resume food/drink.

POLST—Provider Orders for Life-Sustaining Treatment
MOLST—Medical Orders for Life-Sustaining Treatment
VSED—Voluntarily Stopping Eating and Drinking
LST—Life-Sustaining Treatments
DNAR—Do Not Attempt Resuscitation
DNI—Do Not Intubate
LTC—Long-Term Care

Adapted for use by permission of *The Journal of Palliative Medicine* and Mary Ann Liebert, Inc., New Rochelle, NY (Gruenewald 2018).

VSED or assistance hastening death who reside in non-institutional settings, residents of care facilities require a comprehensive assessment of the reasons underlying the person's request and vigorous efforts to remediate causes of suffering (Block and Billings 1994; Quill 1993; Quill and Byock 2000). The approach to responding to requests for hastened death is discussed in Chapter 2 (Section 2.3). In institutional care settings, concerns about protecting vulnerable adults from harm and promoting resident safety are essential and appropriate. At the same time, person-centered care requires that residents are offered choices about their care and encouraged to make their own decisions about matters that personally affect them (Koren 2000). Furthermore, resident satisfaction with care depends on having the ability to choose from options the resident finds satisfactory (Bangerter et al. 2017).

To minimize risk of harm while maximizing resident self-determination and choice, LTC facilities should respond to resident requests to VSED by following best practices in resident-centered care planning. In skilled nursing facilities, care planning involves the use of the Resident Assessment Instrument/Minimum Data Set (RAI/MDS) (Centers for Medicare and Medicaid Services 2019). The RAI/MDS identifies required areas of resident assessment including functional and nutritional status. The overarching goal of care planning is to ensure that residents attain or maintain their highest practicable physical, mental, and psychosocial well-being (Centers for Medicare and Medicaid Services 2017). This normally includes efforts to maintain stable weight and optimize functional status. But residents undergoing VSED will of course experience weight loss, declining function, and eventual death as expected outcomes.

Interdisciplinary care planning is indicated to maximize well-being and quality of life in anticipation of these changes. LTC facility staff must document the reasons for apparently adverse clinical outcomes related to VSED, including weight loss, declining function, pain, and delirium, along with interventions to mitigate these adverse outcomes. Awareness of specific guidance for LTC surveyors around nutrition and hydration issues will aid LTC administrators, providers, and staff to avoid pitfalls when caring for residents choosing VSED. To demonstrate that weight loss, poor nutritional status, or dehydration are unavoidable, the facility must "prove it has assessed/reassessed the resident's needs, consistently implemented related care planned interventions, monitored for effectiveness, and ensured coordination of care among the interdisciplinary team" (Centers for Medicare and Medicaid Services 2017). Facilities are still expected to provide other care that allows the resident to maintain his or her highest practicable physical, mental, and psychosocial well-being, "even if [the] resident has refused food and fluids and is nearing death" (Centers for Medicare and Medicaid Services 2017).

Ethical concerns or moral distress may arise in LTC staff, providers, and administrators working with residents requesting VSED. Although VSED has become more widely acknowledged as a valid last-resort option to relieve suffering near the end of life, the practice remains ethically controversial (Quill et al. 2018). Facility staff with moral or ethical objections to VSED are not obligated to participate in practices that hasten death. A rule issued in 2019 by the U.S. Department of Health and Human Services Office of Civil

Rights gives health care workers latitude to refuse to provide services such as abortion or MAID if they cite a religious or conscientious objection (U.S. Department of Health and Human Services 2019, Sanger-Katz 2019). Similar latitude is provided by Title VII of the Civil Rights Act of 1964 and analogous statutes in most states (Sawicki 2020).

However, to promote resident self-determination and quality of life, LTC providers must inform their seriously and terminally ill patients who request hastened death about all legal care options. This view, supported by the American Nurses Association (2017, Code of Ethics), attempts to balance conscience-based rights with the duty to provide care: " . . . A nurse is justified in refusing to participate in a particular decision or action that is morally objectionable, so long as it is a conscience-based objection and not one based on personal preference, prejudice, bias, convenience, or arbitrariness" (Cipriano 2018). At the same time, "[n]urses are obliged to provide for patient safety, to avoid patient abandonment, and to withdraw only when assured that nursing care is available to the patient."

Additionally, when residents continue to request legal interventions that are unacceptable to the LTC facility, they must be offered the option to transfer care to another provider or care facility (Quill, Lo, and Brock 1997). Effecting such a care transfer, however, may be very difficult in reality. To deal with the challenges of accommodating staff and resident rights within the practical realities of long-term care, strategies to address staff moral distress and conscientious objections are discussed in the next section.

5.7. Specific Care Issues for Residents Who VSED in Institutional Settings

LTC facility practice recommendations for residents requesting VSED are outlined in Box 5.2 (Gruenewald 2018). Interdisciplinary care planning should include not only core disciplines such as nursing, social work, and chaplaincy, but also palliative care and hospice support. Consultations with ethics and mental health specialists may be indicated, especially if there are staff and/or family conflicts around care, or concerns about mental health issues, suicidality, coercion, or decision-making capacity. The care plan must be established together with the resident and involved family, and discussed in an interdisciplinary resident care conference. Any questions and concerns from stakeholders should be addressed, and the results of the care conference rigorously documented.

Documentation of resident care preferences must include a properly completed advance directive that includes: (1) a clear description of the intent and reasons to VSED, (2) a statement that other approaches short of hastened death by VSED do not meet the resident's needs, (3) indication of whether hospitalization is indicated under any circumstances, and (4) designation of supportive surrogate decision maker(s) should the patient lose decision-making capacity after initiation. Video recording of the resident's care preferences is invaluable (see Chapter 2, Section 2.6). "Do not resuscitate" code status must be established in all cases (Schwarz 2019).

Front-line staff must receive training in caring for persons undergoing VSED, and the questions and concerns of all participating staff including evening, night, and weekend shifts must be fully addressed. Using practices discussed elsewhere in this volume, LTC staff must carefully attend to care issues affecting the well-being of residents during VSED, including skin care, management of symptoms such as severe dry mouth and delirium, hygiene, bowel and bladder care, and activities of daily living. The potential use of palliative sedation for management of severe agitated delirium should be discussed in advance.

Facility administrators should bear in mind the potentially harmful effect on other LTC facility residents of witnessing the VSED process. Concerns that witnessing VSED may undermine confidence in care should be addressed by caring for residents undergoing VSED in a private setting.

5.8. Moral Distress and Conscience-Based Objections

LTC facility staff are trained to encourage food and fluids, and offering fluids and food is a potent symbol of caring. It is therefore not surprising that requests to VSED may cause distress among staff who are asked to care for a resident choosing VSED. Staff need training on how to respond to resident requests to resume fluids after VSED has begun, as discussed in Section 5.6 above (Gruenewald 2018; Quill et al. 2018; Wax et al. 2018).

As noted in Section 5.6, facilities with limited staffing may have difficulty accommodating staff conscientious objections to participation in VSED. In practice, it may not be possible to find alternative caregivers to cover all shifts for a resident choosing to VSED. Additionally, it may not be possible to secure an alternative placement for residents wishing to VSED when a LTC facility has religious or other objections to participating in VSED, even with support from a health care agent and the interdisciplinary care team.

Steps that can help to address staff concerns include obtaining specialty consultation(s) from palliative care, hospice, ethics, or psychiatry as indicated. Enrolling the resident in hospice may help staff to focus on quality of life concerns and make loss of weight and function more understandable. Staff may benefit from the knowledge that VSED is supported by position statements issued by the American Nurses Association, AMDA—The Society for Post-Acute and Long-Term Care Medicine, and others (AMDA 2019; American Nurses Association 2017; Appendix D).

Other steps include ensuring comprehensive resident-centered care planning, involving all stakeholders including nurses' aides in care planning and in resident/family conferences, reaching out to staff covering weekends and on all shifts, and training front-line caregivers in approaches to managing common problems encountered during VSED such as dry mouth, delirium, and requests to resume oral intake after VSED is initiated (Gruenewald 2018).

Additionally, it may be invaluable for staff to view video documentation of a resident's wishes regarding VSED if available (Pope 2020; Wax et al. 2018). If facility administrators have intractable objections to participation in hastened death at the system level (e.g., a religious objection based on facility ownership), persons seeking placement in a care facility are advised to assess the facility's willingness to support a VSED request before committing to placement.

5.9. Conclusion—Institutional Care Issues

When residents of LTC facilities with serious debilitating or terminal illnesses request VSED to relieve intractable suffering, or to avoid a prolonged dying process or years of severe debilitation or poor quality of life, resident-centered care planning is fundamental to honoring both residents' right of self-determination and the interests of facilities and staff in ensuring resident safety and protection from harm. This process is interdisciplinary, involving all key stakeholders to comprehensively address the resident's care needs in physical, psychological, social, and spiritual dimensions of care.

5.10. Case Comments from an Institutional Perspective

Case 1.1. Al, the Biker with ALS

Admission to an inpatient palliative care or hospice unit may facilitate VSED while minimizing its obstacles common in other settings. Al's admission to a palliative care unit, in effect, released his home caregivers from the responsibility of participating in VSED. Palliative care unit staff frequently encounter requests for hastened death and are trained to respond in an individualized way, whereas home caregivers, who are often unlicensed aides, are typically trained to offer and encourage oral food and drink routinely as an expression of caring.

Case 1.2. Bill with Indolent Cancer

Bill's palliative care provider and palliative care unit staff worked with him extensively to understand his long-held and passionate desire to control the timing and circumstances of his death. They were unable to support his preference for MAID, which was illegal in his jurisdiction, but they ultimately reached an understanding with Bill that VSED was the best of the "bad options" available to him.

Unfortunately, inpatient palliative care and hospice units are not available or affordable for many patients who wish to VSED. Due to staff scarcity, the extensive and ongoing evaluation and caregiving efforts that Bill received would probably not be possible in many institutional LTC environments without ongoing advocacy and support from others outside the facility. Furthermore, many LTC facilities (and even some home hospice services, as illustrated in Case 1.4, with G.W.) lack expertise regarding VSED. Therefore, hospice and/or palliative care (and perhaps other) consultations must supplement the care provided in these settings.

Hospital-based palliative care and hospice units may face fewer administrative barriers to VSED than units based in skilled nursing settings governed by LTC regulations. Staff in hospital-based units must develop a comprehensive care plan, but they are not required by regulation to complete the RAI-MDS care planning process as in LTC skilled nursing facilities. Given the emphasis on maintenance of function, weight, and nutrition that is usually a part of RAI-MDS based care planning, LTC facilities may be more concerned than hospital-based palliative care and hospice units that a surveyor would view loss of weight and function as evidence of neglect or poor quality of care. In any case, such concerns in LTC facilities can be mitigated by comprehensive patient-centered care planning and documentation.

Disclaimer

This work was supported in part by the Department of Veterans Affairs. The views expressed herein are those of the author and do not necessarily reflect the views of the Department of Veterans Affairs or the U.S. Government.

References

AMDA—The Society for Post-Acute and Long-Term Care Medicine. 2019. "Ethics Committee White Paper: Stopping eating and drinking by advance directives (SED by AD) in the ALF and PALTC setting" (April 2019). https://paltc.org/amda-white-papers-and-resolution-position-statements/stopping-eating-and-drinking-advance-directives.

American Bar Association. 2017. "State Statutory Provisions Related to Orally Provided Food and Fluids and Comfort Care" (July 2017). https://www.americanbar.org/content/dam/aba/administrative/law_aging/2017_Food_%20Fluids_%20Chart.pdf.

American Nurses Association. 2017. "Position Statement: Nutrition and Hydration at the End of Life." https://www.nursingworld.org/~4af0ed/globalassets/docs/ana/ethics/ps_nutrition-and-hydration-at-the-end-of-life_2017june7.pdf.

Bangerter, Lauren R., Allison R. Heid, Katherin Abbott, and Kimberly Van Haitsma. 2017. "Honoring the Everyday Preferences of Nursing Home Residents: Perceived Choice and Satisfaction with Care." *Gerontologist* 5, no. 3: 479–486.

Block, Susan D., and J. Andrew Billings. "Patient Requests to Hasten Death: Evaluation and Management in Terminal Care." 1994. *Archives of Internal Medicine* 154, no. 18: 2039–2047.

Bolt, Eva E., Martijn Hagens, Dick Willems, and Bregie D. Onwuteaka-Philipsen. 2015. "Primary Care Patients Hastening Death by Voluntarily Stopping Eating and Drinking." 2015. *Annals of Family Medicine* 13, no. 5: 421–428.

Centers for Medicare and Medicaid Services (CMS). 2017. "State Operations Manual, Appendix PP—Guidance to Surveyors for Long Term Care Facilities (Rev. 173, 11-22-17)." https://www.cms.gov/Regulations-and-Guidance/Guidance/Manuals/downloads/som107ap_pp_guidelines_ltcf.pdf.

Centers for Medicare & Medicaid Services (CMS). 2019. "Long-Term Care Facility Resident Assessment Instrument 3.0 Version 1.17.1." October 2019 (online). https://www.cms.gov/Medicare/Quality-Initiatives-Patient-Assessment-Instruments/NursingHomeQualityInits/MDS30RAIManual.html.

Chabot, Boudewijn E., and Arnold Goedhart. 2009. "A Survey of Self-directed Dying Attended by Proxies in the Dutch Population." *Social Science and Medicine* 68, no. 10: 1745–1751.

Cipriano, Pamela F. 2018. "ANA responds to the HHS announcement of the New Conscience and Religious Freedom Division" (January 18, 2018). https://www.nursingworld.org/news/news-releases/2018/ana-responds-to-the-hhs-announcement-of-the-new-conscience-and-religious-freedom-division/.

Gruenewald, David A. 2018. "Voluntarily Stopping Eating and Drinking: A Practical Approach for Long-Term Care Facilities." *Journal of Palliative Medicine* 21, no. 9: 1214–1220.

Hospice Foundation of America. "What is Hospice?" https://hospicefoundation.org/Hospice-Care/Hospice-Services.

Hospicare.org. 2020. "Death and Dying." https://www.hospicare.org/education/death-and-dying/.

KNMG (Royal Dutch Medical Association) and V&VN (Dutch Nurses Association). 2014. *Caring for people who consciously choose not to eat and drink so as to hasten the end of life.* http://docplayer.net/10054859-Caring-for-people-who-consciously-choose-not-to-eat-and-drink-so-as-to-hasten-the-end-of-life.html.

Pope, Thaddeus M., and Lindsey E. Anderson. 2011. "Voluntarily Stopping Eating and Drinking: a Legal Treatment Option at the End of Life." *Widener Law Review* 1, no. 2: 363–428.

Koren, Mary J. "Person-centered Care for Nursing Home Residents: The Culture-change Movement." 2010. *Health Affairs.* 2, no. 2: 312–317.

Oklahoma Statutes. 2018. Title 63, § 3101.8. Citation: 63 OK Stat § 63-3101.8 (2018).

Pope, Thaddeus M., and Amanda West. 2014. "Legal Briefing: Voluntarily Stopping Eating and Drinking." *Journal of Clinical Ethics* 25, no. 1: 68–80.

Post, Linda Farber, and Jeffrey Blustein. 2015. *Handbook for Health Care Ethics Committees, 2nd ed.* Baltimore: Johns Hopkins University Press.

Quill, Timothy E. 1993. "Doctor, I Want to Die. Will You Help Me?" *JAMA* 270, no. 7: 870–873.

Quill, Timothy E., Bernard Lo, and Dan W. Brock. 1997. "Palliative Options of Last Resort: A Comparison of Voluntarily Stopping Eating and Drinking, Terminal Sedation, Physician-assisted Suicide, and Voluntary Active Euthanasia." *JAMA* 278, no. 23: 2099–2104.

Quill, Timothy E., and Ira R. Byock. 2000. "Responding to Intractable Terminal Suffering: The Role of Terminal Sedation and Voluntary Refusal of Food and Fluids." *Annals of Internal Medicine* 13, no. 5: 408–414.

Quill, Timothy E., Linda Ganzini Linda, Robert D. Truog, and Thaddeus M. Pope. 2018. "Voluntarily Stopping Eating and Drinking among Patients with Serious Advanced Illness: Clinical, Ethical, and Legal Aspects." *JAMA Internal Medicine* 17, no. 1: 123–127.

Sanger-Katz Margot. 2019. "Trump Administration Strengthens 'Conscience Rule' for Health Care Workers." *New York Times*, May 2, 2019. https://www.nytimes.com/2019/05/02/upshot/conscience-rule-trump-religious-exemption-health-care.html.

Sawicki, Nadia N. 2020. "The Conscience Defense to Malpractice." *California Law Review* 108, no. 4: 1255–1316.

Schwarz, Judith K. 2019. "Lessons From New York's Dementia Directive and Applications to Withholding Oral Feedings." *American Journal of Bioethics* 19, no. 1: 95–97.

Stängle, Sabrina, Wilfried Schnepp, Daniel Büche, and André Fringer. 2020. "Long-term Care Nurses' Attitudes and the Incidence of Voluntary Stopping of Eating and Drinking: A Cross-sectional Study." *Journal of Advanced Nursing* 76, no. 2: 526–534.

U.S. Department of Health and Human Services. 2019. "Protecting Statutory Conscience Rights in Health Care; Delegations of Authority," *Federal Register* 84: 23,170, May 21.

Washington Revised Code § 70.129.140 (2008).

Washington State Long-Term Care Ombudsman Program. 2020. www.waombudsman.org.

Wax, John W., Amy W. An, Nicole Kosier, and Timothy E. Quill. 2018. "Voluntary Stopping Eating and Drinking." *Journal of the American Geriatrics Society* 66, no. 3: 441–445.

6

Best Practices, Enduring Challenges, and Opportunities for VSED

Timothy E. Quill, Paul T. Menzel, Thaddeus M. Pope, and Judith K. Schwarz

The previous four chapters explored VSED from clinical, ethical, legal, and institutional perspectives. In this chapter we offer key summary points in three sections. First, we recommend *best practices* when considering or implementing VSED. Second, we describe *enduring challenges* and suggest ways to overcome them. Third, we identify *opportunities* that VSED offers for patients and families interested in a wider range of end-of-life options.

6.1. Best Practices

Always Provide Palliative Care. Always ensure that good palliative care consistent with the patient's values and preferences is available, offered, and delivered unless the patient refuses such care. Most (though not all) symptoms associated with VSED can be adequately managed with skillful palliative or hospice care.

Patient Control and Commitment. VSED is almost entirely under a patient's own control. It requires neither a diagnosis of terminal illness nor any changes in the law or institutional policies. It does require considerable patient commitment, and there should be thorough conversation with the patient and designated caregivers about this before initiating VSED.

Understand the Process. All those involved in the VSED process—patient, family, and other caregivers—must have an accurate understanding of what is involved, what to expect, and what to provide regarding effective symptom management as the process unfolds.

Assure Clinician Partnership. Although clinicians are theoretically not required for VSED to be feasible, they should almost always be part of the process to evaluate decision-making capacity up front and to help manage symptoms and challenges that emerge once VSED is initiated. When VSED occurs in a long-term care facility setting, rigorous and well-documented interdisciplinary resident-centered care planning is mandatory.

Relatively Short Duration. If the patient adheres fully with the process of forgoing all fluids, VSED has a beginning, a middle, and an end that usually occur over 10–14 days. This allows patients and families time to come together and have a meaningful process of "thank you" and "goodbye," with a relatively predictable end point. All who are interested in death-hastening options should be aware of this possibility.

Reassurance Even If Not Activated. Patients who fear end-of-life suffering and unwanted life extension are often reassured by the potential availability of VSED and other options for intentionally hastening death. Many will not need these options if they receive adequate palliative care. But knowing that they are available can enable patients to feel less trapped and vulnerable.

6.2. Enduring Challenges

Two-Week Duration. For some, death by VSED can take too long to provide effective relief of acute, unremitting, severe suffering at the end of life. Even if there is no better alternative, this timeframe can be difficult even when symptoms and support needs are managed with skillful palliative care. Furthermore, while the VSED process itself has a relatively short duration (of 10–14 days), it may take the patient much longer to first find a willing and available hospice or palliative care provider.

Considerable Will Power Needed. VSED requires significant will power and determination to hasten one's death. It works best for those who can control the urge to drink despite a physiological drive to do so. Patients also need support from caregivers, especially as they get weaker in the late stages.

Delirium and Incapacity Likely in Late Stages. Some patients become delirious and lose decision-making capacity late in the VSED process. They may then lose the discipline and commitment not to drink in the face of severe thirst. While the patient still has capacity, an approach should be identified (and ideally recorded) regarding how family and caregivers ought to respond to verbal or other apparent non-verbal requests for fluids. *N.B. Before initiating VSED, all patients should articulate how they want caregivers* *to respond if they lose decision-making capacity and subsequently express a desire to resume eating and drinking. Guidance for anticipating and responding to these potential challenges is explored in Part II.*

Committed Caregivers Required. VSED requires committed caregivers to assist in the process as patients inevitably get very weak, debilitated, and potentially confused in the later stages of the process. These caregivers must be fully informed about the process and committed to carrying it through to completion according to the patient's pre-stated wishes. Backup caregivers may be required if the initial caregivers are not able to provide ongoing support.

Patient Distress from Knowing about the Possibility of a Hastened Death. Some patients who fear not getting adequate medical treatment may become distressed by discussions of VSED and other options for hastening death, fearing that these options reflect clinicians' lack of commitment to extending life by offering all possible life-prolonging treatments.

Closing Window of Opportunity. Because VSED requires decision-making capacity, patients who fear losing the requisite capacity may have to act preemptively while they are still finding their lives meaningful. *N.B. In Part II, we discuss Stopping Eating and Drinking by Advance Directive (SED by AD) as an important alternative to VSED that can potentially circumvent this obstacle.*

Risk-Averse Caregivers. To be permissible, VSED does not require any changes in the law, but some professional and family caregivers are risk-averse. While explicit direct permission is legally not necessary, it might help these caregivers feel comfortable enough to provide support. Similarly, few health care facilities have policies and procedures on VSED. Development of such policies would also help provide clarity and guidance to caregivers unfamiliar with VSED.

6.3. Opportunities

Informing About the Possibility of VSED. Patients and families who are interested in a wide[r] range of end-of-life options for hastening death should be made aware of the possibility of VSED.

More Available than MAID. VSED is an especially important option for patients who, while they might prefer a more direct form of assisted dying like MAID, live in jurisdictions where such an option is not legally available.

More Flexible than MAID. Even where MAID is legally available, some patients who are seriously ill and ready for death *now* may have a prognosis that is too uncertain for them to qualify (e.g., terminal illness). They may welcome VSED as an option.

Sometimes Preferred Over MAID. Even where other death-hastening options are legally available, VSED might be preferable to patients, clinicians, or institutions: (1) who morally object to other, more direct death-hastening methods, (2) who find the certification and delay requirements of these other methods unacceptable, or (3) who prefer the flexibility and reversibility of VSED.

Often Faster than MAID. Patients can begin VSED at any time. In contrast, MAID usually imposes waiting periods of 15 days or sometimes more. Getting the required multiple clinician assessments for MAID medication access may take even longer.

Patient-Initiated and Driven. Although clinicians and others are strongly recommended for support, the decision to initiate and carry through with VSED is almost exclusively patient driven, provided they are made aware of the option and have other caregiving support. VSED fits the paradigm of patient control in end-of-life options.

Comforted by the Option. Even when the VSED option is not taken, patients can be comforted by knowing about its availability and their right to control the timing of death.

In sum, VSED provides an opportunity to achieve a relatively peaceful, personally controlled death for patients seeking an escape from the prospect of unacceptable suffering or deterioration in their present condition or foreseeable future. VSED, however, requires that the patient has decision-making capacity. How should caregivers respond when a patient who has started VSED becomes confused late in the process and requests something to eat or drink? What about patients who do not want to hasten their death in any way until *after* they lose capacity? We turn next, in the second half of the book, to explore stopping eating and drinking by advance directive (SED by AD) for patients who have lost decision-making capacity.

PART II

STOPPING EATING AND DRINKING BY ADVANCE DIRECTIVE (SED BY AD) FOR PERSONS WITHOUT DECISION-MAKING CAPACITY

Part II of this book considers stopping eating and drinking by advance directive (SED by AD), where assistance with eating and drinking is limited or withheld after a seriously ill person has lost decision-making capacity to make major life and death decisions. Limiting or withholding food and drink is based on the person's having clearly specified this action in an advance directive.

Part II is divided into six chapters:

Chapter 7. Illustrative Cases, each followed by the editors' views of their most notable characteristics and issues raised that will be followed up from different professional perspectives in the subsequent five chapters.

Chapter 8. Clinical Issues, including whether the withholding of all food and fluids or providing "comfort feeding only" should pertain only to assisted feeding as compared to self-feeding; strategies for making future feeding wishes clear in an advance directive; managing symptoms upon the directive's implementation; and the advantages/disadvantages of such advance directives.

Chapter 9. Ethical Issues, including the potential that the incapacitated patient might have had a change of mind, whether feeding is fundamentally different from other interventions, the extent of caregiver burdens and distress, and the acceptability and potential precedent-setting role of comfort feeding only.

Chapter 10. Legal Issues, including the ability to make valid prior requests to withhold assistance with eating and drinking through statute-based advance directives, other types of directives, "Ulysses contracts," videos, and health care agents.

Chapter 11. Institutional Issues, including those raised by the fact that dementia is common in these settings; worry about prolonged nature of dying with dementia is prevalent; withholding food and fluids is not addressed in most advance directives; and not eating and drinking is hard to initiate in long-term care settings.

Chapter 12. Best Practices, Enduring Challenges, and Opportunities for SED by AD, including a summary of bottom-line points from the previous five chapters and an assessment of SED by AD's future place in end-of-life care.

7

Illustrative Cases

The editors have assembled four previously unpublished cases that illustrate the attractions and challenges of using advance directives to guide the possibility of surrogates assisting in the hastening of death by stopping eating and drinking at a later time of patient incapacity. The cases have different authors, some of whom are not one of the volume's editors. At the end of each case, the editors have added what they view as some of the notable characteristics of the case and the issues raised by it.

Case 7.1—Mrs. H. (Early Alzheimer's): Speculation about the Challenge of Waiting

Living Too Long or Dying Too Soon (continued reflections on Case 1.3 in Chapter 1)

Robert K. Horowitz

During the years after informing my mother about VSED, I vacillated between relief and grief. My relief mirrored hers; we both saw VSED as an escape if Mom's "nightmare" of dementia were ever to materialize. VSED transformed the suffocating cave of dementia into a tunnel; it could provide a way through the darkness, and out the other side. Knowing this, she was able to live with more vigor and hope.

My grief was more complicated. It was grounded in part by the recognition that, because she learned about VSED through me, Mom's potential implementation of it would make me an agent in her death. But the real anguish came after she was actually diagnosed with early dementia, converting VSED from abstraction to reality, and forcing our confrontation with dementia's "closing window" of cognition.

The decisional calculus—not whether, but when to enact VSED—was staggering, because, devastating though it was, the dementia diagnosis alone did not inform Mom's decision to die. Rather, it marked the beginning of our struggle to discern when her accumulating losses became unbearable enough, before undermining her capacity to implement VSED. If she waited too long—that is, if she chose to defer VSED and keep living too long— she would lose the capability to "successfully" carry it out. The resultant fear of missing the closing window could conceivably accelerate her decision to die before she was ready. And yet the desire to keep living could risk postponing that decision past her ability to see it through. Hence, the dueling fears of living too long or dying too soon.

Further, since dementia obscures its recognition, Mom would become progressively less able to reconcile the competing wishes to keep living and to prevent her identity's dissolution by dementia. This job fell to me and my siblings. Gratefully, our load would be eased by a trusted physician colleague who could offer a more objective view. He would meet with Mom three times over a few months to explore her hopes, fears, and preferences, and to assess her decisional and functional capacity. I was profoundly relieved when he emerged from their first session and announced, "Your mother is serious about VSED, but not ready." I was also apprehensive, wondering how long Mom had before surrendering the VSED option to dementia's advance.

This possibility was brought to life by one of my palliative care patients. "M" was my mother's age, and living with dementia unhappily in a nursing home. She had been admitted to the hospital with a heart abnormality that was expected to kill her within days unless she had a pacemaker inserted. But M was actually pleased by her short prognosis, and she rejected the pacemaker. To her surprise, she lived on, disappointed by her heart's resilience.

M was familiar with VSED, and interested in using it as her way to die. With her family's backing, she asked for consultation with my palliative care team. She had clear decisional capacity to choose to die by VSED, although we wondered whether she would have sufficient cognition to see it through. After lengthy deliberations we agreed to support her decision, with plans to offer prompts if she lost track. We also were explicit that we would not deny her food and fluid if she expressed a persistent interest despite our reminders.

As it turned out, every morning M forgot her plan, and we responded with the promised prompts, but she vetoed them and demanded breakfast and coffee, which we provided. Later each day she somberly recognized her morning lapse and declared an invigorated commitment to never eat or drink again. However, day after day, her habits and drive to eat and drink overrode her fading cognition, and ultimately she was discharged back to the nursing home. M's cognitive window had closed, dementia the victor.

M's story loomed ever larger in my mind as Mom's losses mounted. The "closing window" became a frequent refrain in our discussions. Mom was famously risk-averse, so it was natural that in the midst of her multiplying worries about losing the VSED option, she requested a second visit from the physician. Remarkably, despite her anxiety about deferring too long, she continued to adapt to her losses better than she or we had imagined possible. The physician emerged from their second session to announce, "She has some more living to do."

This time my relief was clouded by fear. I was scared by Mom's delay, which threatened a recapitulation of M's excruciating dilemma. And I felt torn. Whose wishes was I bound to honor? Those of the pre-dementia Mom, who with furious intentionality would never have sanctioned her current condition, let alone its continued progression? Or those of the fading Mom before me, who had adapted to her losses, and whose deferment seemed to announce, "I'd rather be alive like this awhile longer than dead forever."

Over the subsequent weeks, I offered Mom both wholehearted validation of her desire to enjoy the modest pleasures that remained in her life, and rational encouragement to proceed with VSED while she could. In one of our surreal deliberations she asked that I promise to deny her food and drink once she commenced VSED, even if she begged. I was repelled by this image, and I firmly rejected her request. She looked surprised, and I think hurt. I softened, and assured her I would offer reminders of her decision, but I would not—I could not—withhold food or drink if she wanted either, let alone if she begged. I suspect in this moment came Mom's recognition that her window was about to close.

She requested a third meeting with the physician. It was shorter than the others. This time he emerged to announce, "Your Mom is serious about VSED. And she's ready." I cried with relief and grief. The prospect was real now.

Mom was giddy from that meeting forward, relieved by her decision and the protection it promised from the horror which had loomed for decades. She did not need any reminders during her nine days of VSED. But once, nearly a week in, she felt "parched" and asked me if she could "sneak" a sip of water. As agreed, I told her yes, she could, but even a sip might prolong her life, and her dying. I assured her, "I'm okay with that, Mom," my heart aching with hope and fear that she might drink. She paused, looked into my moist eyes, and smiled, "That's all right, Robby. I'll be okay without it." And she was okay. And serene, poised, gracious, and comfortable until she died three days later. It had been nearly four months since her first physician visit to discuss VSED.

A few weeks afterward, the pathologist escorted me into his office to review Mom's brain biopsy. He informed me solemnly, "Your mother did the right thing." He told me his own mother had advanced dementia, and she was miserable. "She doesn't know me anymore," he said. "I only wish she could have known what your mother did, and acted while she could." As we sat at the microscope, he showed me Mom's neurons, littered with plaques and tangles. I wondered which of them might have held a shared memory, lost. "Alzheimer's," he declared, "for sure." I was relieved by the certainty of the diagnosis. And proud of Mom, now vindicated for knowing and acting when she did. Mixed with relief and grief, I felt amazed by my mother, who consciously, wisely, and courageously confronted her most fearsome adversary, and beat it down.

Notable Characteristics

- Emerging dementia obscured Mrs. H.'s ability to recognize when to initiate VSED—not too soon, not too late. When the job of discerning that time fell to her son and his siblings, they called on a trusted physician to offer a more objective view of when Mrs. H. was ready. He met with her three times to do that. The reports after his first two visits—that she still had "more living to do"—created both relief and fear.
- In anticipation of starting VSED soon, Mr. H. asked her son to promise that once she had begun VSED, he would deny her food and drink even if she begged for it. He firmly rejected her request ("I could not . . . "); he would only remind her of her decision.
- Once VSED started, Mrs. H. did not need reminders. At one point she asked if she could "sneak" a sip of water; she could, her son said, noting that even a sip might prolong her dying but adding, "I'm okay with that, Mom." She replied, " . . . I'll be okay without it." In fact, she was, and she died serene and comfortable three days later.
- Subsequent brain biopsy confirmed advanced Alzheimer's.

Issues Raised

- How many patients pursuing preemptive VSED to avoid living into severe dementia have access to a physician who can visit them to discern when they are "ready"? How many patients with such intentions miss their window of decisiveness?
- Should society permit arrangements for SED by AD, arrangements that could theoretically avoid many of the difficult dilemmas between "dying too early or living too long"?
- Should the son have accepted his mother's request to promise that he would withhold food and drink if she later wanted it? Was he ethically correct is responding, "I could not [do that]"? Should she have written a directive that her later entreaties be refused?
- In what other ways than reminding a patient of her decision can caregivers respond to a request for food and drink while still honoring the VSED plan?
- How would these issues play out in a family where communication was not nearly so open? What can caregivers do to foster helpful communication?

Case 7.2.—Steve (Early Dementia): Patient and Family Challenges

"I've always been a little forgetful"

Judith K. Schwarz

Steve always cared passionately about "death with dignity" and his right to die in a manner consistent with his personal values. This was one of the things he and Jennifer (his second wife) had in common when they first met and married almost 20 years ago. Now 79 years of age and still physically sturdy, he had begun to experience increasing difficulties with his short-term memory and ability to speak cogently about his concerns. His son wasn't surprised when Steve told him he had begun to draft a new directive regarding his current end-of-life wishes and concerns. Steve had completed a "5 Wishes" values statement and tried to explain how his son would "know when to do something to end my life if I have dementia." This was rather concerning for his son, who asked his father to explain what he meant by such a statement. Steve was unable to articulate more detail about his wishes and expectations other than to repeat what he had requested of his son.

Both this son and his wife knew that Steve had recently seen a neurologist who did a thorough evaluation and informed Steve that he had mild cognitive impairment (MCI), the earliest stage of Alzheimer's disease. Steve firmly rejected that diagnosis and assured the neurologist that he had always been a little forgetful, likening it to being an "absent-minded professor." Steve shared this view with his family.

Jennifer began attending several Alzheimer support groups and reported they helped her enormously. She felt less angry at Steve as she learned more about Alzheimer's disease and his disease-related behavior. Sharing common experiences with other caregivers was also comforting and supportive for her.

At this early stage, Steve's two sons did not confront their father with their awareness of his diagnosis. Because they were unable to visit him more than two or three times a month, they were unaware of the daily challenges that Jennifer experienced as Steve's "forgetfulness" increased. Steve has two additional daughters from his first marriage who live in the Midwest; they have a strained relationship with Jennifer. They were unable to visit more than twice a year due to family and professional obligations, but they spoke with him several times a month by phone.

Jennifer learned about the consultation program I lead at End of Life Choices NY that focuses on increasing end-of-life options for those with cognitive impairment. She and I began to speak regularly by phone regarding her concerns about how she could implement Steve's choices if and when he lost decision-making capacity in the future. He had two great fears—developing dementia and experiencing pain.

I invited Jennifer to bring Steve in for a face-to-face meeting. My primary purpose was to try and understand more about what Steve expected his family to do in the event he was "ever" diagnosed with Alzheimer's or another terminal illness. Before this meeting took place, I agreed with Jennifer's request that we discuss dementia as a fearful but *future* possibility, and not a current reality.

Steve was unable to expand on his 5 Wishes statement that someone "should just end my life at an appropriate time." In addition to the vagueness of his overall request, Steve seemed unaware of the limitations imposed by the absence of any kind of medical aid in dying (MAID) legislation in our state. Furthermore, even if he lived in a state with legal access to MAID, he would not qualify because he would be either not terminally ill, or, if he progressed far enough to be deemed terminally ill, he would not be decisionally capable of making a real-time request for MAID. I also told him that anyone who directly assisted him in "ending his life" would assume great legal jeopardy. Steve did not want to put his family at risk.

I encouraged Steve to write down his thoughts about future quality of life issues and the circumstances under which his life would no longer be worth living. This was a difficult assignment for him, but he began to think about the things that currently provide him pleasure. In addition to closely following his much-loved Yankees, he enjoyed gardening, met regularly with a group of male friends, read newspapers, and watched TV. I suggested that he and Jennifer explore the Functional Assessment Staging Test for Alzheimer's disease (FAST—see Table 8.1 in Chapter 8) *in case* he developed dementia. I hoped he might be able to incorporate his thoughts about a particular stage of cognitive and physical decline into an advance directive.

Because he had always been quite healthy, Steve was not taking any life-prolonging medications nor was he dependent upon any treatments that could legally be stopped to hasten his death. The only legal option in New York to hasten dying in his current situation was to stop all oral intake. We discussed the possibility of completing a written directive that would stipulate when oral intake should be limited as a means to hasten dying should he lose decision-making capacity in the future due to dementia. Following some research about the FAST stages of dementia, Steve decided that he would want all oral intake withheld at Stage 6 of the FAST scale. He was adamant that he did not want to have to endure the increasing deterioration associated with the "terminal" (Stage 7) of the disease. It seemed important to arrange a family meeting that would include his four adult children, so he could explain to them in person the choice he made about limiting oral intake in the future.

The meeting was very emotional. Steve told his family about his fears of losing his autonomy and independence and explained that he had given a great deal of thought to his plan. He asked them to respect and support his plan, part of which was to stay at home if and when he ever developed advanced Alzheimer's disease. (He was adamant about never being placed in a nursing home.) He instructed his family to withhold all oral intake from him should he lose capacity in the hope of speeding death by dehydration. He wanted to receive good pain management so he would not suffer, and he specifically instructed his family to simply ignore any requests for food or fluids he might make once oral intake was stopped. He did not want to consider how difficult it would be to pick an actual moment to start the process of fasting once he lost capacity and could no longer participate in reflective decision-making. His daughters began to sob, and his sons and wife looked worried.

I described the option of comfort-focused feeding as another approach to hastening death under circumstances of advanced dementia. Steve rejected that option because he believed it would prolong his dying. He seemed unconcerned about any difficulties his family might experience in their attempt to honor his request that all food and fluids be stopped under those circumstances. His wife, who would be the primary caregiver, said little during the meeting but seemed concerned.

I have continued to meet annually with Steve, Jennifer, and the two sons for three years now. The daughters join our meetings by speaker phone, and I speak often to Jennifer by phone. The question of Steve's decision-making capacity looms large, although he seems currently capable and able to describe his values and wishes regarding his end of life. The approach Steve wants to follow at the very end of his life seems consistent with his long-held values, and he has not wavered in what he wants, despite the burden it will likely place on his wife and family.

In subsequent conversations I have had with Jennifer, she has reiterated her commitment to try to honor Steve's choice to hasten his death by fasting. She is aware of the importance of arranging for good palliative symptom management for Steve while he fasts. She is concerned about how she can ensure that he receives palliative care in their home. In particular, she hopes to obtain sufficient sedating medications, so Steve doesn't suffer and she will be better able to manage his physical care. I am unsure whether that is a realistic expectation given the current challenges of securing home palliative care.

Steve's primary care physician is trained in both geriatrics and palliative care. He received a copy of the dementia directive that Steve signed, indicating his decision to stop all oral intake if he ever reaches Stage 6 of advanced dementia, but they have never had a direct conversation about the topic. The directive stipulates that the patient's appointed health care agent, Jennifer, together with the primary care physician would implement his decision to stop oral feedings once Steve could no longer feed himself, had lost decision-making capacity, and was in an advanced stage of dementia. Presumably, this physician would provide palliative medical oversight for Steve at that time. As of now, I am unsure how aware this physician is of the role that Steve and his family hope he will assume if Steve ever develops advanced dementia. Clearly, this topic should be explored in advance of implementation with his primary treating physician. Three years after the initial diagnosis of MCI, Steve continues to resist accepting that diagnosis. This is an ongoing case and I am not at all clear about how it will play out.

Notable Characteristics

- Despite resisting his diagnosis of mild cognitive impairment (MCI), Steve is clear about what he wants to have happen were he to reach an advanced stage of dementia: stop all oral intake sometime in Stage 6, when he can no longer feed himself. He has written his AD to that effect and expects it to be carried out by wife Jennifer and his primary physician.
- Jennifer arranged for family discussions with Steve, facilitated by an experienced consulting nurse. Some of these exchanges have been very emotional. Steve is adamant that he never be placed in a nursing home and that, in carrying out his directive, his family must ignore any requests for food or fluid he might make once oral intake is stopped. He shows little concern for difficulties his family might experience in attempting to honor his requests.
- Comfort-oriented feeding was suggested as an alternative. Steve rejected it because it would unduly prolong his dying.
- Three years after his initial diagnosis with MCI, Steve continues to resist any explicit dementia diagnosis. At the same time, he has not wavered in his insistence about what should happen if he does become severely demented. The case is ongoing.

Issues Raised

- Should Steve reasonably expect his family and primary care physician to carry out his directive to halt oral intake of food and fluid at FAST Stage 6? Is he underestimating the difficulties they will likely confront?
- Will palliative care and/or hospice support be available for him *at home* after his oral intake is withheld?
- Does Steve's continuing resistance to the dementia diagnosis call into question how competent and clear-headed he is in writing his AD for SED?

Case 7.3.—Patricia (Moderate Dementia): Hastening Death by SED versus Preemptive Suicide

"I used to be smart!"

Judith K. Schwarz

Patricia was a 91-year-old retired professor and a nationally recognized expert in her field who had been the chair of her department for many years at a large university on the east coast of the United States. One of the first things she said during our initial conversation was, "I used to be really smart." She told me she was diagnosed with Alzheimer's disease about five years earlier by a neurologist following clinical examination and imaging. She also said she was very afraid of "becoming a cabbage" and dying slowly and miserably of this disease as her two older sisters had. She recently moved from her university-provided housing into a high-end continuous care facility in another part of the city. She said she hoped to find a new community of "like-minded academics" with whom she could develop relationships, but that had not occurred. She was not able to make new friends because her short-term memory deficit had become an increasing social barrier that was difficult to work around. In addition, she now suffered from "face blindness," and thus, when she dined with other residents in the communal dining room, she was unable to remember with whom she had spoken, what was discussed, or even who they were. We agreed to meet.

We met in her pleasant one-bedroom apartment with her niece Donna, who took notes of our conversation. Donna lived nearby and visited regularly to help with a wide array of personal care tasks. Patricia said her memory had really begun to deteriorate about a year ago. She wanted to be in charge of her dying and hoped to take steps to do so before she became cognitively incapable of completing the task. I explained the VSED process to them in detail because it was the only legally accepted option recognized in the state. They wanted me to repeat this description by phone to her health care agent, a nephew, who was a retired physician and lived in the South. I agreed to do so.

Patricia had a number of concerns about the VSED process. She was particularly fearful about the possibility of suffering once she realized she might have to fast for two weeks or more before dying of dehydration. She made it clear that she did *not* want to experience any pain or suffering during the dying process. She told me that, years ago, she had acquired a lethal amount of barbiturates that she kept in her refrigerator. I told her that taking that medication might put her family at legal risk if they were present and helped in any way. All deaths that occur outside of hospice oversight are investigated by the police in that jurisdiction. After I left her apartment, I wondered how much she would remember of this very fraught discussion. I called her the next day and asked her to describe what she remembered. I was relieved to learn that her recall seemed comprehensive. We entered into a relationship that consisted of frequent phone calls, email exchanges, and family meetings in her apartment and the facility dining room with members of her extended family. The relationship was warm and endured for almost nine months.

Because her memory and executive function were rapidly deteriorating, I suggested she also complete a written directive that would limit future assisted hand-feeding if her dementia became advanced and she lost the ability to make decisions or self-feed. Both she and her family members were supportive of this idea. She said she particularly liked the idea of comfort-focused feeding, as she so enjoyed eating, and she made that option her preferred choice. Her family explored the facility's rules about hospice en-rollment. I informed Patricia and her family that if she chose to VSED, she would need access to hospice medical oversight to ensure that any symptoms of suffering associated with fasting were aggressively managed. Some prelim-inary discussions were begun with the medical director of one of the local hospices about obtaining palliative support in the event she chose to begin to VSED.

Patricia continued her independent life—including taking public trans-portation to visit old friends or attend musical performances in the city (much to her family's distress, as she frequently got lost, misplaced her purse, and lost cash and credit cards). She had "good" days and "bad," but inexo-rably, the bad days began to outnumber the good. Still she retained decision-making capacity and continued her vigorous pursuit of life's pleasures, while remaining resolute in her desire to control the timing of her death.

Several months before she died, she asked me to come to her apartment to meet with her and her niece Donna, as she had something important to dis-cuss. When we assembled, she told me she had given a great deal of thought to her decision about the manner of her death, and had come to the con-clusion that she simply would not be able to fast unto death. She said she enjoyed eating and drinking too much to give it up. Indeed, enjoying a meal and sharing a bottle of wine with her family or other old friends remained a source of great joy. Plus, she had a very hearty appetite. She decided that she would use the accumulated barbiturates to end her life at some point in the future. With that decision made, she continued to live her life fully for several more months until she recognized that her decision-making ability was waning and her "window of opportunity" was about to close.

She knew that no one could be present when she drank down the lethal drugs. Even with very specific written instructions and other assistance provided by her family, it was not clear to any of us that she would be successful in following the necessary steps when she was alone. She chose a day of the week when her regular cleaning person was expected the following morning. If she didn't answer the door, management would arrive with a key and then find her. We all held our breath and waited. Her family was called the next morning by the management and was told that she had died and that the police were present. The family was able to indicate that, while they were "shocked," they were "not surprised." Her memorial was attended by many old friends and members of her extended family who laughed a lot and cried a bit. They told wonderful stories of this indomitable woman who had lived her life fully, and died on her own terms and at a time that she chose.

Notable Characteristics

- At 91, Patricia had already been in Stage 4 of Alzheimer's Disease for five years. Her hope to find a like-minded community of academics in a high-end continuous care facility was disappointed as her growing short-term memory deficit inhibited social interaction. She was now determined to be in charge of her dying.
- VSED was daunting to Patricia, however, both from the suffering she envisioned it would involve and from the recognition that she had always greatly enjoyed eating and drinking. Meanwhile she had previously acquired a stash of barbiturates for potential use in an intentional overdose. She understood that her family could not be present when she swallowed them, as that would potentially put them in legal jeopardy. There was some anxiety that she might not remember all the necessary steps and precautions.
- Patricia eventually determined that for her, taking a lethal dose of barbiturates was the preferred way to control her dying. Aware that her decision-making ability was waning and that her window of opportunity would soon close, she acted, carefully and effectively, without her family present. When her family and friends found out what she had

done, they were "shocked" but "not surprised." Her memorial, attended by many, was rich with positive memories.

Issues Raised

- VSED is "not for everyone." When VSED is not an option because decision-making capacity has been lost and there is no clear AD to guide SED on behalf of the now incapacitated person, what other "last-resort" options might be considered? Clearly all non-comfort-oriented, potentially life-prolonging treatments should be stopped if there is any evidence that the patient would not want such treatment, and all uncomfortable symptoms should be aggressively managed. Proportionate palliative sedation should be considered to treat all physically or psychologically painful symptoms. MAID (defined as clinician prescribed, patient self-administered lethal medication) could be considered depending on its legal status where the patient lives, but would not be an option as defined once decision-making capacity is lost. Euthanasia by advance directive is a possibility in a few Western European countries, but otherwise is generally prohibited.
- Should society provide alternative avenues, such as SED by AD, for those who like Patricia are determined to control death but unwilling to use preemptive VSED?
- How should persons who are accumulating sufficient drugs for a lethal overdose in an environment where MAID is prohibited be counseled about effective doses and self-administration strategies?

Case 7.4.—Charles (Severe Dementia): Refusing Assistance with Oral Feeding

Conflict over Patient Best Interest

Stanley A. Terman

In 2009, Charles was diagnosed with early-stage dementia, probable Alzheimer's type. He and his wife—also his proxy/agent—knew that many advanced dementia patients face this challenge: They have "no plug to pull"; that is, they do not depend on high-tech medical treatment to sustain their lives. Assistance with hand-feeding and hand-hydrating can prolong dying, sometimes for years. Both Charles and his wife dreaded that prospect.

Charles wanted to complete an advance instructional directive that could effectively answer two questions: *when* (for what specific conditions) would he want to implement *what* (an intervention to stop others' assistance with hand-feeding and hand-hydrating). His wife had read a book I authored that offered one possibility (Terman 2007). She contacted me through my psychiatric practice.

Charles completed a patient decision aid that described four dozen conditions of patients with advanced dementia and other terminal illnesses (Terman 2020). For patients who could no longer eat and drink independently due to irreversible cognitive impairment, the format was: "If I reach a condition that causes *severe enough suffering*,[1] **then** I want others to stop assistance with putting food and fluid in my mouth." For each condition, Charles made an advance treatment decision between two alternatives: Either allow him to live by continuing assistance with feeding and hydrating, or allow him to die by foregoing all assistance with food and fluids. His completed advance instructional directive could someday inform physicians and others about when he considered dying timely based on his personal values.

As his advance care planning counselor, I conducted two telephone interviews two weeks apart. The interviews had three purposes: (1) to affirm Charles was sure about each life-determining decision. As a psychiatrist, I would not accept merely checking a box as adequate to reveal Charles' thinking. (2) to assess Charles' mental capacity to make these decisions. And (3) to record Charles' oral testimony on audio in the event a dispute arose later.

I began the interview by informing Charles what it was like to die from medical dehydration. Some patients are hungry for a day or two, but this moderate discomfort can usually be relieved by medications. Almost all patients need extra comfort care to reduce the symptom of thirst, for which over-the-counter aids are usually effective. All patients fall into a deep sleep eventually, although the number of days until this happens varies. Other symptoms that occur can usually be addressed with standard symptom-directed palliative treatments.

I concluded that Charles understood the two treatment options for each condition of advanced dementia and appreciated their consequences.

---

[1] For the various conditions the patient is queried about, the decision aid requires fulfilling the criterion "severe enough suffering" to forego all food and fluid.

Charles also answered another question I posed in both interviews: "Are you willing to endure whatever discomfort medical dehydration might cause, in order to die when you want?" His responses were clear, consistent between the two sessions, and stated strongly. Basically, he said: "Yes, I'm willing to suffer for several days if I can avoid years of dying with suffering and burdening others."

Charles used logical reasoning to arrive at a decision for each condition. He explained, for example, why he did not want to depend on others to change his diapers and why he did not want to burden family members with making sacrifices to provide him total care after he had lost the ability to recognize them.

I concluded that Charles possessed capacity to give his informed, advance conditional consent. I wrote this opinion and sent it to Charles and his wife, along with his printed advance instructional directive that displayed his decisions for each condition, and the audio CD recording of our interview.

Conflict Over Implementing the Plan

Seven years later, Charles met criteria for advanced-stage dementia, including having lost the ability to self-feed and self-drink. He also met specific clinical criteria for more than one condition for which he previously had decided he wanted help with hand-feeding and hand-hydrating to stop. His wife helped arranged his admission to a local inpatient hospice.

Conflict emerged when Charles' wife showed the attending physician his directive and asked him to honor his wish to die by medical dehydration. The physician initially refused, explaining that it was in Charles' "best interest" to continue "comfort feeding only" (Palecek et al. 2010). According to the wife, his approximate words were: "Medical dehydration would cause Charles great discomfort as it destroys his internal organs." The physician justified overriding Charles' prospective autonomy by stating he needed to prioritize the ethical principle, "Do No Harm."

Resolving the Conflict

At this point Charles' wife called me for advice. I recommended she meet with Charles' physician and bring (1) a printed copy of his advance directive, (2) the

CD of his recorded oral testimony, (3) my written psychiatric opinion that Charles had possessed decision-making capacity, (4) a copy of an article that revealed hospice nurses judged the dying of alert patients via medical dehydration to be "good" and "peaceful" (Ganzini et al. 2003), and (5) an invitation to discuss Charles' treatment options with me by phone. I also encouraged her to state she had heard Charles repeatedly express his wish to be allowed to die if he reached certain conditions of advanced dementia even if medical dehydration caused discomfort, which he consistently explained: he valued a timely dying as more important than some temporary discomfort.

Two days later, the treating physician acquiesced by stating, "If this is really what Charles wants, okay."

Charles died peacefully after a fast of nine days. According to his wife, he experienced no uncomfortable or complicating side effects as he died from medical dehydration.

His wife and I discussed how the effort Charles had made years before by completing advance care planning had apparently served him well. At that time, his capacity had been sufficient to make advance treatment decisions. His cognitive functioning subsequently continued to deteriorate. Thus, there were no further opportunities to revisit his decisions. Yet, having two interviews that were consistent, which I noted in his chart and recorded on audio, made his treatment refusal convincing. His clarity regarding his willingness to endure moderate discomfort from medical dehydration in the short term, paired with his abhorrence to a prolonged dying while living with some conditions of advanced dementia, likely seemed compelling to his last treating physician.

Looking Back

Subsequently Charles' wife and I had a debriefing telephone conference about what factors may have led the treating physician to reverse his position and honor Charles' directive. She reported that the treating physician read the directive and saw, but did not listen to, the CD. I revealed that his physician did not call me to discuss the options. While the physician had by now seen Charles die peacefully by medical dehydration, it was not clear what factors had led him to change from his original position.

To speculate, some of these factors may have had an impact: (1) the consistency and certainty with which the proxy/agent and advance instructional directive stated that Charles wanted to be allowed to die if he reached his current conditions; (2) wanting to avoid direct confrontation with me since I likely had more experience in this area; (3) reduced fear of a lawsuit based on the totality of the presented arguments; and (4) pointing out that the law in his state grants physicians immunity for relying on the directive's and proxy/agent's instructions, as long as physicians act in good faith. Therefore, he had both an ethical imperative and low to no legal risk.

Notable Characteristics

- This is one of the few documented cases of successful implementation of an AD for SED.
- Charles developed his AD by responding to a lengthy series of choices for various conditions in severe dementia, between continuing manually assisted feeding and completely withholding food and fluid. Charles' capacity to make these choices and his understanding of them were verified in recorded telephone interviews with his advance care planning counselor and psychiatrist. He was clearly informed about what it would be like to die from dehydration if good palliative support were provided.
- Years later, the stated conditions of Charles' directive having been met, his wife asked the attending physician to honor his directive. The physician initially refused, alleging that this "would cause Charles great discomfort as it destroys his internal organs" and that it would be in Charles' best interest to continue "comfort feeding only." After being presented with a copy of the AD, the recording of Charles' testimony, several other documents, and the willingness of the psychiatrist to be consulted, the physician acquiesced in the decision to follow Charles' directive.

Issues Raised

- When an AD for SED is not as detailed as Charles' was in the way it speaks specifically to severe dementia and withholding food and fluid, and there is no audio recording of the patient's testimony to supplement the directive, will caregivers be as willing as they were with Charles to implement the directive as professionally, ethically, and legally permissible?

- The detailed conditions for which Charles made the choices that constituted his directive were presented to him by asking when a condition would cause him "severe enough suffering" to stop assisted feeding. Is sufficient *suffering*, however, the right category of reason why many patients want not to have their lives extend into years of severe dementia? Should we trust Charles' responses if he thought the choice for each condition concerned degree of suffering, when perhaps the issue is that when the time he has stipulated for withholding assisted feeding arrives, he will be only severely deteriorated and not suffering?
- When Charles would say, for a given condition, that he preferred to "continue the feeding," did he mean at the level of comfort-oriented feeding or at a higher level of feeding adequate for longer term survival?
- When an AD is as specific and its qualifying conditions are as clearly met as they were in Charles' case, and when the patient is not asking for any food or fluids that his AD says should be withheld, should clinicians see following the directive as "standard of care"?

The chapters that follow pursue in depth the clinical, ethical, legal, and institutional aspects of using ADs for SED, independent of the particular cases presented above. They will at many points, however, refer to these cases.

References

Ganzini, Linda, Elizabeth R. Goy, Lois L. Miller, Theresa A. Harvath, Ann Jackson, and Molly A. Delorit. 2003. "Nurses' Experiences with Hospice Patients Who Refuse Food and Fluids to Hasten Death." *New England Journal of Medicine* 349, no. 4 (July): 359–365.
Palecek Eric J., Joan M. Teno, David J. Casarett, Laura C. Hanson, Ramona L. Rhodes, Susan L. Mitchell. 2010. "Comfort Feeding Only: A Proposal to Bring Clarity to Decision-making Regarding Difficulty with Eating for Persons with Advanced Dementia." *Journal of the American Geriatric Society* 58: 580–584.
Terman, Stanley A. 2020. *My Way Cards* © 2009–2020. Carlsbad, CA: Life Transitions Publications.
Terman, Stanley A. 2007. *The Best Way to Say Goodbye: A Legal Peaceful Choice at the End of Life*. Carlsbad, CA: Life Transitions Publications.

8

Clinical Issues

Timothy E. Quill and Judith K. Schwarz

Imagine yourself in the shoes of Mrs. H., our patient with early Alzheimer's disease, who has mild cognitive impairment but is still enjoying herself and having meaningful time with family and friends. Although she would like to live as long as this level of enjoyment continues, she fears that if she waits too long she may lose the cognitive capacity to carry out VSED, and become trapped in a terminal phase of her dementing illness without means of escape. She views VSED as her "safety valve" to avoid living into the late stages of the disease, which she imagines would clearly be worse than an earlier death. Does she have to initiate VSED before she really wants to? Or could she empower others to initiate SED on her behalf once she clearly loses the capacity carry it out on her own and is actually in the condition that she is trying to avoid?

8.1. General Approach When Capacity Is Lost

How should clinicians respond to this dilemma faced by Mrs. H. and so many others who want to avoid the late stages of their illnesses, in part because they will likely lose decision-making capacity before death? One of the first steps in this process is to "stage" the patient's degree of cognitive impairment according to one or both of the commonly used scales (Dementia Care Central 2020; Medical Care Corporation 2020; Reisberg 1996; Sclan 1992):

- Global Deterioration Scale for Assessment of Primary Degenerative Dementia (GDS)
- Functional Assessment Staging Test (FAST)

These widely employed and well-validated scales use the symptoms and functional abilities that the person is experiencing to predict their prognosis as well as to gauge their abilities to participate in medical decision-making. (See Table 8.1 for more details.) Patients like Mrs. H. in early stages

Table 8.1 Stages of Progressive Dementia and Stopping Eating and Drinking Options

Global Deterioration Scale for Assessing Primary Degenerative Dementia (GDS)	Functional Assessment Staging Test (FAST)	Stopping Eating and Drinking Option
Stage 1. No Cognitive Decline. Stage 2. Very Mild Cognitive Decline (no dementia). Forgets names. Misplaces familiar objects. Symptoms not evident to loved ones or doctors. Stage 3. Mild Cognitive Decline (no dementia). Increased forgetfulness. Slight difficulty concentrating. Gets lost more frequently. Difficulty finding right words. Loved ones begin to notice. *Average duration: 2–7 years*	Stage 1. Normal Adult. Stage 2. Normal Older Adult. Personal awareness of some functional decline. Stage 3. Early Alzheimer's. Noticeable deficits in demanding job situations. *Average duration: 7 years.*	Voluntarily Stopping Eating and Drinking (VSED) Write and/or record Advance Directive for Stopping Eating and Drinking (AD for SED) for later loss of capacity.
Stage 4. Moderate Cognitive Decline (early-stage dementia). Forgets recent events. Difficulty concentrating and completing tasks. Cannot manage finances or travel alone to new places. In denial about symptoms. Socialization problems: withdraws from friends or family. Physician can detect cognitive problems. *Average duration: 2 years* Stage 5. Moderately Severe Cognitive Decline (mid-stage dementia). Major memory deficiencies. Needs assistance with ADLs (dressing, bathing, etc.) Forgets details like address, phone number. Does not know time, date, or one's location. *Average duration: 1.5 years.*	Stage 4. Mild Alzheimer's. Most ADLs increasingly affected (bill paying, cooking, cleaning, traveling, etc.). *Average duration: 2 years.* Stage 5. Moderate Alzheimer's. Requires assistance in choosing proper clothing. Continuing loss of ability to perform other ADLs. *Average duration: 1.5 years.*	VSED option depends on careful assessment of patient's current wishes and past statements in this domain, as well as their current capacity to understand the consequences of this decision. Writing or recording an AD for SED may be possible in Stage 4, but likely not in Stage 5. Careful assessment is required in both.

Table 8.1 Continued

Global Deterioration Scale for Assessing Primary Degenerative Dementia (GDS)	Functional Assessment Staging Test (FAST)	Stopping Eating and Drinking Option
Stage 6. Severe Cognitive Decline (mid-stage dementia). Cannot carry out ADLs without help. Forgets names of family members, recent events, major events in past. Difficulty counting down from 10. Difficulty speaking. Personality and emotional changes. Delusions, compulsions, and anxiety. Incontinence. *Average duration: 2.5 years.* Stage 7. Very Severe Cognitive Decline (late-stage dementia). Cannot speak or communicate. Requires help with most activities. Loss of motor skills. Cannot walk. *Average duration: 1.5 to 2.5 years.*	Stage 6. Moderately Severe Alzheimer's. Requires assistance with dressing, bathing, toileting. Urinary and fecal incontinence. *Average duration: 3.5–9.5 months.* Stage 7. Severe Alzheimer's. Speech ability declines to 5–6 intelligible words/ day, one word clearly. Can no longer walk or sit up. Can no longer smile or hold head up. *Average duration: 1–1.5 years.*	Stopping Eating and Drinking by Advance Directive (SED by AD). Should be based on clearly articulated statements about initiating SED if and when capacity is lost. Comfort Feeding Only (CFO) or Minimal Comfort Feeding Only (MCFO) should be the back-up plan if SED by AD is not possible.

Sources: Dementia Care Central 2020 and Medical Care Corporation 2020 (see reference list). GDS and FAST are two of the most well-known stage scales; others include the Clinical Dementia Rating (CDR) and the Mini-Mental State Exam (MMSE). Two influential articles in the founding academic literature for GDS and FAST are Reisberg et al. 1996 and Sclan and Reisberg 1992.

of dementia must decide (1) whether they should act preemptively while decision-making capacity is still clearly present, or (2) whether they could risk waiting for the onset of the condition that they know will be unacceptable, and then count on others to act. If they do choose to wait, how can they provide those around them with enough information about their future wishes and preferences that they will be clearly empowered to enact them? These are some of the many challenges addressed in Part II of this book.

Because "voluntarily" stopping eating and drinking when a patient has lost contemporaneous decision-making capacity raises a host of additional practical, ethical, legal, and institutional issues around agency, we begin by distinguishing similar but distinct practices in this domain:

1. **Stopping Eating and Drinking by Advance Directive (SED by AD)** is the practice of withholding oral feeding (food and drink) from persons with advanced dementia or other conditions causing permanent loss of decision-making capacity—ideally, based on a prior decision documented in a written advance directive by the person on whom the process is being initiated, having been completed while she had decision-making capacity. The patient's preferences in this domain may have been previously communicated verbally to surrogate decision-makers, but preferably also communicated in writing and even with a videotaped recording (Pope, 2020). This decision must be based on clear evidence of the patient's prior desire that their eating and drinking not be assisted in their current incapacitated circumstance.

2. **Comfort Feeding Only (CFO)** involves offering as much or as little food and drink as the patient appears to enjoy without regard to the "adequate hydration and nutrition" that might be required if the goal was long-term survival. CFO is standard of care in hospice circles when a patient is dying of some kind of terminal illness, whether or not they have contemporaneous decision-making capacity. CFO is also an acceptable practice in most (but not all) circles for patients with advanced dementia. Several subgroups of CFO practice that might have been specified in a formal advance directive (relevant details regarding CFO limits written down) or an informal one (explicitly discussed with surrogate decision-makers but specific details not written).[1] If not specifically discussed, surrogate decision-makers may still be able to make these determinations based on "substituted judgment" (what they believe the patient would want under current circumstances but were not specifically discussed). These options are commonly utilized in the context of a clearly defined terminal illness, but they might also be

---

[1] Clinicians should and generally do consider *any* evidence of patient wishes even if not memorialized in a legally binding document (Barnsley Hospital NHS Foundation Trust v. MSP 2020).

considered in circumstances such as advanced dementia, where surrogate decision-makers may have evidence to support their belief that the patient would not want his life prolonged by medical measures of any kind.[2] Two sub-categories of CFO are defined as follows:

2a. **"Self-feeding"** *and* **"caregiver-assisted" feeding**: CFO by mouth where, in addition to facilitating self-feeding, caregivers also directly assist the patient with intake of food and fluids if self-feeding becomes difficult, as long as he appears to easily accept and enjoy the assisted feeding—no more and no less. This practice is standard of care in most hospice programs when a patient is terminally ill. This practice is also usually acceptable for non-terminally ill patients with advanced dementia or other progressive, eventually fatal illnesses when oral intake is declining.

2b. **"Self-feeding only"** but *not* **" caregiver-assisted" feeding**: The CFO is limited to what food or fluids the patient can independently self-administer when placed in front of her. In this instance, no direct assistance in eating and drinking (i.e., no hand-feeding of the patient by a family member or health care provider) should be provided other than preparing food and drink and making it accessible to the patient if she appears to be interested and is capable of self-feeding. Because this restriction on caregiver-assisted feeding is generally not standard of care in this situation, "self-feeding only," even if it qualifies as CFO for self-feeding, should be based on a patient's clearly articulated prior directive (verbally, but preferably also in writing) stating something to the effect of "no assisted feeding" and clearly articulating when that choice should be implemented.

3. **Minimum Comfort Feeding Only (MCFO)** would be a modification on more standard CFO for those patients who had expressed a clear preference for SED under their current circumstance but now do not have the capacity to carry it out. This might apply to one or more of three circumstances:

3a. Patients who were clearly planning to VSED, but lost decision-making capacity while waiting to implement it. Despite meeting the clearly agreed-upon triggering conditions, the now incapacitated

---

[2] There is likely more flexibility about limited CFO decisions based on substituted judgment without direct evidence of the patient's explicit wishes if the patient is under the family's care at home than there is if the patient resides in a nursing facility. In the latter, much more concrete, situation-specific information about the patient's preferences about CFO might be required to limit feeding in this way.

patient still expresses an apparent interest in consuming some food and fluids.

3b. Patients who have initiated VSED while having capacity, but lost that capacity during the process and now express an apparent interest in some food or fluids despite diligent attention to sprays and mouth care to alleviate dry mouth and the sensation of thirst, and also despite being reminded of their prior decision.

3c. Patients who, while capacitated in the past, had completed a clearly articulated AD for SED that they wanted implemented on their behalf after decision-making capacity is lost and any other previously defined criteria have been met, but the now-incapacitated patient still expresses an apparent interest in some oral intake. An exception might be if they had a binding "Ulysses clause" in their AD that strongly suggested their desire that their future self's request to be fed is not to be listened to under this circumstance (see Chapter 9, Section 9.2 and Chapter 10, Section 10.9). In any case, renewed diligence should be paid to mouth care and moisturizing that may minimize sensation of thirst.

In such circumstances, provided previously agreed-upon criteria are clearly met, the amount of food and fluid given (either offered for self-feeding or caregiver-assisted) should be the *minimum amount needed for comfort*. Unlike usual CFO, where the patient is also allowed *as much as is still compatible with comfort*, the MCFO approach is also trying to honor the patient's prior plan for VSED or SED by AD, once stipulated conditions are met, as a way of hastening death in that circumstance. This approach must be carefully discussed with family members as well as clinical personnel and caregivers in advance, to ensure their understanding and comfort with participation in this process. For some who would have to act on the AD for SED, this MCFO approach may be too subtle and ambiguous in terms of intent, in which case standard CFO would be the alternate default.

4. **Maintaining Adequate Hydration and Nutrition** would be standard goal of treatment in most circumstances where a person is acutely ill, has significant potential for future recovery, and has not previously set limits on this aspect of treatment. This practice is also standard for persons with chronic illness, full decision-making capacity, and an acceptable quality of life (by their own personal definition) provided

they have not personally set other limits on treatment or expressed more limited goals. When this practice is based in a patient's current verbal directives, on a previously completed Provider Orders for Life-Sustaining Treatment (POLST) (National POLST 2019), or Medical Orders for Life-Sustaining Therapies (MOLST) (Bomba 2015), or on their clearly articulated advance directive that applies to the current circumstances, then it would not be controversial. For persons who had decision-making capacity in the past and have now lost it without prospect of recovery, every effort should be directed to making current medical decisions using what is known about their past values and preferences, focusing especially on any advance care planning documents they completed while they had capacity (Lang and Quill 2004). If patients themselves made it clear when they had decision-making capacity that they would want CFO, MCFO, or even SED by AD in their current circumstances where they have now lost decision-making capacity, then their care plan should transition as much as possible to their previously articulated desire.

For never-capacitated patients and for previously capacitated patients who are now incapacitated and left no clear articulation of their preferences about the kind of treatment they would and would not want under their current circumstances, trying to maintain "adequate hydration and nutrition" would be the usual initial standard of care unless they were otherwise terminally ill. If such patients are approaching the end of life, or if they appear to be suffering in ways that are difficult to adequately palliate, then the standard of care could potentially shift to CFO depending on any potential inferred evidence that suggested the patient would or would not want this approach based on prior statements and prior values. If there is no relevant evidence about the patient's previously articulated values with regard to eating and drinking under their current circumstances (or if they were developmentally disabled and never had decision-making capacity), then the approach should be based more on the family's, guardian's, and staff's views of the patient's "best interests," and on the statutes or relevant laws protecting such vulnerable patients. In-depth discussion of recommended approaches to these difficult questions and patient circumstances is beyond the scope of this book, except to say that neither VSED nor SED by AD would have any role in these latter circumstances, where there is no clear evidence that the patient himself would want them.

8.2. Background Issues

Palliative care, with its focus on pain and symptom management, enhancing quality of life, and ensuring fully informed decision-making, should be part of the treatment plan for all seriously ill patients, and certainly for those who have lost decision-making capacity (Quill et al. 2019). Many but not all patients who lose decision-making capacity want a focus on treatment that is primarily if not exclusively directed toward enhancing quality of life. Some incapacitated patients would still want to receive some or all potentially effective life-prolonging therapies alongside these palliative treatments. Others have let it be known that they want "comfort measures only" under their current circumstances, including CFO with no life-prolonging or disease-directed therapies.

These latter patients should be transitioned to hospice care, provided they are in the terminal stage of illness and thus would qualify according to prognostic requirements. In addition to accepting and supporting a treatment plan focusing entirely on comfort and not on disease treatment, hospice also requires that the patient be more likely than not to die in the next six months if the disease follows its usual course. If a patient with relatively early or moderate-stage Alzheimer's disease, for example, is not also functionally or nutritionally impaired, this six-month prognostic requirement may be a barrier to timely hospice referral in some programs despite the fact that the program would otherwise seem ideally suited for their care. If there is more than one hospice program available in the patient's region, it would be worthwhile exploring the openness on this question in advance of signing up (NHCPO 2020), as the added support of a hospice program can enhance the comfort and success of the process.

One of the many challenges of Alzheimer's disease is its very long clinical course lasting 10 or more years from its pre-clinical stages to its very advanced stages (Fisher Center 2019). The first three "pre-clinical" stages, lasting on average two to seven years, include "normal aging forgetfulness" through "mild cognitive impairment," where executive function is becoming mildly impaired and performance begins to subtly decline.

Stages four and five last an additional one to five years on average, with gradually growing "moderate impairment in instrumental activities of daily living (IADLs)" including maintaining home, managing money, preparing meals, and shopping.

The last two stages (six and seven), which usually last one to three years or longer, involve "moderately severe to severe impairments in activities of daily living (ADLs)," including the inability to independently bathe and toilet, get dressed, walk, and eventually even to feed oneself, as well as severe impairments in recognizing and communicating with others.

The uncertainty about where the person is in this spectrum, especially from mild through moderate cognitive impairment, and about how rapidly the disease will progress in any particular case, makes end-of-life decision-making very challenging for these patients. On the one hand, an individual might not want to initiate a legally available escape like VSED "too early" when one is still finding life to be meaningful and enjoyable. On the other hand, if one waits "too late," then the cognitive capability to carry out the VSED process might be lost, and one might become trapped inside the late stages of the disease with no ability to escape through controlling the time of one's own death. It would help to have a written advance directive or, even better, one supplemented with an audio or videotaped statement articulating one's wishes about limiting or refusing future hand-feeding if decision-making capacity is lost in the future (Case 7.4; Pope 2020). We list recommended elements of such an advance directive in Appendix A.

Mrs. H. felt she had to initiate VSED while she still had the cognitive capacity to do so, but she was still enjoying many aspects of her life and lamented leaving them behind. If she knew that an escape was still possible when she further lost capacity in the future, perhaps she would have chosen to postpone her decision to initiate VSED while she clearly still had decision-making capacity and would not have missed out on what could have been added meaningful time. Might an AD for SED (including a videotaped record of her wishes) have allowed her this added time? Perhaps it could have, but only if she felt confident her directive could be acted upon when she had lost decision-making capacity later in the process.

8.3. Advance Care Planning

So when patients lose decision-making capacity in the late stages of a serious illness, how should clinicians caring for them proceed? If patients have left any clear indication of their wishes under their current circumstances, those wishes should be followed to the extent possible. The clearer, more specific, and applicable to the circumstances in which the now-incapacitated patient finds herself these instructions are, the more explicitly such advance directives can and should be followed. As outlined in Chapter 2 (Section 2.6) and reviewed in Box 8.1, all adults should be aware of these documents and consider completing all four. If one loses decision-making capacity in the future, then having completed such documents when capacitated will help ensure that one's values and preferences will be honored.

Box 8.1 Care Planning Documents

ADVANCE DIRECTIVES
Activated in the *future* if and when the person losses contemporaneous decision-making capacity.
Should be reviewed and considered by all adults.
Durable Power of Attorney for Health Care—(aka Health Care Proxy or Agent)—designation by a person with decision-making capacity of someone to make health care decisions on her behalf should she lose that capacity in the future—ideally this designation of a future decision-making surrogate is communicated in advance in a written, properly witnessed, and signed document that should ideally be combined with the other documents below.
Advance Instructional Directive—(aka Living Will)—written instructions by a person with decision-making capacity about what kinds of health care interventions she would and would not want should she lose that capacity in the future.
Advance Directive Video—a videotaped statement by a person with decision-making capacity specifically addressing the kinds of health care interventions she would and would not want should she lose that capacity in the future.

CURRENT DIRECTIVES
Activated in the *present* upon completion to guide *current and future* medical treatments.
Should be reviewed and considered in all adults with serious potentially fatal illnesses.
Provider Orders for Life-Sustaining Treatment (POLST) (also **Medical Orders for Life-Sustaining Treatment, MOLST**)—these are forms for recording actual medical orders about the kinds of treatment a person would and would not want under their current medical circumstances, potentially including cardiopulmonary resuscitation, mechanical ventilation, feeding tubes, other disease-directed treatments as well as comfort measures.

If there are no formal advance care planning documents and the patient has lost decision-making capacity, then the clinician's job is to sit down with close family members and friends and try to have them imagine what the patient would want under her current circumstances (Bischoff et al. 2013; Sharma and Dy 2011). Sometimes there is a clear consensus about the patient's overarching values and views. This consensus might provide a guide to what she would or would not want under her current condition, in which case those inferred directives should be followed, especially if they fall within usual standards of practice (such as "comfort measures only" or "treat easily treatable problems").

If there is no document and no clear direction based on prior discussions, medical decisions must still be made. These decisions should be ethically based on the patient's "best interests," with all the hazards of potential misperception inherent in these decisions (Fritsch et al. 2013). For these cases, formal ethics and palliative care consultations should be considered if there is uncertainty about how to move forward clinically.

In meetings with families of patients who have now lost capacity to participate in decision-making, we are continually trying to use all available data to imagine the patient's own view of her current quality of life and treatment preferences. This process is much more complex than one might intuitively think, because of what we have learned about how adaptable humans can be under potentially life-threatening circumstances. Some patients, who thought they would immediately enter hospice if they develop cancer, end up choosing the most aggressive disease-directed treatments available. Others, who thought they would use medical technology to medically fight against the disease all the way through until their deaths, transition to hospice relatively quickly when they learn just how physically demanding many cancer treatments are. These very major medical decisions are made by the patient himself, with assistance from medical providers and family, when the patient has decision-making capacity. But if that capacity is lost, then "substituted judgment" (making decisions as one imagines the patient would if he could understand his current clinical circumstances) should be the guiding principle.

Substituted judgment decisions apply to major invasive treatments like cardiopulmonary resuscitation, mechanical ventilation ("breathing machines"), and aggressive treatments like chemotherapy for cancer treatment. But they also apply to ordinary treatments like the provision of food and fluids. Although many (but not all) medical providers would consider intravenous fluids and nutrition a "medical treatment" that can be withheld if it is not serving a medical purpose, some consider adequate hydration and nutrition by whatever route needed to be a basic human necessity in all clinical circumstances. Still others would limit the provision of food and liquid to the oral route in advanced irreversible illness, offered only as long as the patient seems to enjoy and tolerate it (Chessa and Moreno 2019; American Nurses Association 2017; Meier and Ong 2015; Cavanagh 2014).

Of course, patients with decision-making capacity can and should be asked about their preferences in this domain, including how much intake they want and what routes are acceptable. For patients who are not capable of decision-making, clinicians and family members would consider evidence of enjoyment or pleasure with being fed and offered fluids, especially if the previously capacitated patient had not left any kind of advance directive or had not been clear in their prior directive about their preference to avoid assisted feeding under their current circumstances. If there are differing opinions about the patient's pleasure or desire in this domain among family and professional caregivers, there might be value in obtaining consultation from psychiatry, palliative care, medical ethics, or someone from the patient's spiritual or religious community. On some occasions, there may even be value to patient and family in temporarily postponing a decision to withhold oral feeding, or even to provide a brief course of intravenous fluids to keep the patient alive for an important occasion such as the return of a close family member to "say good-bye" or to participate in an important family event.

8.4. Practical Aspects of Stopping Eating and Drinking by Advance Directive (SED by AD) and Comfort Feeding Only (CFO)

The most important requirement to initiate SED by AD is that a patient clearly made it known that she would not want any food or drink under her current circumstances. Such orders for withholding food and fluids based on a patient's wishes are not routine options within POLST (or MOLST) forms completed by a health care provider in collaboration with the patient or her designated surrogate decision-maker. Therefore, the order and its justification should be carefully written into advance care planning forms for easy access by other health care providers, along with a more detailed note in the patient's medical record. If surrogates are representing the patient, every effort should be made to ensure that the surrogate is representing what is known about the patient's wishes in this regard, rather than what the surrogate personally prefers for the patient or for himself.

In circumstances where non-standard treatments such as SED by AD are being seriously considered, there must be clarity about the patient's own wishes and preferences in this domain. Although permissible under the right circumstances, withholding even CFO from an incapacitated patient is ethically, legally, and practically different from providing CFO but not attempting to provide enough food and drink to indefinitely sustain life. Similarly, decisions about withholding hydration and nutrition, whether artificial or "natural," are morally distinct from medical decisions to withhold mechanical ventilation, cardiopulmonary resuscitation, or other life-prolonging interventions under similar circumstances (Meisel 1991). The ethical and legal dimensions of these questions are addressed in Chapters 9 and 10.

From a clinical perspective, providing CFO is usually considered a quality of life measure which, if withheld, might increase suffering as well as shorten life, especially if the patient was verbally or nonverbally expressing enjoyment with comfort-level food. The decision to withhold CFO ought to be based on clear information the that patient had previously indicated he would like his death hastened in this way under his current circumstances. The withholding itself is likely to increase suffering in the short run, and the now-incapacitated patient will likely not be capable of participating in the "swish and spit" method to keep his mouth relatively moist, which is used during VSED with capacitated patients. Other disease-directed medications and treatments that have little if any quality of life benefits are also generally withheld, as they would not be a part of any usual "comfort-oriented" plan of care.

CFO could be an alternative "back-up" plan for either capacitated or now-incapacitated patients who had previously indicated their desire for VSED but whose basic drive for food and drink seems too strong to overcome, or if the indication to fully implement SED by AD was not clear enough at the point it was being considered in earnest. CFO in one of the two forms below would be standard of care for dying patients who accept that they are dying, subject to discussion with any designated health care proxy or other family representatives. Options within CFO include the following:

- **Comfort-oriented *self*-feeding** involves putting small amounts of the patient's favorite foods and liquids within easy access, and allowing her to self-administer as much or as little as she is interested in. There is no assessment for "adequate hydration and nutrition," because the only metric of interest is short-term pleasure from eating and drinking.

- **Comfort-oriented** *assisted* **feeding** can be considered for a patient who is too physically or mentally incapacitated to self-administer food and fluids, but still appears to be enjoying eating and drinking when fed by others. The purpose of this form of feeding is not to maintain "adequate hydration and nutrition," but rather to respond to verbal and non-verbal cues that the patient is enjoying the food and fluids being provided. There should be an ongoing conversation among family, caregivers, and clinicians to ensure agreement about how to assess the patient's comfort and enjoyment with the process and when, perhaps, to stop the comfort-oriented assisted feeding in the future (see Section 8.5 below).

Other elements of a more general **"Comfort-Oriented Care"** approach (McCann, Hall, and Groth-Juncker 1994) during this phase of treatment include the following: (1) Treatments acceptable to the patient that potentially enhance her quality of life should be offered and implemented. (2) Treatments not geared to the patient's immediate comfort should be stopped, deactivated, or discontinued. This includes all disease-directed medications that are not contributing to the patient's immediate comfort, all blood work, and other potentially life-prolonging treatments such as implantable defibrillators. Medical problems that develop subsequently should only be evaluated and treated if they are causing immediate discomfort. The patient's POLST form should be reviewed to reflect "comfort measures only," and any other dimensions of active patient suffering should be addressed. The patient should be referred to a formal hospice program for added support and follow-up if that has not already occurred. The family should be prepared that death may be coming soon, and they should be encouraged to spend as much time as possible with the patient and share expressions of love and connection. Consideration should be given to contacting the patient's faith community and other social supports for added support.

8.5. Limits of Palliation with Comfort Feeding Only (CFO)

When CFO is initiated for an incapacitated patient, it should be continued as long as it is associated with the patient's apparent experience of pleasure (comfort) from the process. In all probability, a point will be reached when the patient is too weak to participate in eating and drinking at all, or when what has been a comfort-enhancing process now becomes associated with too much physical distress from aspiration of food and fluids into their lungs. At this time, CFO should be minimized or discontinued.

Clinicians should actively guide and warn families and caregivers as to the future potential timing of this decision, emphasizing that losing interest and ability to eat and drink is a natural part of the very end of life. Careful mouth care, skin care, regular turning, and other purely comfort measures should be continued. Most hospice programs are very comfortable with this phase of the process, and they should become formally involved, if that is not already the case, to help support patient and family through the final stage of the dying process.

Death is the inevitable end point for the patient receiving CFO, and a period of bereavement naturally follows for family and close friends. Hopefully the family has been fully prepared for the patient's death, and, with the help of the palliative care or hospice team, the process has gone peacefully and smoothly. However, second-guessing and anguish around decisions made, or periods of possibly preventable suffering during the dying process, can emerge. Ideally, talking to the patient's family right after the death and making one or more additional bereavement phone calls within two weeks of the death should be standard practice. If the patient had been formally enrolled in hospice, meaningful bereavement services, follow-up phone calls, and family visits and support groups are generally offered. Particularly if a decision was made to stop artificial hydration and nutrition, or any measures perceived to have intentionally or unintentionally hastened death were used, such as VSED or SED by AD, the family may experience uncertainty about the entire process after the patient's death that will need subsequent exploration and support.

8.6. Advantages of SED by AD

Some patients with early dementia (Mrs. H.) and other slowly progressive conditions like end-stage Parkinson's disease or recurrent progressive cerebrovascular accidents may want to give watchful waiting or some forms of disease-directed treatment a time-limited trial to see how effective and tolerated they are. Nonetheless, they may not want to live for prolonged periods of time if their illness continues to gradually progress to a state of significant cognitive impairment or physical dependence.

SED by AD is potentially attractive to such patients because it allows them to avoid initiating VSED earlier than they would like out of fear of losing capacity. They can instead have VSED carried out later if and when they clearly reach the condition they find unacceptable. Such patients potentially would have more time to enjoy their lives. If they miss their "window of opportunity" to make a real-time decision themselves to initiate VSED, they could still have food and fluids stopped or limited on their behalf later, provided they had made their wishes clear enough through an advance directive. Thus, the possibility of SED by AD is an added level of reassurance for all patients considering VSED that they may not have to initiate the process before they really want to. The clinician's role in hastening death with SED by AD is still mediated by the patient's wishes, though it lacks the reassurance of patient self-initiation of the process in real time that characterizes VSED by a fully capacitated patient. Thus, the practice could be supported by some hospice programs and many palliative care and hospice clinicians.

Although palliative measures needed to treat the added suffering associated with SED by AD are imperfect, the dry mouth can be relieved to some degree by a fine water mist without providing amounts of fluids that would prolong the dying process. Unfortunately, the ability to effectively participate in the "swish and spit" method of palliation will probably be lost if decision-making capacity is seriously compromised. If delirium contributes to agitation as the dying/dehydrating process evolves, any associated discomfort should be managed with anti-anxiety and anti-psychotic medications, including potentially sedating doses if they are needed, as is the tradition in hospice and palliative care under similar circumstances.

Actually initiating and carrying through SED at the time called for in the person's AD may end up being too difficult for a variety of reasons, including patient discomfort that cannot be adequately managed with minimal amounts of oral intake offered as MCFO, or resistance of caregivers or institutions to the overall SED process itself. In such circumstances, less contentious CFO may serve as a "back-up plan" of sorts. While it will likely not accomplish as early a death as the person envisioned in their AD for SED, CFO may accomplish part of their goal not to live long into a deteriorating condition. Depending on how little or how much added food and fluid are taken in for comfort, the last phase of the dying process may not be prolonged at all (if MCFO), or it may be prolonged for several weeks to many months (if the patient desires large amounts of food and fluids as part of more standard CFO.)

CFO has a long tradition in palliative care and hospice, and is within the standard of care for people in the last phase of life who accept they are dying. People have died by gradually stopping eating and drinking since the beginning of time. CFO allows for the smell, taste, and touch of eating and drinking real food, along with the human contact and connection with the debilitated person around feeding, without a dominating focus on medical interventions. Most (but not all) dying people want natural eating and drinking for pleasure provided during this phase of life, and most do not want this process expanded by medical interventions such as feeding tubes and intravenous fluids. Neither do they want caregivers pressuring them to eat and drink more than is comfortable and pleasurable to "maintain hydration and nutrition."

Minimal Comfort Feeding Only (MCFO) as outlined above is a variant of CFO where caregivers err of the side of giving the minimum amount of food and drink needed for basic comfort in an attempt to both respond to the patient's immediate desire for and pleasure from food and drink, while at the same time trying to honor her prior AD for SED. To restate, standard CFO has goals of providing pleasure/enjoyment from eating/drinking, and neither hastening nor postponing death, as is the case with standard hospice care. MCFO also has the goal of providing pleasure/enjoyment from eating/drinking, but in this case hastening death is also intended based on the patient's clearly articulated AD for SED. For this reason, the amount of intake with MCFO is kept to the *minimum needed* for comfort instead of up to *as much or as little as is compatible with* achieving comfort, as would be the case for CFO. For example, a patient on hospice receiving CFO might be given a full plate of her favorite food with frequent offerings for more if she seems to be enjoying the meal, or allowed to stop after one or two bites if that seems enough. On the other hand, a patient receiving MCFO would be given a small amount of her favorite food for immediate comfort, but offered more *only* if she expresses (verbally or nonverbally) a clear interest in more.

Almost all hospices are willing to enroll patients who have initiated CFO providing they also (1) have a progressive, potentially terminal illness; (2) have stopped other life-prolonging therapies; and (3) otherwise want a purely comfort-oriented approach to additional medical problems that inevitably will emerge. Some hospices may have discomfort admitting patients who would like MCFO, because it potentially violates their position of not supporting actions intended to hasten death. In the future, if any such patients receiving either CFO or MCFO appear to have stabilized such that they are no longer "more likely than not to die in the next six months if their underlying disease follows it usual course" (as required to remain on hospice), they may have to be discharged from hospice. They may subsequently be re-enrolled as their condition deteriorates, and they then meet the prognostic requirements. Such discharges should be relatively infrequent, especially for the MCFO patients, if they are carefully selected up-front. Provided the patient has a serious underlying progressive illness, most physicians accept CFO because of its long tradition in hospice and because the physician's role in potentially hastening death is unintended and indirect, if it exists at all. Some physicians may be more hesitant about accepting patients desiring MCFO because part of the intention behind the approach is to hasten death.

8.7. Disadvantages of SED by AD

In comparison to real-time consent, all medical decisions based on advance directive planning lose the anchor of contemporaneous consent. Many people contemplate the future possibility of "last-resort options" should their suffering become unacceptable in the future (Quill, Lo, and Brock 1997), but relatively few activate them even when they still have capacity to make their own decisions. The clearer the past expression of the now-incapacitated person's wishes about not being hydrated or fed in the circumstance in which he now is situated, the less the possible death-hastening aspects of this practice are likely to be a major issue for surrogate decision-makers and health care providers. But the burden of an AD for SED directive on family members and medical decision-makers, when the now-incapacitated patient does not understand why he is not being fed or not allowed to drink, can be substantial.

The usual palliation for the dry mouth caused by VSED involves using saline mist spray that does not provide enough hydration to prolong the dying process. If the saline mist spray does not provide adequate relief from the sensation of dry mouth, the usual back-up plan is to have the patient "swish and spit" artificial saliva or other kinds of fluids. But these methods are probably not within the capabilities of an incapacitated, very thirsty patient. Swallowing a substantial volume of artificial saliva intended to be a "comfort measure only" could unintentionally prolong the patients' dying process while simultaneously relieving some of his suffering. Proportionate doses of sedating medications to help indirectly relieve the distress associated with thirst and dry mouth are also possible, especially if the distress is severe and if the patient, when still capable of decision-making, had made her wishes clear that she would rather be sedated than fed under such circumstances.

The back-up plan of CFO could also potentially help relieve these symptoms. But, as mentioned above, it may have the unwanted potential effect of substantially prolonging the dying process. With CFO, the patient is offered food and fluids by mouth in small amounts according to interest and tolerance. The family and other caregivers should be clearly informed that the main purpose of feeding is patient comfort and pleasure, and that it is explicitly not intended to prolong life. With MCFO, there is a higher likelihood of death occurring in a shorter period of time, which would make sense as a back-up if the original plan was to achieve a hastened death through VSED or SED by AD. On the other hand, the relatively clear intent to hasten death may make MCFO unacceptable to those whose initial intent was to "neither hasten nor postpone" death, as in standard CFO in hospice. In either a CFO or MCFO context, family should be encouraged not to push or force more volume or calories than the patient appears to want or enjoy. As the patient's intake gets less and less, artificial saliva can be provided in the amount needed to keep his mouth moist, no more and no less. For the patient who was exploring VSED earlier in their course of illness but lost capacity before fully activating it, MCFO as outlined above would be a potential way of simultaneously honoring the patient's views and values, while also working within the usual standards of care for the dying.

8.8. Return to the Cases

Case 7.1. (Originally Case 1.3).
Mrs. H. with Early Alzheimer's

Rob Horowitz, Mrs. H's palliative care physician son, reflected on his recollection of the patient and family struggles between waiting too long and acting too soon as they prepared for her to initiate VSED. On the one hand, she and her family might miss out on what could be valuable time together by acting while she still had sufficient intellectual capacity and will power to carry out the process. On the other hand, if she had waited until her current life was truly unacceptable to her, she risked that she would no longer have the cognitive ability and discipline not to drink in the face of significant thirst. Once she initiated VSED (which she did while she still had decision-making capacity), Mrs. H wanted her son and family to promise not to give her food and fluids "even if I ask for it." Her request in this regard felt like a very heavy burden to the family, taking away the possibility that she could "change her mind" about initiating the process. A subsequent post-mortem brain biopsy reassured the family that they acted at the "right time." But the uncertainty of whether the time was right can still weigh heavily on those involved.

Bottom Line Points
- The very unclear timeline of Alzheimer's creates tremendous uncertainty for patients and families who are considering an escape through VSED about when to initiate the process. Second-guessing the timing of initiation is common and potentially haunting, even when there is strong clinical evidence that the patient was truly on the verge of losing decision-making capacity.
- The possibility of SED by AD might have given Mrs. H. the reassurance needed to risk living longer without the fear that if she waited too long she might have to live a prolonged last phase of her life in an incapacitated state from which there would be no escape (which was her worst nightmare).

Case 7.2. Steve: Mild to Moderate Cognitive Impairment that Complicated All Aspects of Decision-Making

Steve, in mild to moderate cognitive impairment, both feared and was personally in denial about the extent of his own dementia. He wanted his family to stop all oral intake when he reached Stage 6 on the FAST scale (significantly advanced dementia). Not only did he want his family to stop oral feeding at that point, but he also wanted them to "ignore any of his future requests" to be fed, without any acknowledgment of how difficult that would be psychologically for the family. Steve rejected the possibility of CFO as a potential future approach because he feared a prolonged dying process, and instead wanted family to completely stop feeding him even if he expressed a desire to eat and drink when he reached that stage. His genuine underlying hope was and is that someone could "just end my life at an appropriate time." This case is currently still ongoing.

Bottom Line Points

- Writing and then activating an advance directive when a person has mild to moderate cognitive impairment is fraught with hazard. Because of the human tendency toward denial of difficult subjects, major gaps may emerge: (1) how cognitively impaired a person perceives himself to be, and the potentially different perceptions of his doctor and other members of his family; (2) how able patients are to facilitate their own plans in this domain; and (3) how much they must trust others to implement them. Similar levels of denial and differing perceptions may be also be present among family members.

- Many patients facing such major life and death decisions avoid these difficult discussions, preferring instead that their families take on a central role and responsibility in medical decision-making without acknowledging or understanding the profound and lasting potential psychological burdens such decisions may have. Ideally, these subjects should be discussed with family members while the patient still has decision-making capacity, and the family gains a clear sense of the patient's views and preferences. But the human tendency to avoid painful topics means that the discussion is often avoided until the patient can no longer participate.

Case 7.3. Patricia: SED by AD versus Preemptive Suicide

Patricia, a 91-year-old retired university professor, was a national expert in her field who had been living with relatively early Alzheimer's (Stage 4 on both FAST and GDS scales) for about five years. She had significant short-term memory problems as well as "face blindness" such that she could not recognize those around her whom she had previously known. Patricia was prepared for her death and did not want to suffer in any significant way during the final dying process. She contemplated VSED, but she enjoyed eating and drinking too much to give them up entirely during the last phase of her life. Her advance directive stated that she wanted "comfort feeding only" if she became fully incapacitated.

Although she lived in a state where MAID is illegal, in the past she had acquired a "stash" of barbiturates to allow her an escape to death at a time of her own choosing. Patricia eventually died after taking an intentional overdose of the medication. Her death was briefly investigated as a "suicide," but there were no legal repercussions for her or her caregivers around the manner of her death.

Bottom Line Points
- Although VSED may be a legally permitted option of last resort for those who would prefer MAID but live in states where it is not permitted, the process of successfully completing VSED is sometimes difficult and beyond the abilities of many seriously ill patients. It is especially difficult for those for whom eating and drinking are essential human pleasures who are looking for an escape through death. If the pleasure coming from eating and drinking prohibited a patient desperately looking for an escape from initiating the VSED process while still decisionally capable, imagine how hard it would be for a family to initiate SED by AD after such a patient has lost decision-making capacity.
- An underground practice of MAID and voluntary active euthanasia exists in places where either or both are illegal (Cohen 2019; Magnusson 2004). In these circumstances, where these legally prohibited death-hastening interventions are carried out in secret, there is generally not an investigation if the patient is otherwise near death and the act is not discovered by the medical practitioners or legal authorities. However, knowledgeable family members are left with a "secret" that may complicate their bereavement. In this case, the cause of death, suicide, was discovered by assisted living administrators, and the case was preliminarily investigated by the police without legal consequences to the family. Her family also was very accepting of Patricia's final act, which she accomplished without directly involving them. Even if she lived in a state where MAID were legal, Patricia would probably not have qualified because she was not terminally ill (prognosis of six months or less).

Case 7.4. Charles: A "Successful" SED by AD

Charles developed signs of early Alzheimer's disease and was very fearful of a prolonged dying with "no plug to pull." He met with a psychiatrist, Dr. Stanley Terman, who helped him to explore his future options including the circumstances when he would want others to stop feeding him. As part of his assessment, Dr. Terman carefully evaluated Charles' capacity for medical decision-making, as well as his level of commitment to not being fed in the future when his decision-making capacity would be lost. Together they created an audio recording of Charles' thinking process and wishes as a lasting record of his commitment to the process.

Seven years later, Charles lost the ability to self-administer food and drink from his progressive dementing illness. He then met the criteria he had previously committed to for withholding assisted feeding. He was admitted to an inpatient hospice facility, where there was initially conflict and uncertainty with the medical director over whether it was permissible for the staff to withhold assisted "comfort-oriented feeding" or whether it should be administered as the standard of care. There was also conflict over whether the directive clearly reflected the patient's wishes. Eventually, the hospice doctor and staff accepted the plan to withhold all assisted feeding. They were swayed by Charles' written advance directive, audiotaped prior testimony, and psychiatric evaluation of capacity at the time those wishes were expressed. Charles died peacefully nine days later.

Bottom Line Points
- Comfort Feeding Only (CFO), offering food and drink in amounts that the patient appears to enjoy without regard to overall hydration and nutrition, should be the standard of care for patients with advanced cognitive impairment. This practice is clearly comfort and pleasure driven, distinct from attempting to enable long-term survival. In the context of a severe, progressive illness, "adequate hydration and nutrition" rather than CFO should only be provided if there is clear indication (such as through an advance directive) that the previously capacitated patient would want such an intervention under her current circumstance.
- Withholding assisted CFO from a patient who can no longer self-feed and is no longer capable of consent or refusal should be permitted, as in this case, when a patient has made it very clear through prior directives (verbal, written, and/or audio or videotaped) that he would not want even comfort-oriented feeding under his current circumstances. While CFO can enhance short-term quality of life, it can also substantially prolong life. That is a "good" outcome if prolonged life is what the patient would want under current circumstances. But CFO can also prolong dying for an indefinite time. That is a "bad" outcome for those who would prefer to die more quickly under current circumstances. This patient and one of his treating clinicians went to great lengths to clarify his wishes not to receive assisted feeding if he lost capacity in the future.

Treating clinicians should do their utmost to honor that clearly articulated prior request.

References

American Nurses Association. 2017. "Position Statement: Nutrition and Hydration at the End of Life." https://www.nursingworld.org/~4af0ed/globalassets/docs/ana/ethics/ps_nutrition-and-hydration-at-the-end-of-life_2017june7.pdf.

Barnsley Hospital NHS Foundation Trust v. MSP. 2020. EWCOP 26.

Bischoff, K.E., R. Sudore, Y. Miao, W.J. Boscardin, and A.K. Smith. 2013. "Advance Care Planning and the Quality of End-of-Life Care in Older Adults." *Journal of the American Geriatrics Society* 61, no. 2: 209–214.

Bomba, Patricia A., and Katie Orem. 2015. "Lessons Learned from New York's Community Approach to Advance Care Planning and MOLST." *Annals of Palliative Medicine* 4, no. 1:10–21.

Cavanagh, Maureen. 2014. "How Should a Catholic Hospice Respond to Patients Who Choose to Voluntarily Stop Eating and Drinking in Order to Hasten Death?" *Linacre Quarterly* 81, no. 3: 279–285.

Chessa, Frank, and Fernando Moreno. 2019. "Ethical and Legal Considerations in End-of-Life Care." *Primary Care* 46, no. 3: 387–398.

Cohen, Lewis M. 2019. *A Dignified Ending: Taking Control Over How We Die.* Lanham, MD: Rowman & Littlefield.

Dementia Care Central. 2020. "Stages of Alzheimer's & Dementia: Durations & Scales Used to Measure Progression" (last updated April 24, 2020). https://www.dementiacarecentral.com/aboutdementia/facts/stages/.

Fisher Center for Alzheimer's Research Foundation. 2019. "Clinical Stages of Alzheimer's." Based on *The Encyclopedia of Visual Medicine Series: An Atlas of Alzheimer' Disease,* by Barry Reisberg, MD. Pearl River, NY. https://www.alzinfo.org/understand-alzheimers/clinical-stages-of-alzheimers/.

Fritsch, Jenna, Sandra Petronio, Paul R. Helft, and Alexia M. Torke. 2013. "Making Decisions for Hospitalized Older Adults: Ethical Factors Considered by Family Surrogates." *Journal of Clinical Ethics* 24, no. 2: 125–134.

Lang, Forrest, and Timothy Quill. 2004. "Making Decisions with Families at the End of Life." *American Family Physician* 70 (4): 719–723.

Magnusson, Roger. 2004. "Euthanasia: Above Ground, Below Ground." *Journal of Medical Ethics* 30: 441–446.

McCann, Robert M., William J. Hall, and Ann-Marie Groth-Juncker. 1994. "Comfort Care for Terminally Ill Patients. The Appropriate Use of Nutrition and Hydration." *JAMA* 272, no. 16: 1263–1266.

Medical Care Corporation. 2020. "Functional Assessment Staging Test," https://www.mccare.com/pdf/fast.pdf.

Meier, Cynthia A., and Thuan D. Ong. 2015. "To Feed or Not to Feed? A Case Report and Ethical Analysis of Withholding Food and Drink in a Patient With Advanced Dementia." *Journal of Pain and Symptom Management* 50, no. 6: 887–890.

Meisel, Alan. 1991. "Legal Myths about Terminating Life Support." *Archives of Internal Medicine* 151, no. 8: 1497–1502.

National POLST. 2019. "National POLST Form: Portable Medical Order, Information for Professional, Patient Guides." https://polst.org/national-form/.

NHCPO 2020. "Find a Care Provider." https://www.nhpco.org/find-a-care-provider/.

Pope, Thaddeus M. 2020. "Video Advance Directive: Growth and Benefits of Audio Recording." *SMU Law Review* 73, no 1: 163–179.

Quill, Timothy E., Periyakoil, Vyjeyanthi S., Erin M. Denney-Koelsch, Patrick White, and Donna S. Zhukovsky. 2019. *Primer of Palliative Care, 7th Ed*. Chicago: American Academy of Hospice and Palliative Medicine.

Quill, Timothy E., Bernard Lo, and Daniel W. Brock. 1997. "Palliative Options of Last Resort: A Comparison of Voluntarily Stopping Eating and Drinking, Terminal Sedation, Physician-Assisted Suicide, and Voluntary Active Euthanasia." *JAMA* 278, no. 23: 2099–2104.

Reisberg, Barry, Emile H. Franssen, Maciej Bobinski, Stefanie Auer, Isabel Monteiro, Istvan Boksay, Jerzy Wegiel, et al. 1996. "Overview of Methodological Issues for Pharmacological Trials in Mild, Moderate, and Severe Alzheimer's Disease." *International Psychogeriatrics* 8, no. 2: 159–193.

Sclan, Steven G., and Barry Reisberg. 1992. "Functional Assessment Staging (FAST) in Alzheimer's's Disease: Reliability, Validity, and Ordinality." *International Psychogeriatrics* 4, Supp. 1: 55–69.

Sharma, R.K., and S.M. Dy. 2011. "Documentation of Information and Care Planning for Patients with Advanced Cancer: Associations with Patient Characteristics and Utilization of Hospital Care." *American Journal of Hospice & Palliative Medicine* 28, no. 8: 543–549.

9

Ethical Issues

Dena S. Davis and Paul T. Menzel

9.1. Introduction

For a person with decision-making capacity, VSED may be the least legally restricted way to assuredly hasten death. It is not limited to fatal illness or the opportunity to refuse lifesaving treatment, nor does it require a "terminal" prognosis. VSED poses a hard choice, however, for anyone with a progressive condition like dementia who faces the prospect of losing capacity and badly wants life not to extend into the condition's later stages. One option is to pursue VSED while still decisive and sacrifice some time that would still be valuable. An alternative is to try to achieve a hastened death at a later time by writing an advance directive for stopping eating and drinking (AD for SED) and communicating it clearly to one's proxy and primary physician.

Many would likely prefer the AD strategy if successful implementation of the directive could be reasonably assured, but assistance with SED to the point where death occurs can hardly be guaranteed once capacity is lost. Faced with this dilemma, Mrs. H., whose case is featured in both parts of this book, chose to preempt any need for others to act later on her behalf and stopped eating and drinking while she still could. Given the challenges for implementing a directive later, she felt such preemptive VSED was only the reasonable choice. She embraced it without complaint and attended carefully to not missing any window of decisive decision-making capacity that could be her last.

Should people like Mrs. H. have a more realistic likelihood of accomplishing SED by AD? In this chapter we pursue the ethical dimensions of this question. Is it morally permissible for proxies and caregivers to implement such a directive? Can the dilemmas that will likely be encountered be resolved by more explicit, detailed attention to them in the directive itself? Given the likely difficulties, is it fair for the person who writes such a directive to expect implementation from her proxies and caregivers?

In pursuing these questions we make certain moral assumptions about ADs generally.

1. ADs have normative force when they are reasonably clear (regarding the sorts of measures to be withheld, in what circumstances, and for essentially what reasons). People do not lose their rights when they lose decision-making capacity (generally hereafter referred to as "capacity"); their rights just need to be exercised for them by appropriate others.

2. Even when valid and sufficiently clear, a directive's normative weight is not absolute. Genuine "then-self vs. now-self" problems can still arise (Dresser and Robertson 1989). These do not, however, pose an insurmountable barrier to ADs. The life at stake is still *the individual's* life, and a life that extends over time. Even when the person no longer has decision-making capacity, he is still a person who previously had capacity. We do not respect him as this person if we ignore his directives and treat him as if he had never had capacity (Rhoden 1990, 860; Cantor 2017).

3. That said, any AD can be revoked or revised by the person who wrote it, though as we shall see, what constitutes valid revocation/revision can be a complex matter.

With normative weight for ADs thus established, we assess the special difficulties facing directives specific to withholding food and water by mouth. Unlike contemporaneous VSED, where a person "starves" herself, the food and drink in SED by AD is ultimately denied to the person *by someone else*. To be sure, this difference should not be overdrawn. VSED by persons with contemporaneous capacity will likely rely on the cooperation and assistance of others in the later days of the process and even before, and SED by AD is directed by the will of the patient through their AD. Nonetheless, we can still ask whether the remaining difference is morally relevant.

As with the term "suicide" applied to VSED (see Chapter 3, Section 3.3), terminology here is contentious. "Starvation" in its usual context, when people want to live, denotes a sad and terrible process. Things are very different for those who choose to "starve" themselves by VSED. The resolute determination that VSED requires provides more assurance that it is voluntary, and people do it for arguably good reasons. VSED may literally be self-"starvation," but it does not carry the word's usual negative connotation. Similarly, if food and drink are withheld by someone else from a person who has lost capacity, because of that person's clear directive, it may literally be "starving" and "dehydrating" the person to death, but the meaning in this context is different.

That is hardly, though, the end of the greater controversy about SED by AD than about VSED. Respecting the autonomy of a person to control the end of her life may be paramount, but the distress of proxies and caregivers who feel constrained to implement a directive is also morally relevant. Can writing a directive to withhold food and water by mouth be the right thing to do if the directive will very likely create distress, including moral distress, for caregivers and family? Or may people take little account of such distress because caregivers should accept their distress out of respect for the patient's wishes? In our subsequent treatment we will use "moral distress" carefully and not see it as simply psychological or emotional distress more generally. One experiences moral distress when one knows the right action to take but is constrained from doing it. If I believe, for example, that supporting my mother's VSED is the right thing to do, I would not feel moral distress if I tried to talk her out of eating when she gets hungry—I am not prevented from doing that—but I would probably still experience psychological stress.

Writing ADs to withhold oral feeding is often driven by the desire to avoid living years into the severe stages of a debilitating condition. Is that desire itself subject to ethical critique, or is it morally protected as part of the patient's prerogative to decide how his life should end? It could, of course, be both— I can be critical of someone's reason for not wanting to live in this condition and still believe they have the right not to. Moreover, is avoiding being a burden to others an ethically appropriate reason for such a desire?

Some comparisons will be significant in our assessment. A primary comparison is with conventional ADs to refuse lifesaving treatment. A relevant comparison is also "comfort feeding only" (CFO), a practice in which an incapacitated patient is not fed at a level adequate to sustain survival but only in amounts that the patient seems to enjoy.

9.2. Change of Mind

Advance directives are valid when written by a person with appropriate decision-making capacity, and a directive can be revised or revoked as long as the person still has that capacity. (On legal criteria for revocation, see Chapter 10, Section 10.8.) Decision-making "capacity," of course, is relative to what is being decided. Revising or revoking a directive will normally require an understanding of both what is being revised or revoked and what is being put in its place. Very few if any dementia patients who have reached the triggering conditions of their ADs have such capacity. By then, they likely no longer think of the reasons they had for their directive, especially one to withhold oral feeding in severe dementia, and they are probably not aware they even have a directive. If they also seem to experience some minimal enjoyment in living, are not suffering, seem content to continue living, and are willing to eat and be fed (perhaps even appearing to enjoy it), we may see them as having changed their mind. Yet as Ron Berghmans notes, by then "you don't have enough mind left to change" (Berghmans 2000, 107).

We might then quickly conclude that once the person is well along in progressive dementia, no valid change of mind about the person's directive is possible. As correct as this conclusion may be, though, it hardly settles the matter. Even if one does not have the appropriate capacity to revise or revoke a directive, certain expressions and behavior may be reason to set prior instructions aside. A classic case is the patient who stipulated that she is to receive no manually assisted feeding in the condition that she's now in, but who now seems to want to eat.

Various questions can be asked in such a case:

1. Does the person have capacity *to revise or revoke the directive*? By the previous analysis, she does not.

2. Does the person have capacity *to decide to eat*? The bar for an activity as basic as eating is lower than the bar, say, for consenting to medical treatment or for writing or revising a previously articulated directive. If a person sees and smells food and seems to want to eat, she presumably has some basic understanding of food and eating and therefore has the necessary capacity for deciding to eat.

3. But is this the relevant capacity? Perhaps we should modify the question: Does the person have the capacity to decide to eat *in the actual situation in which the eating will occur*? The person may understand food and eating, alright, but does he understand *what he is doing in his current real context if he eats*—namely, not only prolonging life, but doing that when he has said not to in his AD? Approaching severe dementia

or already being there, he almost certainly does not. We are then back to the previous point: change of mind is no longer possible when there is "not enough mind left to change." Analogous situations regarding the relevant level of decision-making capacity might be eating before surgery or when eating risks aspiration; the patient might understand normal eating but not understand the risks eating now poses in a specific situation.

4. At some point we might also ask: Is the patient's behavior merely *a reflexive physiological reaction to the presence of food*, not a decision and desire to eat? Suppose the patient is in the last stages of Alzheimer's, not communicative or engaged in any discernible way with things around her. She gives no indication of recognizing food before it gets very close to her nose or touches her lips, but she will then usually open her mouth if the food is patiently held there and will swallow when it is tipped into her mouth. That is reflexive behavior, arguably, not a decision or even a "desire." But modify the case slightly to that of Margot Bentley, for example, who lived her last four years in the most advanced stage of dementia before dying in 2016. Mrs. Bentley would often open her mouth and swallow some foods, but not others (Bentley 2015, paras. 1–3; Bentley 2014, paras. 18–20, 23–24; Hammond 2016; Pope 2015). Did her "discriminating" behavior indicate cognition and desire beyond mere reflex? In some sense her behavior constituted "willingness" to eat, but we hesitate to say she *consented* to eat.[1]

---

[1] Beyond what is highlighted by the four questions in these paragraphs, there is another kind of arguably relevant change of mind. Even if people no longer have the capacity to revise or revoke the directive itself, *they may make new and different judgments about the very matters that were reasons for their directive.* Suppose one of a person's important reasons for her AD for SED in late-moderate/early-severe dementia was her expectation that she would then no longer experience any enjoyment in living, or that she would even be miserable. Now that she is in that stage, she seems to have some minimal, perhaps even considerable, enjoyment and is not miserable. She has not revised or revoked the directive, but isn't her unexpectedly greater enjoyment or contentment a relevant change? An AD's moral authority is rooted in respect for the person who wrote it, with the reasoning and values she brought to it as a person with the ability to reason and value. If one of her primary reasons, an expectation about the condition, turns out not to be the case (not yet, at least), then respect for the person who wrote the directive arguably calls for not yet implementing it. She may have written a different directive had she known she would still enjoy life at this stage (Menzel 2017a, 131–133).

That said, many who write ADs for advancing dementia will not be vulnerable to this sort of change of mind. Their reasons focus on how they see their life in its whole arc best ending, not on expected misery or lack of contentment once they get to a certain stage.

Willingness to eat thus covers a spectrum of behavior, from capacity to decide in the action's full context to reflexive mouth-opening. The strongest cases for following a patient's directive to withhold oral feeding occur when there is no evident desire or willingness to eat at all. Similarly strong cases occur when acceptance of food appears to be merely reflexive. Much more difficult will be cases where the patient seems happy to eat or expresses frustration when not fed.

Those difficult cases are not likely to be resolved by referring to "decision-making capacity." Even if we deem the person to have the requisite ability to decide to eat, does such minimal capacity justify pushing aside his directive? We are thrown back to the basic then-self vs. now-self problem—the need to help the patient before us, but also to respect the patient as a person who previously had decision-making capacity and left a directive. The directive shouldn't automatically control, but neither should the current desire to eat. (For a different conclusion reached by the Society for Post-Acute and Long-Term Care Medicine, see the discussion in Chapter 11, Section 11.4.)

One strategy for dealing with the problem would be to address it explicitly in the directive. The directive might say to feed when there are such expressions of desire to eat, or it might say not to feed even if there are (perhaps administering anxiety-relieving drugs as well). Such explicit instructions, however, may only perpetuate the then-self/now-self problem: the conflict would now be between the then-self with just a more detailed directive and the current willingness to eat. On the other hand, a directive that specifically addressed this very problem would convey more clearly and powerfully the patient's convictions about what to do. A proxy's attempt to discern what the patient would have wanted will involve less guesswork.

Another plausible strategy is to address the problem with "sliding scale" or "balancing" reasoning at the time of possible implementation: weigh the enduring interests of the patient to have the directive followed against her current apparent interest in survival. The clearer, more knowledgeable, more insistent, and more recently affirmed the directive is, the stronger are the enduring interests of the once-capacitated person that the directive conveys. At the same time, the less the current person can anticipate tomorrow or remember yesterday, the weaker is the subjective value to her of surviving (Menzel and Steinbock 2013, 492–496; Menzel and Chandler-Cramer 2014, 28–29). We may disagree about just when the balance tips toward following the directive, but at some point in a disease like progressive dementia, it almost certainly will.[2]

This array of considerations about change of mind can be summarized:

- Valid revocation or revision of the AD is no longer possible once the level of decision-making capacity needed to write a directive is lost. (For legal qualifications to this claim, see Chapter 10, Section 10.8.)

- Expressions of apparent willingness to eat may be considered grounds for saying the person has capacity to decide to eat, but whether that capacity is sufficient to generate a relevant change of mind is highly questionable.

- As conditions like dementia progress into their final stages, any behavioral willingness to eat becomes so reflexive that it no longer reflects even the capacity to *decide* to eat.

- Provisions in an AD that specifically stipulate that any apparent urge or desire to eat should not be taken as sufficient grounds for setting aside the directive's instructions add considerably to the directive's moral weight, but they do not definitively resolve the conflict between the long-term interests conveyed by the person's directive and his currently experienced interest in survival. Eventually in the progression of a chronic condition like dementia, however, the interests conveyed by the directive win out because of the diminishing subjective value of survival to the patient.

- ADs to withhold oral feeding do not attempt to bind someone from changing their mind later when they still then have decision-making capacity. ADs for SED sometimes do mean to bind a person against their later objections when they are *no longer capacitated*, but such "Ulysses" contracts are not inherently objectionable. (See Chapter 10, Section 10.8, for legal considerations.)

---

[2] A related objection is that ADs to withhold oral feeding are "Ulysses contracts" (see also Chapter 10, Section 9). Ulysses contracts—contracts that prevent one from changing one's mind in the future—are often said not to be enforceable. A distinction, though, must be made between directives that would overrule "future *capacitated* objections" (objections made with decision-making capacity) and "directives to overrule future *incapacitated* objections" (Pope 2015, 392). The latter are true Ulysses contracts, and they are not objectionable. Only the former are objectionable, dismissing, as they do, later changes of mind when the person still has decision-making capacity. If ADs to withhold oral feeding are interpreted as denying patients the prerogative of changing their minds when they still have the appropriate capacity to do so, of course they are objectionable, but we are then just thrown back to the previous analysis of what kind of capacity is involved when patients with such directives later exhibit contrary desires. Dismissal of ADs to withhold oral feeding because they are allegedly all "Ulysses contracts" fails to make the relevant distinctions.

9.3. Is Feeding Fundamentally Different?

We have pursued this discussion of what constitutes valid change of mind with the implicit presumption that oral feeding lies within the legitimate scope of an AD. Is there something about oral feeding, however, that makes it relevantly different from the health care that patients ought to be able to control in their future incompetence?[3]

One view focuses on oral feeding as basic *personal care*, as distinct from health care (Bentley 2014, paras. 62–84; Menzel 2017, 690, ftn. 26). Advance directives may be appropriate for health care, extending as they do the basic right to refuse medical treatment. Perhaps refusal of oral feeding is no different, since a competent person has the right to refuse food and fluid, not just treatment. When people lose capacity, however, they often require assistance with the most basic and universal of human needs, independent of any health care. Food and fluids are among those needs, if anything is. When someone no longer has capacity and is unable to procure food and self-feed, one of the most basic caregiver obligations is to assist in feeding.

This argument, though initially attractive, is incomplete. Caregivers (whoever they are designated to be) may have an obligation to provide basic lifesaving health care measures, too, as meeting basic human need. Yet if a person refuses such care, either when competent or by an AD, the obligation is modified, if not removed. Why should the life-sustaining care of assisted feeding be any different? It will not do just to insist that "feeding is different." *How* is it ethically different if the person has refused it beforehand and has not had a valid change of mind?

It is important to keep in mind the context for oral feeding in the situations addressed by an AD. Usually such directives focus on withholding *manually assisted* feeding, not the preparing and offering of food for self-feeding. If that is the substance of the directive—not to spoon-feed appropriately prepared food when a person has reached a specified deteriorating condition— we may reasonably regard the directive as aimed at a basic health-sustaining measure. Medicine itself, after all, often pays a great deal of attention to adequate nutrition. Nursing home assistants who patiently and artfully spoon-feed and coax residents to swallow are doing more than just "feeding." The case for regarding assisted feeding of those who cannot self-feed as care

---

[3] Significant parts of the substance of this section were articulated in Menzel 2017, 690–695.

within the legitimate scope of advance refusal *is based on the same princi-*
ples of respect for individual persons, continuous ownership of a life, and self-
determination that undergird any advance directive.

A more contentious domain within the spectrum of feeding would be the
simple provision of food to a person who can still self-feed. Some may write
ADs to withhold that, too. One might argue that no non-arbitrary line can
be drawn between any of these different kinds of food provision, and that if
one kind may be refused by AD, any of them may be. We leave that question
open, contending only that the delicate, manually assisted feeding appropriate for most patients who cannot self-feed is truly life-sustaining care, not
the basic offering of food to someone who can self-feed.

In any case, advance refusal of food and water by mouth runs into other
objections. One concerns the legitimacy of a common reason for ADs for SED,
to lessen burdens on family and loved ones. Another concerns the distress, including moral distress, that withholding oral feeding from a non-capacitated
person can create for caregivers, beyond the distress that withholding basic
lifesaving treatment pursuant to a directive may create. We pursue each in turn.

9.4. Burdens of Survival on Family and Family Caregivers

A common reason people give for wanting to shorten their lives should they
become demented is the fear of burdening families and loved ones. This fear
is not unrealistic (Levine 2005).[4]

Some degree of burden on loved ones is inevitable. If my mother is suffering from dementia, no amount of the best care in the world is going to substitute for me, her daughter, visiting her. And some of that burden is going to
be emotional, especially if the person becomes abusive (Kleinman 2019) or
forgets who you are.

Some ethicists (Meilaender 1991) believe that the concern itself is illegiti-
mate, that just as children should not feel guilty for burdening their parents,
parents should not try to avoid burdening their children. Burdening each
other is simply part of being a family. From this perspective, refusing to
countenance dependency is a symptom of our over-individualistic culture.

---

[4] 83% of the care for older adults in the United States is provided by unpaid family and friends, and
half of that care goes to people with Alzheimer's. More than 1 million Americans provide unpaid care
for people with Alzheimer's (Alzheimer's Association 2020).

Some of the concern about "being a burden" reflects the difficulties of living in a less than ideal society. It thus reflects a larger problem for practical ethics generally: *how does one act justly in an unjust society*? Can we allow someone to sell a body part when they are driven to it by financial desperation? Do we say to the poor person, "Sorry, you can't sell your kidney, even though you are out of work and are about to be evicted from your home, because you are really being coerced by your poverty, but, no, we have no idea how we are going to actually change the system to get you the help you need." There is something very odd about this stance. The poor person is no better off because of our ethical concern, but they are constrained from making the choice they want to because, to tell the truth, allowing them to do that would make the rest of us too uncomfortable.

With respect to a decision to end one's life, be that with MAID, VSED, SED by AD, or some other method, we may find ourselves stuck in the same structural quandary. Most Americans would welcome a world in which aging people, and especially those with dementia, were not an overwhelming burden. However, people will continue to get older and life expectancy will likely continue to increase. Large families will become rarer, so that the typical aging parent will not be spreading the burden among numerous children. And women will continue to enter the workplace and to want careers, not just jobs, so they will be less available for caregiving. The only way to address the problem is through taxpayer-supported social services, plus welcoming immigrants who will fill the functions daughters used to perform and paying them a just wage to do it. None of this seems remotely on the horizon.

This problem was a large part of the debate about the first "Death with Dignity" laws. Some feminist writers and disability rights activists argued that the people who took advantage of those laws would come disproportionately from already marginalized populations: the poor, the elderly, the underinsured, and the lonely, who had nowhere else to turn. These commentators argued that the laws would allow us to push these people and their problems under the rug, under the guise of respecting their rights (Wolf 1996).[5]

It is fundamentally unfair to react to society's failings by denying autonomous choices to people who already have too little choice. Yes, it would be better if we found a cure for dementia. Yes, it would be better if people with dementia had access to really great care regardless of ability to pay. We

[5] However, statistics from the State of Oregon and from research studies showed that this concern was not borne out by the facts (Battin et al. 2007).

should get busy on those goals. But meanwhile, let people themselves decide how much of a burden they are willing to be.

Moreover, even if we were to make major progress to high-quality care that lifted financial and logistical burdens on family members, some people would strongly not want to live in a condition of great dependency. Thus, when people who prefer not to live into those conditions are forced to do so, family and caregivers will be emotionally burdened by the pain of witnessing their loved one's desires about the end of life left unsatisfied.

9.5. Caregiver and Proxy Distress

Moral distress occurs when a person knows the course of action she believes she ought to take, but is constrained from doing the right thing—or forced to do the wrong thing—by legal, institutional, financial, or other obstacles (Jameton 1992). Moral distress can cause acute discomfort, leading to burnout, lack of job satisfaction, and physical symptoms (Hamric 2012).

Just as it is prima facie wrong to cause physical distress to others, it is prima facie wrong to cause moral distress. After all, moral distress stems from the sincere desire of the person suffering it to do the right thing. Callous or cruel people do not experience moral distress. Avoiding causing moral distress is an important ethical goal, not only because we should attempt to avoid suffering, but because it seems especially wrong to inflict suffering based on the other person's conscience.

Most accounts and examples of moral distress explicitly or implicitly cast the distressed professional as a hero, who wants to do what everyone agrees is the right thing, but who is stymied by a callous, indifferent, or money-grubbing system. However, just because the distressed professional is motivated by compassion and may deserve our sympathy does not automatically mean she is right.[6] There are a number of scenarios in which moral distress appears to be pitted against an equally important value: autonomy at the end of life, especially in the case of people wishing to avoid dementia. What follows is a hypothetical scenario in which moral distress of health

---

[6] Legally, the need to take account of a health care provider's moral distress is limited. What a clinician thinks is "right" is personally value laden unless the patient is asking the provider to deviate from settled standards of care. The patient is asking her only to deviate from her own personal standards. Why should her values trump the patient's? Typically, they should not, though the clinician may assert a conscience-based objection (Chapter 4, Section 4.9).

professionals and caregivers threatens to derail respect for the patient's stated wishes.

The Case of Ms. Snyder

Ms. Snyder is 90 years old, diagnosed with Alzheimer's disease, and has lived in a nursing home for the last five years. She has outlived her siblings and close friends, and never married nor had children. Ms. Snyder had a long career as a foreign correspondent and could often be seen on television news, as she reported from some of the world's most dangerous "hot spots." Ms. Snyder fought to stay in her home as long as possible, but as her dementia progressed, her nephew Larry intervened and arranged the nursing home placement.

Before dementia struck and while still living on her own, Ms. Snyder had written a detailed advance directive, naming her nephew, Larry, as her health care proxy. She stated clearly that if she were ever to become cognitively compromised, she wanted to die as soon as possible. Specifically, she would not wish to live if she had to live in a nursing home. She gave some examples, such as not receiving antibiotics should she contract pneumonia and not being coaxed to eat should she lose her appetite.

Ms. Snyder took some months to adjust to the nursing home, but she eventually settled in quite well. She does not appear to be in physical pain. She likes the staff, although she cannot remember their names, and often smiles at them and strokes their arms. She especially enjoys the music sessions, where she claps to the music and moves in time in her wheelchair. One day, as an experiment, her nephew showed her a clip of herself on television, and she showed no recognition whatsoever that the intrepid reporter was her younger self.

Now, Ms. Snyder has come down with pneumonia. Larry reminds the staff that by the terms of her directive, she should be given no antibiotics. He feels a bit uncomfortable about this, because he appreciates that her current life is quite a pleasant one, but he is sustained in his course of action by his decades of memories of his fiercely independent aunt, and by the promises he made when he agreed to be her proxy.

The nursing staff and other caregivers are outraged by Larry's refusal. They have no experience of the independent, younger Ms. Snyder, but they do have five years' experience of this pleasant woman, enjoying her life and making personal connections. They see Ms. Snyder on a daily basis, whereas

Larry, who lives in another city, visits once a month. Were Larry refusing a burdensome therapy such as surgery or dialysis for his aunt, they would understand, but a simple antibiotic? They are sure that the present Ms. Snyder would prefer to go on living, and that their professional and moral duty is to support her health. When a temporary physician takes over the night shift, they simply tell him that Ms. Snyder has symptoms of pneumonia and request that he order an antibiotic. She recovers and enjoys two more years in the nursing home until dying of a stroke.

Ms. Snyder's situation could easily have unfolded with loss of appetite occurring before pneumonia, in which case Larry, following her directive, would have rejected any assistance that involved coaxing her to eat and drink. Accomplished as her facility's caregivers were in successfully getting residents to eat and drink, they would likely have been distressed by and resistant to that, too.

In this scenario the moral distress of the nursing staff is a challenge to the efficacy of Ms. Snyder's advance directive in two ways. First, Ms. Snyder, while she still had decision-making capacity, may have resisted writing a directive that had the likelihood of causing severe moral distress in others. She could realize that, if she is to spend any time in a nursing home before disease overtakes her, she wants to be treated with compassion and tenderness, even if she becomes irascible and difficult to care for. She wants to be cared for in that future by staff who are exceptional in their devotion, despite probably being overworked and underpaid. Is it fair to take steps that will almost certainly lead to the staff's moral distress?

Second, even if the competent Ms. Snyder is willing to risk causing moral distress to her caregivers, she has good reason to worry that once she becomes demented, her wishes will not be carried out. Moral distress may stop caregivers from acting according to her directives, especially if her values are not those of the mainstream. Ms. Snyder, after all, is now their responsibility, under their professional care, and it may be extremely difficult for them to accept withholding such basic and non-intrusive medication as an antibiotic or such basic care as artfully getting a person to eat and drink, even if providers may be obligated to respect a patient's clear directive regardless of their distress. Here again, if Ms. Snyder really wants to be sure that she will not spend many years in a nursing home, her best bet would seem to be preemptive suicide or VSED early enough in her dementia for her still to be capable of such a decision and carrying it out.

We also need to take into account the moral distress experienced by health care proxies when their loved ones become trapped in dementia. An agreement to act as someone's health care proxy, to hold their durable power of attorney, is a solemn pledge to do everything possible to help that person live or die in a manner consistent with their wishes and values. If Larry gives in and agrees to the antibiotic, he ought to feel moral distress for breaking his promise. We speak often in our society about the guilt people feel when they have to admit that they can no longer care for family members with dementia at home and must take them to some sort of "memory care" facility (Kleinman 2019). We ought to be able to speak more openly about the guilt one feels when one is unable to help that person attain their goal of a shorter life.

Thus some degree of moral distress is likely inevitable in this sort of situation, one that is becoming more and more common as people live longer and are more likely to have dementia. Not only is moral distress inevitable, but more than likely it will be experienced in more than one direction, both from those who support and those who oppose following the directive.

It is facile to say that professional caregivers should just be converted to the cause of patient autonomy and align their feelings to cohere with the principles laid down in an advance directive. Certainly, as a daughter and as her mother's health care proxy, one of us (Dena Davis) felt great moral distress throughout her mother's decade of dementia, even when her mother seemed to be enjoying herself. Davis was distressed when she imagined how her "real" mother would react could she suddenly see herself in the situation she was now in. It also helped that Davis and her mother shared fiercely autonomy-focused values. Although Davis's mother became a much nicer, sweeter woman with dementia than she had been while competent, Davis mourned the loss of her brusque, acerbic mother and would not have been distressed by implementing a directive that would hasten death. But that is partly because Davis had a lifetime in which to experience her "real" mother before dementia set in, which is not the case for most professional caregivers.[7] Someone who had not shared such time with the patient might

---

[7] The lack of staff familiarity with the pre-dementia person can be remedied to some degree if various mementos of the person's life are displayed or made available where they are being cared for—pictures, cover pages of any writing, a favorite letter, a craft the person made, perhaps even a video of some memorable or particularly indicative moment. Also enlightening, of course, would be articulation of the person's essential reasons and values for their directions in the AD, as would a video-directive. Family and friends might wisely attend to providing such material about their loved one.

be greatly distressed in feeling obliged to follow a death-hastening directive when the patient was still experiencing some enjoyment.

Moral distress should be acknowledged, explored, and addressed with sympathy and support, not cast off by advocates of ADs for SED as the avoidable problem of those who are distressed. At the same time, though, it ought not to be allowed to divert caregivers from following the person's wishes; if they cannot follow those clearly stated wishes, they should at least be obligated to refer to other caregivers. An advance directive is useful to the extent that people have good reason to believe that it will be followed when the person no longer has capacity. If people cannot count on that, fatalism or preemptive suicide become attractive options despite their own disadvantages.

9.6. The Odds of Implementation and the Attraction of Preemptive Measures

It is important to understand at what stages of dementia SED by AD would likely be carried out (see Chapter 8, Section 8.1, Table 8.1). The discussion here focuses primarily, as noted above, on the person who can no longer feed herself, has lost apparent interest in food, and is spoon-fed soft or puréed foods. According to the Mayo Clinic, requiring "total assistance with eating" is typical of the advanced stage of Alzheimer's, the stage at which one usually loses the ability to communicate coherently, be continent and go to the toilet, recognize family or caregivers, dress oneself, and so on. This final stage may follow a long progression, since the average person lives three to eleven years after diagnosis, with some people surviving more than 20 years (Mayo Clinic 2019).

If SED by advance directive is most likely to be feasible in the late stages of Alzheimer's when people cannot feed themselves, how useful is it in helping people to assert their autonomy and meet their goals once they no longer have decision-making capacity? Davis argues that it is not. To make that point, let us contrast what most people fear about dementia, with what SED by advance directive tries to promise, always remembering that in practice, implementation of an AD for SED will not likely be considered until a stage of dementia when the person is no longer able to self-feed or even express interest in food.

Why do people fear dementia, to the extent that it is now more feared than even cancer, and rated by some as a state worse than death (Patrick et al.

1994)? People who express interest in ending their lives rather than enduring advanced dementia usually do so from a mixture of motivations related to autonomy (distaste for a life of dependence), non-maleficence (a wish to avoid burdening others), and beneficence (preservation of assets to hand on to others). From the perspective of the not-yet demented person, impending dementia threatens some of one's most precious interests: (1) conservation and control over assets, (2) not burdening family, (3) independence and autonomy, and (4) preserving how one is remembered by others so that the final chapter does not distort the preceding narrative arc of one's life. Losing control over these interests is plausibly seen as a loss of dignity. Let us look at these four interests as they are threatened by enduring advanced dementia, and then compare them to the reality of a successful SED by AD when one becomes demented.

Conservation and Control over Assets. First, many people wish to conserve their assets to use in ways consistent with their long-held values, for example, to endow a scholarship fund at their alma mater or leave money for their grandchildren. During the final stages of Alzheimer's, the person usually needs round-the-clock care, which can be ruinously expensive. As one person memorably wrote in his advance directive, "Just because I may suffer from a disease that robs me of my cognitive capacity, that doesn't mean that I've made a decision that the prime beneficiaries of my estate shall then become hospitals, nursing homes, doctors, or leasers of medical devices" (Latham 2010).

Not Burdening Family. Second, people may wish to avoid burdening grown children with their care; this might be especially true of the feminists among us, as caregiving so often falls disproportionately on women. Most dementia care in the early and moderate stages is handled "informally" by family members, whose own health, finances, and quality of life often suffer dramatically.

Independence and Autonomy. Third, many people believe that their dignity and sense of self is tied up with at least some degree of autonomy and independence. This is not only a question of being able to drive, to handle one's finances, or to do one's own shopping, although all these mundane tasks can be heartbreaking to give up. There is also a sense of being a moral agent (an aspect of autonomy), which is increasingly lost as dementia progresses. What do we mean by being a "moral agent"? A moral agent is someone who is responsible for her actions, someone to whom one owes the truth and from whom one expects the truth, someone who can be held to a promise.

Everyone whose parent or partner has succumbed to dementia likely has some key moment which, looking back, they see as a turning point. Perhaps it is taking away the car keys, or when a parent no longer calls you by your name. In my case (Davis speaking now), I think of two moments having to do with moral agency. The first occurred in the early stages of my mother's dementia, while she was still living alone. That year, Hanukkah fell only a week after Thanksgiving. My mother wanted me to come home for both events. I resisted flying home two successive weekends, so I told my mother I would come for only one, but that she could choose. She reluctantly agreed, and chose Thanksgiving. I came, we cooked a turkey, we had a nice time, I flew home.

But two days later she was imploring me to come for Hanukkah. When I reminded her of our "deal," she insisted she had no memory of our bargain, and I am sure she was right. How does one hold someone to the terms of a promise she cannot remember? Would it have been cruel to have had her write it down and sign and date it, so I could show it to her later as evidence? Somehow that does not sit well. And yet, can one be a moral agent if one cannot make a promise? Should I have treated my mother like I would a four-year-old who promises to make her bed every day for the rest of her life if she can only have a lollipop now?

The second event, a few years later, involved lying. My mother had always detested even "social lies," and was incapable of lying herself. She hated people lying to her more than anything else, even cruelty. This presented a problem when the furnace in my mother's house died. The live-in caregiver arranged for the emergency installation of a new furnace, but my mother was beside herself with anxiety. A product of the Great Depression, she was always vulnerable to financial fears, although she was now well-off. How, she wondered, could she possibly pay for a new furnace? Her caregiver had no qualms about telling my mother that my brother had offered to pay, and insisted that I go along with the lie. Reluctantly, I did so. I knew the caregiver was right, that I could never convince my mother that there was enough money in the bank for a plethora of furnaces. But that day remains fixed in my mind as the day when my mother became "demoted" as someone to whom it was appropriate to lie.

Preserving How One Is Remembered by Others. Fourth, many people care a great deal about how they are remembered and wish to preserve the narrative arc of their lives. Ronald Dworkin writes, "We worry about the effect of [our] life's last stage on the character of [our] life as a whole, as we might worry about the effect of a play's last scene or a poem's last stanza on the entire creative work" (Dworkin 1993, 199). When that final scene lasts an average of eight years, one can reasonably fear that it will obscure the path of one's life. As legal scholar Norman Cantor declared, ending life with substantial dementia would be "a stain on my memory" (Cantor 2018).

If we think of how long the average victim of Alzheimer's takes before arriving at the final stage, it is clear that most if not all of these goals will have been defeated by the last severe stages. Over the course of three to eight years or longer, family members have likely been burdened with caregiving; daughters have perhaps lost their jobs or even their marriages. At least $5,000 a month is one estimate of the average cost of care in a memory loss facility, an expense few families can afford. The person's independence has been entirely eroded; she can no longer take herself to the toilet, dress, shower on her own, move about independently, or even identify the people who visit and care for her. And if she is someone who has always valued independence and autonomy, then, to paraphrase Dworkin, the narrative arc of her life has been deformed. Any intervention, SED or euthanasia, that comes into play only at the final stages of Alzheimer's does not meet many, perhaps even most, people's goals.

In summary, stopping eating and drinking by way of an advance directive may be an attractive option for those who are primarily concerned not to live into the final, most severe stages of dementia. But for those who are concerned with the issues described above, SED in the final stage (GDS/FAST 7, or perhaps 6) is a highly compromised solution. For them, the only truly realistic and assuring strategy may be preemptive suicide (by VSED or some other means) when one still has decision-making capacity and is decisive, which must always occur in an earlier stage of dementia. Even then, one would need to be careful not to wait too long, as executive function is sometimes significantly impaired in moderate and sometimes even in early dementia.

9.7. Comparison with Comfort Feeding Only

The previous chapter on clinical issues, in addition to addressing ADs for SED, dealt with a closely related, typically less controversial feeding limitation that can also potentially hasten death, "comfort feeding only" (CFO; see Chapter 8, Sections 8.1, 8.4, and 8.5). Defined broadly, CFO is offering as much or as little food and drink as patients appear to enjoy, without regard to what is nutritionally adequate for long-term survival. It can be used by patients with capacity but can also be specified in an AD. Four aspects of such comfort-oriented food and fluid limitation need clarification.

First, in practice CFO is seldom a specific level of food and drink but rather a range, from the minimum that avoids distress or discomfort for the patient to the maximum that the patient can tolerate without distress or discomfort, a level that may or may not be adequate for sustaining life. The conventional sense of CFO is *no more* than is compatible with comfort, *but no less* than what is needed for it—the "no-less/no-more" sense of CFO. The purpose of the CFO that is standard of care in traditional hospice, for example, is to provide enjoyment from eating and drinking but neither to hasten death nor to postpone it.

Second, in an AD for limiting food and drink, some people may direct CFO in a notably different sense, with the goal of not only maintaining comfort but also of gently hastening death. Thus the focus of any CFO included in such an AD would be the *minimum* needed for comfort—not less, but also not more than is needed for basic comfort. We refer to this as Minimum Comfort Feeding Only (MCFO, see Chapter 8, Section 8.1).

Third, if their aim includes hastening death at the appropriate time, those who write ADs may want to extend the limitation to *self-feeding only*—that is, to *not providing any assisted feeding*. Only the food and fluid that patients can self-administer will be provided, presumably in only the minimal amount and kind they can comfortably ingest.

Fourth, the most aggressive death-hastening step would be to *withhold all feeding, while making as comfortable as possible with maximal palliative measures*. One way to understand how such complete withholding from a patient who has lost capacity might be made comfortable is to compare it with VSED, where the dry-mouth, distress, and delirium experienced by capacitated patients who stop all eating and drinking can typically be managed with appropriate palliative care directed at alleviating discomfort without providing any food and fluid. If the non-capacitated person who is given nothing to eat or drink can also be kept comfortable by appropriate palliative care, potentially including proportionate sedation if needed for comfort, then that would be the best way to honor an AD requesting that all feeding be withheld. If withholding all food and fluids becomes too difficult because caregivers are not willing to provide adequate sedation, then MCFO could be the back-up approach.

Regardless of any such distinctions among CFO, MCFO, no assisted feeding, and more complete SED, the relationship between CFO on the one hand, and various degrees of SED by AD on the other, should always be kept clear. In the usual hospice approach, CFO can be clinical standard of care for patients whose interest is judged to be remaining comfortable, not living longer, but without directly or intentionally hastening death either. No formal AD is needed for limiting oral feeding to CFO if the approach for a particular patient is already Comfort Measures Only. Incapacitated patients who had previously indicated their desire for VSED but whose basic drive for food and drink was too strong to overcome, leading them at the time not to initiate VSED, could be managed with MCFO (see Chapter 8, Section 8.4). That basic drive and their comfort can be satisfied by feeding at a level well below what is nutritionally adequate. Since this would limit food and drink more than the usual hospice practice, MCFO would generally need to be supported by an AD reflecting the patient's wishes in this regard, or by a substituted judgment determination by a well-informed and trusted proxy.

All of the more extensive versions of withholding food and fluids beyond conventional CFO—MCFO for manually assisted feeding or self-feeding, no manually assisted feeding, and withholding all feeding—need AD support. An AD that explicitly stipulates any of these limitations will be essential for initiating any SED after decision-making capacity is lost. In any case, all of these options at the time of implementation should be accompanied by optimal palliative care.

Though CFO and ADs for even further limitations on food and drink need to be kept distinct, long-term support for ADs for SED may be boosted even by a conventional, no-less/no-more variety of CFO. CFO has already arguably achieved "standard of care" status in hospice (Fischberg et al. 2013, 597). Where it has achieved that status, comfort strongly dominates life extension as a goal of treatment. But if patients can also be kept comfortable when provided with MCFO, or with no assisted feeding, or when not fed at all, how much different in terms of patient well-being—and how much different morally—are any of these compared to conventional, standard-of-care CFO?

These points should not be misinterpreted as claiming that if CFO becomes standard of care in appropriate stages of severe dementia, it will have made ADs for more extensive withholding of oral feeding likely to be followed. ADs for SED may have a realistic likelihood of being implemented *if all of the person's relevant bases are covered.*[8] The implementation of an AD for limiting food and drink in such cases should be regarded as ethically legitimate, but undoubtedly, both ethically and practically, SED by AD will remain problematic compared to CFO that is standard of care. And it will certainly remain problematic compared to virtually any VSED by capacitated patients.

9.8. Conclusions

- A clear, competently written AD can have normative force for SED just as it does for refusing lifesaving treatment (RLST). The rights to VSED and RLST are established and grounded in the same values, and the essential principle behind ADs—one's rights are not lost when one loses decision-making capacity—applies to both. *Manually assisted* feeding, especially, is so similar to basic life-sustaining treatment that refusing it, too, should come within the legitimate scope of ADs.
- Change of mind is potentially an issue in implementing any AD, and especially ADs for SED since willingness to eat and drink can easily still be present when the triggering conditions set forth in the patient's advance directive are met. Seldom in the advanced stages of a progressive disease like dementia, however, does mere behavioral willingness to eat constitute a relevant change of mind.
- Implementing any AD—for RLST as well as SED—is vulnerable to the "then-self/now-self" problem. The problem cannot be dismissed, but neither does it destroy the relevance of ADs, including those for SED. Detailed instructions in an AD for SED about what should be done when the directive clashes with the patient's later willingness to eat can bolster the directive's normative force, but they do not completely resolve the then-self/now-self problem.
- Burdens to others from living long into a highly debilitated condition can be a legitimate reason for writing an AD for SED, even when these burdens are exacerbated by unfortunate and unjust social conditions that should be remedied.

---

[8] See the case of Charles, Case 7.4 in Chapter 7, and the recommended elements of an AD for SED in Appendix A. Especially important are clear statements in the AD of what is to be withheld and when, persuasive evidence in the record of decision-making capacity and substantive understanding at the time the directive was written, and appointment of a health care proxy with whom the person has discussed the directive.

- Caregiver and proxy distress, including moral distress, is virtually inevitable in implementing ADs for SED. Such prospective distress should be considered by anyone writing such an AD, but it does not pose an insurmountable ethical barrier to writing or implementing one.
- ADs for SED are useful to the extent that people have good reason to think proxies and caregivers loyal to the patient will follow them. This condition is likely to be met only in implementing such directives in the very late stages of a deteriorating condition. The earlier in the progression of the disease that the person wants to have her life shortened, the less useful ADs for SED become. In turn, the less useful they are, the more attractive preemptive VSED or preemptive suicide become to persons intent on not living long into such conditions.
- Comfort Feeding Only (CFO) can be "standard of care" in the very late stages of progressive conditions, especially if decision-making capacity is irreversibly lost, without needing to be requested in an AD. Minimal Comfort Feeding Only (MCFO) may also be appropriate, though it should ideally be specified in an AD. For less advanced stages of progressive conditions, it may be possible to limit feeding to "self-feeding only" (no manually assisted feeding under any circumstances, even when such feeding is comfortable for the patient), but only by a clear AD. Because it emphasizes comfort, not life extension, as the controlling purpose of care, however, CFO's achievement of clinical status as standard of care may establish significant precedent for SED by AD.
- While ADs for SED are problematic, they may be both ethically permissible and their prospect of being followed not unrealistic in circumstances where all their important ethical bases are covered, including having a demonstrably clear, well considered directive, and an appointed health care proxy who knows the patient well. Charles in Case 7.4 is an instructive example.

9.9. Ethical Issues Review of Initial Cases

Case 7.1. Mrs. H. with Early Alzheimer's: Preemptive VSED

Mrs. H. had known about VSED in detail from its successful use by an acquaintance. When her diagnosis with progressive dementia solidified, she was adamant about remaining at home. Several years later she raised the possibility of VSED. Realizing that SED by AD would be problematic, but being determined not to have her life end in severe dementia, she decided to do VSED while she had decision-making capacity and was sufficiently decisive. Her son (a physician) and other family members were supportive, but anxious about her ability to discern when to initiate VSED. Her conversations with a consulting physician led him first to tell the family that she's "serious about VSED, but not ready," and then, months later, "she's ready now."

Mrs. H. felt liberated from that time forward. Home hospice and VSED followed. Mouth discomfort was competently managed. She wanted her son to promise he would deny her food and drink even if she were to beg for it later; he refused, promising only that he would remind her of her basic VSED decision. When she later asked to sneak a sip of water, her son noted this could prolong dying but that he would satisfy her request, whereupon she said she would be "okay without it." She died nine days after initiating VSED.

Bottom Line Points
- If societal arrangements had allowed Mrs. H. to be confident that an AD for SED would be followed, she may well have chosen to live considerably longer. In the actual situation she saw preemptive VSED as her only reasonable option.
- Mrs. H was fortunate to have exemplary information about the process, clear support from her family, and optimal consultation and hospice care. Without these, clinical and ethical tensions could easily have been extreme, and she might have waited too long, her desire to avoid living into the later years of progressive dementia never satisfied.
- Amid the VSED process, her physician son handled her request to "sneak" a sip of water by reminding her that this could prolong her dying, but allowing her to do so. She seemed to understand and quickly said she would be okay without it. Artful physician response to a still-discerning patient produced a good ending; in other cases with the same issues, things may not work out as well.

Case 7.2. Steve with Early Dementia: Family and Patient Challenges

Despite resisting his diagnosis of mild cognitive impairment, Steve is clear about what he wants to have happen were he to reach advanced dementia: stop all oral intake sometime in Stage 6, when he can no longer feed himself. He has written his AD to that effect and expects it to be carried out by wife Jennifer and his primary physician. He seems to understand VSED well and has completed a "Five Wishes" values statement to explain and supplement his AD.

Jennifer arranged for a number of family discussions with Steve, facilitated by an experienced consulting nurse. Some of these meetings have been very emotional. Steve is adamant that he never be placed in a nursing home and that, in carrying out his directive, his family must ignore any requests for food or fluid he might make. He shows little concern for difficulties his family might experience in attempting to honor his requests. The consulting nurse has suggested comfort-oriented feeding as an alternative, but Steve has rejected it on the grounds that it would come too late and unduly prolong his life.

Three years after initial diagnosis, Steve continues to resist any explicit dementia diagnosis. He has not changed his AD, however, and he has never wavered in his insistence about what should happen if he becomes severely demented. The case is ongoing.

Bottom Line Points
- Given his already emerging dementia and his denial of it at the same time that he writes an insistent AD for SED, how clear is it that Steve has sufficient cognitive capacity to write such a directive?
- Though he has decisional capacity at this point, does he understand the distress and difficulty that following his directive may well cause his family? If he does understand it, is it fair for him to place on his family the responsibility of implementing his directive and discerning just when to do that? Is his wife, to whom he accords primary responsibility, up to the task?
- As the family discussions continue, the lack of any communication with his physician on these matters is unfortunate.
- The discussion process in which Steve and his family have been involved is laudable. Even if it does not eventually resolve their differences, at least they will have aired them, and his family will understand better his views and beliefs.

Case 7.3. Patricia with Moderate Dementia: AD for SED, or Preemptive Suicide?

At 91, Patricia had already been in Stage 4 Alzheimer's disease five years. Her hope to find a like-minded community of academics in a care facility was disappointed as her growing short-term memory deficit inhibited social interaction. She was determined to be in charge of her dying.

VSED was daunting to her, however, both because of the suffering she envisioned it to involve and because she had always greatly enjoyed food and drink. She therefore wrote her AD for "comfort feeding only," though a "no manually assisted feeding" instruction was also attractive to her. Meanwhile, she had a previously acquired stash of barbiturates for a potential overdose. She understood the potential legal jeopardy for her family and that they could not be present when she swallowed the pills. She was also anxious she might not remember the necessary steps and precautions.

Months later, she determined that the barbiturate overdose was the best solution. Aware that her window of opportunity would soon close, she acted, carefully and effectively without family present. Upon finding out, they were "shocked but not surprised." Her memorial was well attended and rich with positive memories.

Bottom Line Points
- Patricia feared the suffering from SED pursuant to an AD, despite the accurate information she received that palliative support would likely manage most of it. While conventional CFO reinforced by an AD was a feasible option, she did not want to have to limit her oral intake. In any case, such a modest limitation of feeding would not, in her mind, hasten death soon enough.
- As anyone resorting to preemptive suicide should do, Patricia carefully protected her family from legal liability.
- After its initial suggestion, the nurse consultant and her family did not further press the SED by AD option. VSED, whether contemporaneous or by AD, is not for everyone. Nonetheless, one wonders whether society could legitimize an inclusive enough version of SED by AD that people like Patricia could live longer into their still-acceptable years and not have to resort to preemptive VSED or suicide.
- Open communication among Patricia and her family was exemplary, facilitated in part by the experienced consulting nurse.

Case 7.4. Charles with Severe Dementia: A Successful Use of an AD for SED

Early in his progressive dementia, Charles developed his AD for SED by responding to a lengthy series of choices about different steps to take in various conditions in advancing dementia, steps ranging from continuing manually assisted feeding to completely withholding food and water. In several recorded interviews, his advance planning counselor and psychiatrist verified his capacity to make these choices and his understanding of them. He was well informed about what it would be like to die from dehydration if good palliative support were provided.

Years later, the triggering conditions stated by Charles in his directive were met, and his wife, as appointed proxy, asked the attending physician to honor his directive. The physician refused, alleging that this "would cause Charles great discomfort as it destroys his internal organs" and that it would be in Charles' best interest to continue CFO. After being presented with a copy of the AD for SED, the audio recording of Charles' testimony, several other documents, and the psychiatrist's willingness to be consulted about the directive and its development, the main treating physician acquiesced in the wife's decision to follow it. Charles died peacefully nine days later.

Bottom Line Points
- Virtually all the pieces of an ideal AD for SED were in place: a sufficiently detailed directive regarding what to withhold and when, recorded lengthy interviews by a psychiatrist verifying Charles' understanding of his choices and the personal values behind them, strong support of his wife for implementing the AD, and no conflict within his family.
- At time of implementation, his primary care physician objected to withholding assisted feeding on the grounds that that would not be in Charles' best interest. The physician's change of mind to follow the decision of his wife/proxy illustrates the clinical and ethical persuasiveness of having not merely a written directive, but additional material to verify the patient's understanding of it. Sometimes conflicting interpretations of patient best interest are resolved by a demonstrably competent and sufficiently clear AD.
- The patient did not in any way plead for food or drink at time of implementation, avoiding one of the most difficult complications for SED by AD. In part because of his behavior, Charles' SED by AD caused little if any moral distress.
- The case illustrates how in the appropriate circumstances, with all pieces in place for ethically implementing an AD for SED, withholding all manually assisted food and drink, not just CFO, can become a more accepted option for hastening death.

References

Battin, Margaret P., Agnes van der Heide, Linda Ganzini, Gerrit van der Wal, and Bregje D. Onwuteaka-Phillipsen. 2007. "Legal Physician-assisted Dying in Oregon and the Netherlands: Evidence Concerning the Impact on Patients in 'Vulnerable' Groups." *Journal of Medical Ethics* 33: 591–597.

Bentley v. Maplewood Seniors Care Society, 2014 BCSC 165 (Feb. 3, 2014).

Bentley v. Maplewood Seniors Care Society, 2015 BCCA 91 (Mar. 5, 2015).

Berghmans, Ron. 2000. "Advance Directives and Dementia." *Annals of the New York Academy of Sciences* 913 (January): 105–110.

Cantor, Norman L. 2017. "Changing the Paradigm of Advance Directives to Avoid Prolonged Dementia." *Bill of Health* (blog by the Petrie-Flom Center, Harvard Law School, April 20, 2017), http://blogs.harvard.edu/billofhealth/2017/04/20/changing-the-paradigm-of-advance-directives/.

Cantor, Norman L. 2018. "On Avoiding Deep Dementia." *Hastings Center Report* 48, no. 4: 15–24.

Dresser, Rebecca, and John S. Robertson. 1989. "Quality of Life and Non-Treatment Decisions for Incompetent Patients." *Law, Medicine & Health Care* 17, no. 3: 234–244.

Dworkin, Ronald. 1993. *Life's Dominion: An Argument about Abortion, Euthanasia, and Individual Freedom.* New York: Oxford University Press.

Fischberg, Daniel, Janet Bull, David Casarett, Laura C. Hanson, Scott M. Klein, Joseph Rotella, Thomas Smith, C. Porter Storey Jr., Joan M. Teno, and Eric Widera for the AAHPM Choosing Wisely Task Force. 2013. "Five Things Physicians and Patients Should Question in Hospice and Palliative Medicine." *Journal of Pain and Symptom Management* 45, no. 3: 595–605.

Hammond, Katherine. 2016. "Kept Alive—The Enduring Tragedy of Margot Bentley." *Narrative Inquiry in Bioethics* 6, no. 2 (summer): 80–82.

Hamric, Ann B. 2012. Empirical Research on Moral Distress: Issues, Challenges, and Opportunities. *HEC Forum* 24: 39–49.

Jameton, Andrew. 1992. "Dilemmas of Moral Distress: Moral Responsibility and Nursing Practice." *Awohnn's Clinical Issues in Perinatal and Women's Health Nursing* 4, no. 4: 542–551.

Kleinman, Arthur. 2019. *The Soul of Care: The Moral Education of a Doctor.* New York: Viking/Penguin Random House.

Latham, Stephen R. 2010. "Living wills and Alzheimer's disease." *Quinnipiac Probate Law Journal* 23: 425–431.

Levine, Carol. 2005. *Always on Call: When Illness Turns Families into Caregivers, 2nd ed.* Nashville: Vanderbilt University Press.

Mayo Clinic Staff. 2019. "Alzheimer's Stages: How the Disease Progresses" (April). https://www.mayoclinic.org/diseases-conditions/alzheimers-disease/in-depth/alzheimers-stages/art-20048448.

Meilaender, Gilbert. 1991. "I Want to Burden My Loved Ones." *First Things* (October): 12–14.

Menzel, Paul T. 2017a. "Change of Mind: An Issue for Advance Directives." In *Ethics at the End of Life: New Issues and Arguments*, edited by John K. Davis, 126–137. New York: Routledge.

Menzel, Paul T. 2017b. "Three Barriers to VSED by Advance Directive: A Critical Assessment." *Seattle Journal for Social Justice* 15, no. 3: 673–700. http://digitalcommons. law.seattleu.edu/sjsj/vol15/iss3/12.

Menzel, Paul T., and M. Colette Chandler-Cramer. 2014. "Advance Directives, Dementia, and Withholding Food and Water by Mouth." *Hastings Center Report* 44, no. 3 (May–June): 23–37.

Menzel, Paul T., and Bonnie Steinbock. 2013. "Advance Directives, Dementia, and Physician-Assisted Death." *Journal of Law, Medicine & Ethics* 41, no. 2 (Summer): 484–500.

Patrick, Donald L., Helene E. Starks, Kevin C. Cain, Richard F. Uhlmann, and Robert A. Pearlman. 1994. "Measuring Preferences for Health States Worse than Death." *Medical Decision Making* 14, no. 1 (January–March): 9–18.

Pope, Thaddeus M. 2015. "Prospective Autonomy and Ulysses Contracts for VSED," one of two sections of Thaddeus M. Pope and Bernadette J. Richards, "Decision-Making: At the End of Life and the Provision of Pretreatment Advice." *Journal of Bioethical Inquiry* 12, no. 3 (September): 389–394.

Rhoden, Nancy. 1990. "The Limits of Legal Objectivity." *North Carolina Law Review* 68, no. 5: 845–865.

Wolf, Susan M. 1996. "Gender, Feminism, and Death: Physician-Assisted Suicide and Euthanasia." In *Feminism and Bioethics: Beyond Reproduction*, edited by Susan M. Wolf, 282–317. New York: Oxford University Press.

10

Legal Issues

Thaddeus M. Pope

10.1. Introduction

In Chapter 4 we established that individuals with decision-making capacity have a legal right to VSED and that clinicians may legally support individuals who VSED. We further established that this right is generally recognized by lawmakers and professional medical societies. But the analysis and discussion in Chapter 4 was premised on the assumption that the individual had decision-making capacity when she began VSED. We now address the rights of incapacitated individuals to have food and drink withheld.

Stopping eating and drinking for an incapacitated individual is fundamentally different from contemporaneous VSED. Therefore, not only the legal analysis but also the terminology is different. Since an incapacitated individual cannot "voluntarily" decide to stop eating and drinking, VSED for these patients is best represented as "SED," without the "V." The individual's incapacity means that the decision to SED must be made by someone else on their behalf. Since authorization for this decision typically (though not always) comes from the patient's advance directive, we refer to this exit option as "SED by AD."

While the advance directive is our primary focus, there are three different mechanisms by which care decisions can be made for individuals when they cannot make them for themselves. First, the instructional advance directive (also known as a living will) allows caregivers to hear from the patient himself.[1] The individual can specify in his own words whether and when he would not want food and fluids. Second, a proxy advance directive (also known as a durable power of attorney for health care) appoints an agent who

---

[1] Increasingly, patients are supplementing their written advance directives with audio and video recordings (Pope 2020). So, the clinician and family may not only read but also listen to and watch the patient's recorded wishes.

can make that decision on the individual's behalf. Third, if the patient has not completed a proxy advance directive, then a surrogate will be appointed for him. Most surrogates are appointed by health care providers pursuant to statutory priority lists. Occasionally, a court appoints a guardian or conservator.

Authorization for every type of substitute decision-making mechanism is typically specified in state statutes. Because this statutory language varies materially from jurisdiction to jurisdiction, so does the permissibility of SED by AD. Individuals may be able to circumvent statutory obstacles in two ways: (1) by completing a non-statutory advance directive, or (2) by completing an advance directive in a state where SED by AD is permitted and having it recognized in their home state. Yet, those are imperfect solutions. As we discussed in Chapter 4 (Section 4.2), there is a gap between technical legal validity and what is recognized and honored as legally valid.

Furthermore, assuring the validity of an AD for SED is not the only challenge. Even in jurisdictions where SED by AD is permitted, there may be challenges in application. Most notably, once they reach late-stage dementia, some individuals may make utterances or gestures that suggest they want food and water. In many states, this constitutes a revocation of the AD for SED even though the patient lacks capacity. Below (in Section 10.9), we extend the discussion of Ulysses contracts from Chapter 9 (Section 9.2). We suggest that individuals may be able to resolve the contradiction between the wishes of their past self and their present self by including "Ulysses clause" language in their advance directives.

10.2. There Is Little On-Point Precedent

In Chapter 4 we summarized nearly a dozen court cases holding that clinicians may (and must) honor a capacitated individual's decision to VSED. In contrast, we have no such explicit judicial guidance on SED by AD (Pope 2018a; Pope 2019a; Pope 2019b). This is no surprise. At least one sample AD for SED was published 25 years ago (Hensel 1996). But that publication was the exception until recently, when SED by AD became more widely discussed and promoted. Because the courts have not yet addressed the permissibility of SED by AD, it remains unsettled whether an individual may use an advance directive or surrogate decision-maker to restrain caregivers from offering her food and fluids when she later reaches a pre-defined state of advanced dementia (Pope and Anderson 2011).

While there is no judicial precedent specifically addressing SED by AD, there is growing authority holding that clinicians must honor advance directives in general (Pope 2017a; Pope 2017b). Health care providers have been increasingly subjected to civil liability and disciplinary sanctions for administering treatment interventions without appropriate authorization. Furthermore, many states continue to refine their cases, statutes, and regulations to better assure compliance with advance directives (Pope 2013).

10.3. Draft the Advance Directive Carefully

Before examining whether SED by AD may be or must be honored, it is important to clarify what constitutes a request for SED by AD in the first place. In two recent cases, North American courts found it unnecessary to address the legal questions concerning the permissibility of SED by AD, because the patients had not clearly requested SED in their advance directives.

Margot Bentley (Canada). Margaret Anne Bentley (Margot) was a retired nurse who cared for patients suffering from dementia during her career. Partially as a result of those experiences, in 1991 she executed an advance directive that stated, "If at such a time the situation should arise that there is no reasonable expectation of my recovery from extreme physical or mental disability, I direct that I be allowed to die and not be kept alive by artificial means or heroic measures" (Bentley 2014; Bentley 2015). Margot also listed specific instructions, including "no nourishment or liquids." She designated her husband and daughter as her surrogate medical decision-makers (Pope 2015).

In 1999, Margot was diagnosed with Alzheimer's disease. Consistent with her advance directive, Margot repeatedly told her family that she wished to be allowed to die when she reached advanced dementia. That soon happened. By 2005, Margot's condition had deteriorated to the point that she needed to be moved to a residential care facility.

In 2013, at age 82, Margot was diagnosed with stage 7 Alzheimer's (severe dementia). She was in a near vegetative state. She did not recognize or respond to her family. She lost all verbal abilities and basic psychomotor skills. She neither spoke nor made more than very limited physical movements. She spent her days "motionless in bed or slumped in a wheelchair" with her eyes closed. Most importantly, she required spoon-feeding by caregivers (Bentley 2014).

Margot's family wanted to honor her advance directive and other instructions. So, once Margot had reached severe dementia, her family asked the care facility to stop providing food and liquids. But the facility refused to stop feeding Margot. The facility also refused to allow the family to transfer Margot either home or to another care facility. Frustrated, in August 2013 Margot's husband and daughter petitioned the court for declaratory relief that would prohibit the facility from providing Margot with oral nutrition and hydration.

The family lost. In February 2014, the Supreme Court of British Columbia denied the family's petition (*Bentley* 2014; *Bentley* 2015). The court was troubled because the meaning of Margot's advance directive was unclear. The court observed that the phrase "no nourishment or liquids" appears under a broader heading, "I direct that I . . . not be kept alive by artificial means or heroic measures." Therefore, the court concluded that the best interpretation of the phrase "no nourishment or liquids" was that it did not refer to oral food and fluid. Instead, this phrase was just a specification of one particular type of "artificial means or heroic measures" that Margot did not want.

Significant evidence from Margot's family indicates that she wanted SED by AD to avoid living in late-stage dementia (Hammond 2016; Fayerman 2016). But Margot's written advance directive was not explicit or clear about that fact. Her advance directive never mentioned or described SED. Nor did it mention any synonymous descriptions like a desire to stop (a) oral food and fluids, (b) nutrition and hydration by mouth, (c) normal feeding, (d) hand-feeding, or (e) spoon-feeding.

Nora Harris (United States). The advance directive of the patient in the second court case suffered from the same defects as Margot's advance directive. In June 2009, 56-year-old Californian Nora Harris was diagnosed with Alzheimer's disease. She drafted an advance directive stating that she did not want nutrition and hydration in an advanced state of dementia. Nora and her husband then moved to Oregon because it had lower health care costs. In 2013, Nora's husband admitted her to Fern Gardens, a memory care facility (*Harris* 2016).

In 2016, Nora's husband discovered that clinicians at Fern Gardens were spoon-feeding Nora, contrary to her wishes. He tried to have the spoon-feeding stopped, but he was overruled by the Oregon ombudsman for long-term care. So, Nora's husband filed a lawsuit asking the court to order Fern Gardens to stop. He argued that "there was overwhelming evidence and testimony that she wouldn't want to be spoon-fed" (*Harris* 2016).

Nora's husband lost. In July 2016, an Oregon trial court refused to issue the injunction. The judge refused to order the nursing home to stop spoon-feeding Nora because her advance directive, like Margot's advance directive, addressed only "artificial" nutrition and hydration. The advance directive never explicitly mentioned food and fluid by mouth. Therefore, the court never addressed the question of whether the facility had to honor Nora's wishes. It was unclear what her wishes were. By this time, Nora lacked capacity to express wishes regarding her care. And her advance directive was too vague to convey whether she would want help eating and drinking in her current state (Aleccia 2017).

Margot Bentley and Nora Harris were unable to SED by AD as they apparently had wanted. But we can learn from their failures. Today, there are more planning tools and strategies that can help individuals avoid drafting pitfalls by better reflecting upon and more clearly documenting their wishes regarding SED by AD. We collect citations or links to nearly a dozen of these in Appendix B at the end of this book.

One widely discussed tool for SED by AD is the End of Life Choices New York "Advanced Directive for Receiving Oral Foods and Fluids in Dementia" (End of Life Choices New York 2020). It includes an option, "If I am suffering from advanced dementia and appear willing to accept food or fluid offered by assisted or hand feeding, my instructions are that I do NOT want to be fed by hand even if I appear to cooperate in being fed by opening my mouth."

In contrast, some dementia directive tools are focused on comfort feeding only (CFO) instead of SED by AD. As discussed in Chapters 8 and 9, these are common alternatives to SED by AD. For example, End of Life Washington designed its "My Instructions for Oral Feeding and Drinking" to allow stopping attempts to give food and water only when the individual "loses interest in eating or drinking" (End of Life Washington 2020).

Whichever tool one uses, it is important to specify at least three separate things. First, be more precise and explicit than Bentley and Harris. Clarify *what* you want. Clarify whether you want CFO (and which type—minimal, usual, or maximal) or SED. Second, clarify *when* you want it to be initiated. Third, specify how your caregivers should measure the satisfaction of that condition. For example, in the case of Steve in Chapter 7, he decided that he wanted SED "at stage 6 of the FAST scale." Stanley Terman's *My Way Cards* are a particularly good tool for reflecting on the "when" question (Terman 2011; Appendix B).

It is no surprise that more SED by AD tools are being developed and disseminated. Many individuals are afraid of living in late-stage dementia when they cannot participate in activities that they find meaningful or enjoyable. For example, by Alzheimer's Stage 7 of GDS or FAST (see Chapter 8, Section 8.1), individuals need constant supervision and frequently require professional care with activities of daily living such as toileting and bathing. They are unable either to recognize the faces of close friends and relatives or to remember most details of their personal history. They lose the ability to communicate or respond to their environment.

A significant number of individuals hasten their deaths with VSED to avoid living with late-stage dementia or other diseases that cause a permanent loss of decision-making capacity.[2] Unfortunately, VSED is often an inadequate solution. Since it requires that the individual act before losing capacity, VSED may necessitate that the individual act earlier than they prefer (Volicer, Pope, and Steinberg 2019). They must act while they still find life worthwhile. As illustrated in the cases of Mrs. H. and Patricia in Chapter 7, the timing of VSED is difficult and fraught. Because it is uncertain when the individual will lose capacity and the "window of opportunity" will close, individuals frequently must err on the side of acting early, as we saw in the case of Patricia.

10.4. Non-Statutory Advance Directives Potentially Allow SED by AD

Now that we have established what constitutes a sufficiently clear request for SED by AD, we can address the legality of such requests. Many commentators start and end their analysis by focusing on whether SED by AD fits within the "four corners" of a jurisdiction's advance directive statute. They do this because statutory advance directive laws are often "perceived as the exclusive legal pathway" for ensuring that one's wishes are known and respected when one loses capacity (Sabatino 2007).

This is wrong. Assessing the legality of an advance directive solely by reference to the jurisdiction's advance directive statute is an unnecessarily restrictive approach (Meisel et al. 2020 § 7.01[B][8]). As we will see below, advance

---

[2] Increasingly, families are documenting these cases in books and films (Brosio 2019; Clevenger 2019). We collect many of these in Appendix E at the end of this book.

directive statutes often impose limits that do not permit SED by AD. But these limits and constraints can be circumvented. There is no requirement that an advance directive satisfy the statutory requirements to be valid and enforceable.[3]

As we saw in Chapter 4, individuals have broad rights to refuse unwanted interventions. These rights are grounded in common law and constitutional law, and they are not constrained by statute (Cantor 2020; O'Sullivan 2017). First, many advance directive statutes include non-preemption language providing that they do not impair or supersede existing rights regarding health care decision-making authority. For example, Florida clarifies that its statutory provisions are "cumulative to the existing law . . . and do not impair any existing rights or responsibilities . . . under the common law, federal Constitution, state constitution, or statutes" (Florida § 765.106).

Second, while state statutes could impair a common law right, without non-preemption language, they could not impair a constitutional right. For example, the Puerto Rico advance directive statute provided that clinicians could honor advance directives only when the patient is terminally ill. The commonwealth's supreme court held this limitation was unconstitutional (Tirado 2010). After all, in 1990 the U.S. Supreme Court ruled that patients have a federal constitutional right to refuse treatment through an advance directive even when they are not terminally ill (Cruzan 1990).

While less commonly discussed than statutory advance directives, non-statutory directives are specifically authorized. For example, Michigan has no statute recognizing instructional advance directives (aka living wills). No statute specifies what elements are necessary to create a binding document. Nevertheless, the state supreme court held that instructional advance directives are valid (Martin 1995). Similarly, while Idaho has an advance directive statute, it requires that "any authentic expression of a person's wishes with respect to health care should be honored" (Idaho § 39-4509(3)).

Michigan and Idaho are not unique. Individuals may complete non-statutory directives in other states, too. For example, Estelle Browning wrote a Florida advance directive stating her desire not to have artificial nutrition and hydration. Estelle later suffered a stroke which resulted in permanent

---

[3] For many years, Oregon required use of the official state advance directive form. In 2018, the legislature amended this requirement to require only that it "be written in substantially" the form specified in the statute (Oregon 2018).

brain damage, making her unable to swallow. Her condition was not terminal, because she could live for an indeterminate time with artificial nutrition. This was a problem because the Florida statute authorized advance directives only when patients are terminal. Consequently, Estelle's surrogate had difficulty enforcing the advance directive.

Ultimately, Estelle and her surrogate succeeded when the state supreme court held that Estelle's advance directive could (and should) be followed. The court explained that following the statute was optional. Estelle's right to complete a statutory advance directive was "cumulative to [her] existing rights . . . by statute, common law, or constitution" (Browning 1990).

Nevertheless, technical legality diverges from practical enforceability. While a non-statutory AD for SED is probably legally valid for the same reasons that VSED is legal, health care providers may refuse to honor it. First, non-statutory directives are not as clearly and obviously valid as advance directives that comply with black and white, bright line statutory requirements (Meisel 1995). There is a material difference between having a constitutional right and being able to exercise that right. For example, the U.S. Supreme Court ruled that Nancy Cruzan had a constitutional right to refuse treatment (Cruzan 1990). But the court did not issue that ruling until December 14, 1990, more than three years after Nancy's parents first requested the withdrawal of treatment (on May 28, 1987).

Second, advance directive statutes offer more than just clarity in validity. They also offer civil, criminal, and disciplinary immunity for good faith compliance (California § 4740). It is less clear that immunity applies to non-statutory directives (Meisel et al. 2020 §§ 7.01[C][3], 7.05[B], 7.03[F], 11.11). This uncertainty is salient to clinicians whose perceptions of the law are often more rigid and defensive compared to what the law actually requires.

In sum, while likely enforceable through judicial action, non-statutory directives may not be practically enforceable with health care providers (Margolis 2020). Nevertheless, while it may not be prudent to use a non-statutory advance directive *instead* of a statutory advance directive, it is prudent to *supplement* a statutory advance directive. Charles' case in Chapter 7 illustrates the value of an audio recording. An audio or video recording helps clarify the individual's intent and that she completed the advance directive with capacity and understanding (Pope 2020). Accordingly, the tools collected in this book's Appendix B are intended to supplement, not replace, traditional advance directives.

10.5. Some Advance Directive Statutes Permit SED by AD

In assessing whether SED is legally authorized by an advance directive, we must first determine whether the statute allows decisions regarding eating and drinking. There are four variations. First, some advance directive statutes explicitly permit SED by AD. Second, some statutes probably permit SED by AD because they allow individuals to leave binding instructions as to both health care and personal care. Third, some statutes specifically prohibit SED by AD. Fourth, in the remaining states that authorize only instructions for "health" care, it is unclear whether SED by AD is authorized.

1. **Explicitly Authorized.** In October 2019, a new Nevada statute became the first to explicitly recognize the legitimacy of SED by AD (Pope 2019b). The law authorizes a new "dementia directive" that includes an "End-of-Life Decisions Addendum Statement of Desires." This Addendum permits the individual to choose "yes" or "no" to the following statement: "I want to get food and water even if I do not want to take medicine or receive treatment" (Nevada § 162A.870).

This "food and water" statement clearly addresses SED, because it is an option framed as an alternative to "medicine" and "treatment." Nevada law considers "artificial" nutrition and hydration as medical treatment. For example, the standard durable power of attorney for health care form refers to artificial nutrition and hydration as "treatment." Therefore, the dementia directive's language contrasting "food" and "water" with "treatment," clearly references hand-feeding or food and fluid by mouth.[4]

2. **Probably Authorized.** While not as explicit as Nevada, advance directive laws in other jurisdictions also probably authorize SED by AD. In Canada, for example, two recent scholarly reviews concluded that most Canadian provinces permit SED by AD (Mader and Apold 2019; Trowse 2019). In the United States, Vermont permits individuals to provide directions about not only their "health care" but also about their "personal circumstances" (Vermont § 9702(a)(12)). Indeed, a statutory Vermont directive may direct whether the individual rejects "services to assist in activities of daily living

---

[4] The framing of the Nevada form suggests the statement of desires is triggered only when the patient is "sick and suffering." Some potential users might be concerned that such prerequisite conditions for SED by AD will not be satisfied because patients in late-stage dementia often do not experience present suffering. But this potential challenge is easily circumvented by eliminating the reference to "suffering." The statute requires only that a dementia directive be "substantially in the . . . form" specified in the statute.

provided by a health care provider or in a health care facility or residential care facility" (Vermont §§ 9702(a)(5), 9701(12)). Eating and drinking are surely "activities of daily living."

3. Prohibited. While some states definitely or probably authorize SED by AD, many others specifically prohibit it.[5] For example, while Colorado permits individuals to "direct that life-sustaining procedures be withheld or withdrawn," it excludes "interventions for nourishment" unless supplied through a tube or intravenously (Colorado §§ 15-18-104(1), 15-18-103(3), 15-18-103(10)). Wisconsin provides that individuals may authorize the withholding or withdrawal of nutrition or hydration "that is administered or otherwise received by the declarant through means other than a feeding tube" only when such "administration is medically contraindicated" (Wisconsin § 154.03(1); Wisconsin Attorney General 2014).

In other states, what appear to be prohibitions may not apply to SED by AD. For example, Maryland requires health care providers to make "reasonable efforts to provide an individual with food and water by mouth and to assist the individual as needed to eat and drink voluntarily." But if the individual has specifically refused such assistance in her advance directive, then this duty is probably discharged. It is not "reasonable" to provide food and water to an individual who has directed SED by AD (Maryland § 5-611(d)).

4. Unclear. In the remaining states the permissibility of SED by AD is unclear because of vague language. For example, in Tennessee an advance directive can direct withholding of "health care" (Tennessee § 68-11-1803). This is defined as "any care, treatment, or service, or process to . . . affect an individual's physical . . . condition and includes medical care" (Tennessee 68-11-1802(a)(6)). While "health" care is broader than "medical" care, it still does not necessarily include hand-feeding. Yet, at least with respect to late-stage dementia patients, their dependence on licensed providers (like CNAs and RNs) in a licensed facility makes the case strong.

Similarly, in Minnesota, the relevant statute defines "health care" as "any care, treatment, service, or procedure to maintain, diagnose, or otherwise affect a person's physical or mental condition" (Minnesota Statutes). This

---

[5] These statutes include Alabama, Idaho, Iowa, and Wyoming (Alabama § 8A-4(a); Oklahoma § 3101.8; Iowa §§ 144B.2, 144A.3(1), 144A.2(8); Idaho §§ 39-4510, 39-4514(4); Wyoming §§ 35-22-402, 35-22-403(a)).

definition may include hand-feeding, because hand-feeding is a "service or procedure" that "affects a person's physical . . . condition." Arguably, since individuals may refuse any "health care" in a Minnesota advance directive, they may direct SED by AD. Yet, this conclusion is not as certain as in Nevada or Vermont.

10.6. Many Advance Directive Statutes Require Triggering Conditions

Even if an advance directive statute permits decisions regarding SED, many of these statutes impose various "triggering" conditions. In other words, advance directive statutes limit not only "what" may be withheld or withdrawn but also "when." One almost universal triggering condition is that the advance directive does not take effect until the patient lacks capacity. This condition is not problematic, because it aligns with the very purpose of advance directives.[6] But other common conditions require that the advance directive (or at least its provisions regarding nutrition and hydration) not take effect until the patient is "terminal" or in a "persistent vegetative state" (Connecticut § 19a-571).[7]

Limiting advance directives to these narrow diagnostic categories is an obstacle to SED by AD for most individuals interested in using it. Even patients with late-stage dementia will probably not satisfy these conditions. While a few courts have held that patients with Alzheimer's were "terminally ill," this conclusion is uncertain. Most dementia patients have years of remaining life and at least some cognitive awareness and ability to interact with their environment.

Fortunately, some states have less demanding triggering conditions. For example, Florida provides that an advance directive is triggered not only when the patient has a terminal condition or is in a persistent vegetative state, but also when the patient has an "end-state condition" (Florida § 765.302). This is "an irreversible condition caused by injury, illness or disease that has

---

[6] In many states an individual can draft their advance directive to take effect before they lose capacity. For example, in California "the authority of an agent becomes effective only on a determination that the principal lacks capacity . . . unless otherwise provided." (California § 4682).

[7] As discussed above, these conditions may be unconstitutional. Nevertheless, they are presumed valid until successfully challenged (Ogden v. Saunders 1827).

resulted in progressively severe and permanent deterioration, and which, to a reasonable degree of medical probability, treatment of the condition would be ineffective" (Florida § 765.101(4)). Progressive dementia qualifies as an end-stage condition. Other states, like California and Tennessee, impose no triggering conditions at all (Reilly and Coppolo 2008).

At this point, it may seem that SED by AD is so complicated, contingent, and variable that it is not a practical option. But that would be an oversimplification. One might summarize the forgoing analysis by analogy to the colors of a traffic light (green, red, yellow). Some jurisdictions have green lights: SED by AD is a solidly authorized option. Some jurisdictions have red lights: SED by AD is prohibited. The remaining jurisdictions have yellow lights: the permissibility of SED by AD is unclear.

10.7. Circumventing Home State Law with Reciprocity Rules

While SED by AD may be authorized in only some states, its legal availability extends beyond those states through reciprocity rules common in advance directive statutes.[8] For example, the California Probate Code provides: "A written advance health care directive . . . executed in another state . . . in compliance with the laws of that state . . . is valid and enforceable in this state to the same extent as a written advance directive validly executed in this state" (California § 4676). This means that a valid Nevada or Vermont advance directive is a valid AD in California.[9]

Many other states follow the same reciprocity rules. For example, a patient in Minnesota could complete a Nevada dementia directive. That document would constitute a valid AD in Minnesota. Therefore, the Minnesota patient may have a clearer right to SED by AD by requesting it in a Nevada dementia directive than by requesting it in a Minnesota advance directive.[10]

---

[8] Even if state statutes lacked reciprocity language, the same result might be required by interstate comity, the legal principle that political entities must mutually recognize each other's legislative acts (Baldwin 1978).

[9] Lawyers use the term "forum shopping" to refer to the practice of choosing the court in which to bring an action based on a determination of which court is likely to provide the most favorable outcome (Garner 2009, 726).

[10] It might seem odd that a person who is not a resident of Nevada could write a "Nevada directive." But most reciprocity rules do not require residency.

10.8. Inadvertent Revocations and Vetoes

Even if an AD for SED were legal and enforceable, there are other challenges. Most problematically, the patient may make gestures or utterances that seem to contradict her prior instructions. We saw in the cases of Mrs. H and Steve in Chapter 7 that both were concerned they might later ask for food and drink. Does such communication revoke the advance directive?

A recent court case from the Netherlands involving an advance request for euthanasia suggests the answer is no (Asscher, Alida, and van de Vathorst 2020; Regional Euthanasia Review Committee 2020). In 2015, a 70-year-old Dutch woman completed an advance directive requesting euthanasia when her dementia advanced. Like Margot Bentley, the Dutch woman had seen others linger for a long time in nursing homes with severe dementia. She knew that was a life she found intolerable. But, in April 2016, when the Dutch woman's physician came to administer euthanasia, the patient made some indications that she had changed her mind. The physician nonetheless proceeded (Miller, Dresser, and Kim 2019; Regional Euthanasia Review Committee 2016). While prosecutors brought criminal charges against the physician, the Dutch court acquitted, holding that once the patient reaches late-stage dementia she is unable to knowingly and voluntarily revoke decisions that she earlier made with capacity.

Many U.S. states follow a similar rule: only individuals with capacity can revoke their advance directives. For example, California allows patients to revoke all or part of an advance health care directive "at any time and in any manner that communicates an intent to revoke," only when the patient has capacity (California § 4695(b)).

But when exactly does a patient have capacity? We addressed this in Chapter 8 from a clinical perspective and in Chapter 9 from the perspective of medical ethics, and now tackle it from a legal perspective. In late-stage dementia, when nursing home staff puts a spoon of food or thickened liquids in the patient's mouth, she may open her mouth and swallow. Since capacity is a decision-specific inquiry, some might argue that even in end-stage dementia the patient knows she wants to eat and is expressing that wish.

If these patients have decisional capacity to consent to hand-feeding, then their manifestation of consent to hand-feeding constitutes a revocation of prior contrary instructions for SED by AD. This is exactly what happened in the Margot Bentley case. Even had her advance directive been clearer about SED, the court held that would not matter because Margot still had decision-making capacity to decide whether to eat. Because she was in stage 7 Alzheimer's, Margot lacked capacity to make most medical and personal decisions. But capacity is not an all-or-nothing concept. It is decision-specific. The court held that Margot retained capacity to accept or refuse food and fluids (Bentley 2014).

This is a remarkably low test for decisional capacity. But it seems to be a peculiar consequence of the limited evidentiary record in the Bentley litigation. Three medical experts testified at trial. Only the two testifying on behalf of the facility had experience with Alzheimer's. They both testified that Margot was capable of consent and that she indicated that consent either by opening or by not opening her mouth. These experts explained that Margot's behavior was not just reflexive, because when a spoon or cup was pressed to her lips, she accepted different types and different amounts of food and liquids on different days. They testified that Margot expressed a preference for certain flavors and stopped opening her mouth, apparently, when she felt full. The trial court explained that it preferred the evidence of these experts to that of the family's expert, a general physician (Bentley 2014).

Having found that Margot had the capacity to give, and was giving, "current consent" to feeding, the court logically concluded that Margot's advance directive and other earlier expressed wishes were all irrelevant. Margot had capacity to consent to assistance with feeding, and she continued to give her consent. Consequently, the court held that her care providers must continue to offer such assistance.

The court's conclusion shocked those familiar with health law and medical jurisprudence. It seems remarkable to hold that, when a spoon or glass is pressed to the lips of someone with severe dementia, the mere opening of his mouth evidences capacity to continue eating and drinking. In fact, this satisfies only the first of four widely accepted elements for capacity. While the patient may be (1) able to communicate a choice, he is not able to (2) understand the relevant information, (3) appreciate the situation and its consequences, or (4) reason about treatment options (Appelbaum 2007).

Ultimately, the capacity question is irrelevant in many jurisdictions. Advance directive statutes in these states impose no requirement that the patient be of sound mind to revoke the directive, and some specifically provide that a directive may be revoked at any time and without regard to the declarant's mental state (Meisel et al. 2020 §§ 7.03[E], 7.08[A][5]). This is a potential problem for SED by AD because it makes it too easy for patient to inadvertently revoke their AD.

For example, the South Australia statute states: "a health practitioner may refuse to comply with a provision of an advance care directive if the health practitioner believes on reasonable grounds that . . . the provision does not reflect the current wishes of the person" (South Australia § 36(2)(b)). The Maryland statute states: "Nothing in this subtitle authorizes any action . . . if the health care provider is aware that the patient . . . has expressed disagreement with the action" (Maryland § 5-611(e)(2)).

10.9. Ulysses Clauses May Solve the Incapacitated Revocation Problem

One way around the revocation problem is with a Ulysses clause (Clausen 2014). This special language in an advance directive specifies the interventions (treatments) to which it applies and includes an explicit statement that the patient does not desire the proposed interventions even over their own apparent desire for them at the time the intervention is being offered.[11] In other words, a Ulysses clause permits agents and clinicians to withhold treatment over an incapacitated patient's demurs and dissents. A Ulysses clause allows the capacitated author of an AD to overrule her own later incapacitated objections.[12]

The term comes from the mythical Greek hero in Homer's *Odyssey* (Homer 2017).[13] Returning home after the Trojan War, Ulysses is warned about the Sirens who lure sailors to their deaths with the sweetness of their song. Ulysses wanted to hear the magical songs yet avoid crashing the ship into the rocks. So, Ulysses ordered his crew to bind him to the mast and sail the ship straight. Knowing that he will come under the powerful influence of the Sirens, Ulysses orders that his men not release him, no matter how earnestly he might later plead. In short, Ulysses wanted his men to follow his earlier orders given with capacity and to ignore his later orders given without capacity.

Ulysses clauses are common in mental health directives. A person with an episode of mental illness, not realizing that they are sick, might refuse

---

[11] Ideally, caregivers would first try to remind the patient of her plan and palliate her symptoms of thirst. That might resolve any apparent requests to "drink" and avoid a conflict between the patient's a past instructions and present desires.

[12] Note that Ulysses clauses do not allow capacitated authors to overrule their later *capacitated* objections. Individuals with decision-making capacity can always revoke their ADs.

[13] Odysseus is the hero and mythological figure's name in Greek. Ulysses is his name in Latin.

help. So, while still capacitated they authorize treatment even over their later objections. Ulysses clauses are less common in advance heathcare directives. In fact, Maryland, Vermont, and Virginia are the only states that explicitly recognize a Ulysses clause (Virginia § 54.1-2986.2; Maryland § 5-604(a)(2); Vermont § 9707(h)(1)). When properly executed, the Vermont statute requires clinicians to follow the agent's instructions "over the patient's objections."

As one might expect, before giving this much authority to an agent, the statute requires satisfying many safeguards (Vermont § 9707(h)(3)). First, the agent must accept this responsibility in writing. Second, a clinician must sign the Ulysses provision and affirm that the patient appeared to understand the benefits, risks, and alternatives to the rejected care. Third, an ombudsman, attorney, or certain others must sign a statement affirming that the patient knowingly and voluntarily signed the Ulysses clause.

While only Maryland, Vermont, and Virginia statutorily provide for a Ulysses clause, patients in other states might achieve the same objective. They may draft a Ulysses clause in a non-statutory directive or in a supplement to their state's statutory directive. While this is an easier and more accessible option, advance directive statutes in most states do not recognize Ulysses clauses. Some of these statutes even expressly provide that incapacitated utterances are sufficient to revoke the advance directive. Therefore, individuals may alternatively (or additionally) consider completing a Maryland, Vermont, or Virginia advance directive (with Ulysses clause). Then, pursuant to common reciprocity rules, their home state will likely recognize the foreign directive as a valid advance directive.

10.10. Appointed Health Care Agents

So far, we have focused on the instructional advance directive because that is likely the most effective mechanism to achieve SED by AD. But it is important to note that instructional directives should almost always include a proxy directive. Because written documents are rarely unambiguous and self-executing, it would be imprudent to have an instructional advance directive without also appointing an agent to interpret and enforce it.

While most instructional directives include proxy directives, many proxy directives do not include instructional directives. These proxy-only directives provide no specific instructions about care that the patient does and does not want. They only appoint an agent (or durable power of attorney for health care). Families and clinicians often ask whether an agent can direct SED without any specific written direction from the patient herself. Again, the answer varies from jurisdiction to jurisdiction.

There are three variations. In some states, agents may direct SED without specific prior direction or permission from the patient. In some other states, they may not. In the remaining states, the answer is unclear.

1. Permitted (California). Some states permit agents to make a wide range of decisions for an incapacitated patient without explicit permission from the patient to make those decisions.[14] For example, California law explicitly authorizes individuals to complete an advance directive that authorizes their agent to make not only "health" care decisions but also "personal" care decisions, including decisions about "providing meals" (California §§ 4615, 4623, 4670, 4671, 4684).

Nevertheless, even if agents in states like California were authorized to direct SED for an incapacitated patient without specific direction from the patient, it is safer to bolster the agent's authority with explicit instructions. An agent must act in accordance with the patient's wishes (California § 4684). Therefore, it is prudent to clarify what exactly those wishes are. Indeed, some statutes presume that agents may not make decisions regarding nutrition and hydration unless the patient specifically granted that authority (New York § 2982(2)).

2. Prohibited (Wisconsin). In contrast, other states specifically prohibit agents from making decisions about SED.[15] For example, the Wisconsin statute defining the powers and duties of health care agents provides that an agent "may not consent to the withholding or withdrawal of orally ingested nutrition or hydration unless provision of the nutrition or hydration is medically contraindicated (Wisconsin § 155.20(4))."

3. Unclear (New York). While agents in states like California have authority to direct SED, and agents in states like Wisconsin do not, in the remaining states the authority of an agent to direct SED is unclear. For example, in New York an agent has the authority to make only "health care decisions"

---

[14] These states include Colorado, Tennessee, Vermont, and Wyoming (Colorado §§ 15-14-506, 15-14-505(7); Tennessee §68-11-1803; Vermont § 9701; Wyoming §§ 35-22-402 35-22-403(b)).

[15] These states include Alabama, Iowa, Massachusetts, Missouri, Nebraska, New Hampshire and South Dakota (Alabama §§ 22-8A-3(3) 22-8A-4(b); Iowa § 144B1; Massachusetts § 201D13l; Missouri § 404.820; Nebraska §§ 30-3418, 30-3402; New Hampshire §§ 137-J:19, 137-J:18, 137-J:32; Oregon § 127.505; South Dakota § 34-12D-1).

(New York § 2982(1)). Those are defined as decisions regarding "any treatment, service or procedure to diagnose or treat an individual's physical or mental condition" (New York § 2980(4)). As we discussed in Chapter 4, it is unclear whether that includes eating and drinking.

10.11. Default Surrogates and Guardians

If the patient has not appointed a health care agent, then a substitute decision-maker will be appointed for him (Meisel et al. 2020 ch.8; Pope 2012; Pope 2017c). Typically, a health care provider does this pursuant to default surrogate laws in almost every state. Occasionally, a court appoints a guardian or conservator. Both types of decision-makers typically have less authority than agents chosen by the patient himself (Shepherd 2014; Meisel et al. 2020 ch.8; Tennessee § 68-11-1806(e)). Therefore, without an instructional advance directive to guide the surrogate, it is extremely unlikely that a default surrogate or guardian could direct SED for an incapacitated patient.

Indeed, statutes in some states specifically prohibit default surrogates from directing SED for an incapacitated patient. For example, the New York Family Health Care Decisions Act provides not only that surrogates may make only "health" care decisions but also that they may make them only "subject to the standards and limitations" in the statute (New York § 2994d(3)). The statute specifically excludes "providing nutrition or hydration orally, without reliance on medical treatment" from the scope of surrogate authority (New York § 2994a(12)).

Without evidence of the patient's wishes (ideally in the written advance directive itself), the surrogate must make decisions in the patient's "best interests." Typically, these seven factors guide the application of the best interest standard: (1) the patient's present level of physical, sensory, emotional, and cognitive functioning; (2) quality of life, life expectancy, and prognosis for recovery with and without treatment; (3) the various treatment options and the risks, side-effects, and benefits of each; (4) the nature and degree of physical pain or suffering resulting from the medical condition; (5) whether the medical treatment being provided is causing or may cause pain, suffering, or serious complications; (6) the pain or suffering to the patient if the medical treatment is withdrawn; and (7) whether any particular treatment would be proportionate or disproportionate in terms of the benefits to be gained by the patient versus the burdens caused to the patient (Pope 2018b).

It is unclear that SED is in a patient's objective best interests. Some courts have suggested it might be (A v. E 2012). But this conclusion is difficult to support when the patient is not now apparently suffering (Dildy and Largent 2021). In 2019, the Society for Post-Acute and Long-Term Care concluded that SED by AD would never be in a patient's best interest. So, the Society recommends a policy of comfort feeding for all those with advanced dementia in residential communities (Wright et al. 2019). Given the uncertainty of a best interest analysis, SED by AD is typically a realistic option only when the patient has left clear and informed instructions.

10.12. Conscience-Based Objection

In Chapter 4, we demonstrated that even if an individual has a legal right to VSED, a clinician or facility may assert a conscience-based objection and refuse participation. Similarly, clinicians and facilities may assert conscience-based objections to SED by AD. Indeed, almost all advance directive statutes explicitly permit providers to "decline to comply with an individual instruction or health care decision for reasons of conscience" (California § 4734). That does not mean the provider may thwart the plan or abandon the patient. Providers asserting a conscience-based objection must inform the patient or agent and make reasonable attempts to transfer the patient to a provider willing to comply (California § 4736).

10.13. Conclusion

Advance directive statutes in several states explicitly permit instructions about eating and drinking or about personal care. While other statutes apply only to "health" care, that often includes eating and drinking. Still, even if an AD for SED is statutorily authorized, individuals should supplement it with a Ulysses clause to prevent their later incapacitated utterances or gestures from inadvertently revoking the directive.

To maximize the chances that an AD for SED will be honored, individuals should take extraordinary efforts to complete the directive carefully. They should thoroughly document: (1) their capacity, (2) their appointment of agent, (3) their understanding of SED by AD, (4) their desire for SED, (5) when they want it, (6) how that triggering condition should be measured, and (7) their Ulysses clause. Furthermore, this ideally should be done not only in writing but also in a video. We offer a more complete summary of recommended elements of an advance directive for stopping eating and drinking (AD for SED) in Appendix A at the end of this book.

10.14. Return to the Cases

Case 7.1. Mrs. H., the Mother with Early Alzheimer's

Recognizing the challenges of SED by AD, Mrs. H. hastened her death by VSED while she still had decision-making capacity. During the process, Mrs. H. asked for water.

Bottom Line Points
- One can never be certain that any type of advance directive will be followed. That uncertainty is greater with respect to ADs for SED.
- SED by AD typically requires the participation of one's health care agent, clinicians, and nursing facility. Where ADs for SED are legally binding, it is more likely that they will be followed.
- Once a patient loses capacity (during either SED by AD or VSED), she may ask for water without realizing that drinking will undermine her plan. Reminding the patient of her plan and palliating the feeling of thirst can avoid difficult questions regarding whether the patient is revoking her advance directive. Ulysses clauses in an AD for SED disallow revocation when the patient is incapacitated.

Case 7.2. Steve, the Husband with Early Dementia

Steve has written a clear AD for SED and has asked his family to ignore any requests for water that he might later make.

Bottom Line Points
- Steve has prudently anticipated that his incapacitated future self may undermine his plan for SED by AD.
- Given that Steve already has early dementia, to best assure the validity of his AD for SED it would also be prudent to document his capacity to complete it.

- In many jurisdictions Steve's later requests for water would constitute a legal revocation of his AD for SED, even if he lacks decision-making capacity when he makes the request.
- Only a few jurisdictions authorize advance directive Ulysses clauses that permit clinicians to ignore incapacitated requests. Patients in other jurisdictions can complete advance directives from these states and have them recognized in their home state. Or they could complete non-statutory directives with Ulysses clauses in their home state.

Case 7.3. Patricia, the Academic with Moderate Dementia

Unlike Mrs. H. and Steve in the first two cases, Patricia already has moderate dementia. She was not comfortable with the prospect of SED by AD, and instead hastened her death with an overdose of barbiturates.

Bottom Line Points
- While hastening death through either VSED or SED by AD is probably not suicide, self-hastening death through a drug overdose is suicide.
- By taking the drugs without her family's assistance or presence, Patricia was careful to protect them from being criminally investigated or charged with assisted suicide.

Case 7.4. Charles, the Early Dementia Patient with Thorough Documentation

The inpatient hospice facility to which Charles was admitted was initially hesitant to allow him to die by SED. But they eventually honored his request, given its careful documentation in writing, on audiotape, and in a psychiatric evaluation.

Bottom Line Points
- Clinicians and facilities have legal obligations under state and federal law to obtain and follow their patients' advance directives.
- Because SED by AD is a lesser known option, many clinicians and facilities are unsure whether rules addressing advance directives require or permit them to honor an AD for SED.

- Because SED by AD seems unusual, clinicians may question whether the patient really understood it or really wanted it. While unusual for traditional advance directives, Charles' extraordinary documentation is prudent for ADs for SED.

References

A v. E, [2012] EWHC 1639 (COP).

Alabama Statutes § 8A-4.

Aleccia, JoNel. 2017. "Dementia Patient at Center of Spoon-Feeding Controversy Dies." *Kaiser Health News* (October 12). https://khn.org/news/dementia-patient-at-center-of-spoon-feeding-controversy-dies/.

Appelbaum, Paul S. 2007. "Assessment of Patients' Competence to Consent to Treatment." *New England Journal of Medicine* 357: 1834–1840.

Asscher, Eva, Constance Alida, and Suzanne van de Vathorst. 2020. "First Prosecution of a Dutch Doctor Since the Euthanasia Act of 2002: What Does the Verdict Mean?" *Journal of Medical Ethics* 46: 71–75.

Baldwin v. Fish & Game Commission, 436 U.S. 371 (1978).

Bentley v. Maplewood Seniors Care Society, 2014 BCSC 165

Bentley v. Maplewood Seniors Care Society, 2015 BCCA 91.

Brosio, Martha Risberg. 2019. *The Last Ten Days—Academia, Dementia, and the Choice to Die: A Loving Memoir of Richard A. Brosio.* Gorham, ME: Myers Education Press.

Browning (In re), 568 So. 2d 4 (Fla. 1990).

California Probate Code § 4615.

California Probate Code § 4623.

California Probate Code § 4670.

California Probate Code § 4671.

California Probate Code § 4676.

California Probate Code § 4682.

California Probate Code § 4684.

California Probate Code § 4695.

California Probate Code § 4734.

California Probate Code § 4736.

Cantor, Norman L. 2020. "Dispelling Medico-Legal Misconceptions Impeding Use of Advance Instructions to Shorten Immersion in Deep Dementia." *SSRN*, https://papers.ssrn.com/sol3/papers.cfm?abstract_id=3712186.

Clausen, Judy A. 2014. "Making the Case for a Model Mental Health Advance Directive Statute." *Yale Journal of Health Policy Law and Ethics* 14: 1–65.

Clevenger, Susan. 2019. *Dying to Die: The Janet Adkins Story.* Maui: Sacred Life Publishers.

Colorado Revises Statutes § 15-18-103.

Colorado Revises Statutes § 15-18-104.

Connecticut Statutes § 19a-571.

Cruzan v. Director, Missouri Department of Health, 497 U.S. 261 (1990).

Dildy, Katherine C. and Emily A. Largent. 2021. "Directing the End of Life in Dementia." In *Living with Dementia" Neuroethical Issues and International Perspectives*, edited by Veljko Dubljević and Frances Bottenberg, 71–89. Switzerland: Springer Nature.

End of Life Choices New York. 2020. "Advance Directive for Receiving Oral Food and Fluids in Dementia." https://endoflifechoicesny.org/.

End of Life Washington. 2020. "My Instructions for Oral Feeding and Drinking." https://endoflifewa.org/choices-and-planning/dementia-directives/

Fayerman, Pamela. 2016. "Margot Bentley Dies, A Finality That Couldn't Come Too Soon for Anguished Family." *Vancouver Sun*, November 11.

Florida Statutes § 765.101.

Florida Statutes § 765.106.

Florida Statutes § 765.302.

Garner, Bryan A. 2009. *Black's Law Dictionary* (9th ed.). Eagan, MN: Thomson Reuters.

Hammond, Katherine. 2016. "Kept Alive—The Enduring Tragedy of Margot Bentley." *Narrative Inquiry in Bioethics* 6, no. 2 (summer): 80–82.

Homer. 2017. *The Odyssey* (Transl. Emily Wilson). New York: W.W. Norton.

Harris (In re), No. 13-017-G6 (Jackson County Circuit Court, Oregon July 3, 2016) (order).

Hensel, William Arthur. 1996. "My Living Will." *JAMA* 275: 588.

Idaho Statutes § 39-4509.

Idaho Statutes § 39-4510.

Idaho Statutes § 39-4514.

Iowa Statutes § 144A.2.

Iowa Statutes § 144A.3.

Iowa Statutes § 144B.2.

Mader, Sarah, and Victoria Apold. 2020. "VSED as an Alternative to MAiD: A Pan-Canadian Legal Analysis." https://papers.ssrn.com/sol3/papers.cfm?abstract_id=3500173.

Margolis, Harry S. 2020. *Elder Law Portfolio* § 16-3.3.

Martin (In re), 538 N.W.2d 399 (Mich. 1995).

Maryland Code, Health—General, § 5-604.

Maryland Code, Health—General, § 5-611.

Meisel, Alan. 1995. "Barriers to Forgoing Nutrition and Hydration in Nursing Homes." *American Journal of Law and Medicine* 21: 335–382.

Meisel, Alan, Kathy L. Cerminara, and Thaddeus M. Pope. 2020. *The Right to Die: The Law of End-of-Life Decisionmaking*. New York: Wolters Kluwer.

Miller, David G., Rebecca Dresser, and Scott Y. H. Kim. 2019. "Advance Euthanasia Directives: A Controversial Case and Its Ethical Implications." *Journal of Medical Ethics* 45, no. 2: 84–89.

Minnesota Statutes §145C.

Nevada Revised Statutes § 162A.870.

New York Public Health Code § 2980.

New York Public Health Code § 2982.

New York Public Health Code § 2994-a.

New York Public Health Code § 2994-d.

Ogden v. Saunders, 25 U.S. (12 Wheat.) 213 (1827).

Oklahoma Statutes § 3101.8.

Oregon H.B. 4135 (2018).

O'Sullivan, Timothy P. 2017. "Drafting Health Care Advance Directives in a Rapidly Changing Legal and Sociological Environment." *Journal of the Kansas Bar Association* 86, no. 8: 32–60.

Pope, Thaddeus M. 2012. "Legal Fundamentals of Surrogate Decision Making." *Chest* 141, no. 4: 1074–1081.

Pope, Thaddeus M. 2013. "Clinicians May Not Administer Life-Sustaining Treatment without Consent: Civil, Criminal, and Disciplinary Sanctions." *Journal of Health & Biomedical Law* 9: 213–296.

Pope, Thaddeus M. 2015. "Prospective Autonomy and Dementia: Ulysses Contracts for VSED." *Journal of Bioethical Inquiry* 12, no. 3: 389–394.

Pope, Thaddeus M. 2017a. "Legal Briefing: Unwanted Cesareans and Obstetric Violence." *Journal of Clinical Ethics* 28, no. 2: 163–173.

Pope, Thaddeus M. 2017b. "Legal Briefing: New Penalties for Disregarding Advance Directives and DNR Orders." *Journal of Clinical Ethics* 28, no. 1: 74–81.

Pope, Thaddeus M. 2017c. "Unbefriended and Unrepresented: Medical Decision Making for Incapacitated Patients without Healthcare Surrogates." *Georgia State University Law Review* 33, no. 4: 923–1019.

Pope, Thaddeus M. 2018a. "Law and Ethics in Oncology: Voluntarily Stopping Eating and Drinking Is a Legal and Ethical Exit Option." *ASCO Post*, June 25.

Pope, Thaddeus M. 2018b. "The Best Interest Standard for Health Care Decision Making: Definition and Defense." *American Journal of Bioethics* 18, no. 8: 36–38.

Pope, Thaddeus M. 2019a. "Whether, When, and How to Honor Advance VSED Requests for End-Stage Dementia Patients." *American Journal of Bioethics* 19, no 1: 90–92.

Pope, Thaddeus M. 2019b. "Avoiding Late-Stage Dementia with Advance Directives for Stopping Eating and Drinking." *KevinMD*, October 6, https://www.kevinmd.com/blog/2019/10/avoiding-late-stage-dementia-with-advance-directives-for-stopping-eating-and-drinking.html.

Pope, Thaddeus M. 2020. "Video Advance Directives: Growth and Benefits of Audiovisual Recording." *SMU Law Review* 73: 161–175.

Pope, Thaddeus M., and Lindsey Anderson. 2011. "Voluntarily Stopping Eating and Drinking: A Legal Treatment Option at the End of Life." *Widener Law Review* 17, no. 2: 363–428.

Regional Euthanasia Review Committee (The Hague, Netherlands). 2017. *Oordeel [Judgment] 2016-2085.* https://www.euthanasiecommissie.nl/uitspraken/publicaties/oordelen/2016/niet-gehandeld-overeenkomstig-de-zorgvuldigheidseisen/oordeel-2016-85.

Regional Euthanasia Review Committee (The Hague, Netherlands). 2020. *Oordeel [Judgment] 2020-118.* https://www.euthanasiecommissie.nl/uitspraken-en-uitleg/p-2020/documenten/publicaties/oordelen/2020/2020-101-e.v/oordeel-2020-118.

Reilly, Meghan, and George Coppolo. 2008. "Living Wills and Health Care Representatives." *Connecticut Office of Legislative Research Report No. 2008-R-0237* (March 28, 2008). https://www.cga.ct.gov/2008/rpt/2008-R-0237.htm.

Sabatino, Charlie P. 2007. "Advance Directives and Advance Care Planning: Legal and Policy Issues." *Report for the U.S. Department of Health and Human Services* (October 2007). https://aspe.hhs.gov/basic-report/advance-directives-and-advance-care-planning-legal-and-policy-issues.

Shepherd, Lois. 2014. "The End of End-of-Life Law." *North Carolina Law Review* 92: 1693–1748.

South Australia Advance Care Directives Act 2013 § 36.

Tennessee Code Annotated § 68-11-1802.

Tennessee Code Annotated § 68-11-1803.

Tennessee Code Annotated § 68-11-1806.

Terman, Stanley A. 2011. *My Way Cards for Natural Dying*. Carlsbad, CA: Life Transitions Publications.

Tirado v. Flecha, 177 D.P.R. 893 (2010).

Trowse, Phillippa. 2020. "Voluntary Stopping of Eating and Drinking in Advance Directives for Adults with Late-Stage Dementia." *Australasian Journal on Aging* 39, no. 2: 142–147. https://doi.org/10.1111/ajag.12737.

Vermont Statutes § 9701.

Vermont Statutes § 9702.

Vermont Statutes § 9707.

Virginia Statutes § 54.1-2986.2.

Volicer, Ladislav, Thaddeus Mason Pope, and Karl E. Steinberg. 2019. "Assistance with Eating and Drinking Only When Requested Can Prevent Living with Advanced Dementia." *Journal of the American Medical Directors Association* 20, no. 11: 1353–1355.

Wisconsin Statutes § 154.03.

Wisconsin Attorney General. 2014. "Opinion AG10-14." (December 16, 2014). https://www.doj.state.wi.us/sites/default/files/dls/ag-opinion-archive/2014/2014.pdf.

Wright, James L., Peter M Jaggard, Timothy Holahan, and Ethics Subcommittee of AMDA. 2019. "Stopping Eating and Drinking by Advance Directives (SED by AD) in Assisted Living and Nursing Homes." *Journal of the American Medical Directors Association* 29: 1362–1366.

Wyoming Statutes § 35-22-402.

Wyoming Statutes § 35-22-403.

11

Institutional Issues

David A. Gruenewald

11.1. Introduction

Patient advocates and medical journalists are beginning to highlight the challenges that patients and their families face in having their advance directives honored to limit assisted hand-feeding in care facilities in the event of advanced dementia and other diseases that permanently impair cognition (Aleccia 2017a). Increasingly, patients and families with concerns about prolonged incapacity due to dementia are being counseled to discuss this issue explicitly with facility administrators before being admitted to a facility.

In this chapter, I discuss concerns that emerge when patients wish to stop eating and drinking by advance directive (SED by AD) in institutional settings. It is in these settings where the ethical tensions between (1) individual autonomy and self-determination and (2) societal obligations to protect vulnerable people are most apt to manifest. I briefly discuss the commonly encountered issue of "dementia worry" in older residents of long-term care (LTC) facilities, the limitations of most advance directives, and the practice of "comfort feeding only" in addressing the concerns of these residents. I discuss the resistance within the professional LTC community to the implementation of dementia-specific advance directives that specify conditions under which oral nutrition and hydration are to be withheld, along with counter-arguments that SED by AD is ethically justified. I conclude both by identifying areas of shared understanding and by proposing ways to address the desire of some older people not to linger in a state of advanced dementia, while recognizing that others find value in caring for older demented people who ultimately appear to accept or even enjoy oral nutrition and hydration.

11.2. "Dementia Worry" Is Common in Older Adults

As noted elsewhere in this volume, worry about living in a state of advanced dementia is very common among older adults. Many people want control over the end of their lives, and they may worry more about prolonged dying with a dementing illness than about death itself. Unlike other diseases such as advanced cancer that typically have a more rapidly terminal course, people with dementia may survive for years in a state of decisional incapacity even with a "comfort measures only" care plan. Some people who are diagnosed with early-stage dementia opt to end their own lives through some form of suicide while still able to do so, rather than face the prospect of living for years with advancing dementia (Volicer, Pope, and Steinberg 2019). Some people who die by suicide while residing in LTC facilities may be similarly motivated by "dementia worry." The result is lost years of satisfactory or even high-quality living, and traumatic consequences for surviving family, friends, and professional caregivers.

Traditional advance directives do not fully address concerns of those with dementia worry. Such directives are often inadequate to guide care in the face of a gradually progressive dementing illness. Without periodic re-assessment of care goals, clinicians may continue to provide the same medical treatments they would have even if dementia were not present. Many people would prefer to change plans for their care as dementia severity progresses, typically stepping down medically aggressive care in favor of interventions aimed at quality of life and comfort.

This conundrum has given rise to proposals for dementia-specific advance directives, in which care plans are adjusted based on cognitive "milestones" associated with dementia stages of increasing severity (Gaster, Larson, and Curtis 2017; Appendix B). As part of a care plan to improve quality of life and minimize the risk of unacceptably prolonged dying with dementia, comfort feeding only (CFO) has been suggested as a best practice in the care of people with advanced dementia (Palecek et al. 2010). CFO involves hand-feeding a demented person as long as the person shows no signs of distress with feeding such as coughing or choking, with the goal of maintaining comfort. It is acknowledged that CFO often fails to keep a severely demented person from losing weight, although oral intake and weight do sometimes stabilize. With CFO, oral feeding is stopped or diminished if it causes distress.

Despite these conceptual advances, CFO and many dementia-specific advance directives may not fully address the worries of people who do not want to live for long periods with advanced dementia and who prefer hastened death to prolonged incapacity. In many cases of dementia, there are no life-sustaining treatments in place that if discontinued would lead to the person's demise. An increasing number of people are turning to advance directives that specifically address limiting oral nutrition and hydration (ONH) in advanced dementia (i.e., implementing SED by AD in advanced dementia).

11.3. Challenges of SED by AD in Advanced Dementia Are Most Apt to Manifest in Institutional LTC Settings

The ethical, legal, and practical challenges associated with AD for SED in advanced dementia are most likely to manifest in institutional LTC settings where care facility staff may face conflict about whether to honor an incapacitated resident's directive specifying conditions under which assistance with oral food and fluid intake should no longer be provided (Aleccia 2020). By contrast, for persons with advanced dementia residing at home and receiving unpaid caregiver support from family and/or friends, it is likely that some cases of SED by AD occur without involving the formal health care system (Aleccia 2020). In other cases, health care providers and staff including hospice workers may provide informal support for SED by AD in advanced dementia at home. To the author's knowledge, the prevalence and incidence of either such supported or unsupported SED by AD in the home setting have not been studied.

Many people with worsening dementia eventually require care in an institutional setting, and in the United States people with dementia are most likely to die in a LTC facility (Cross and Warraich 2019). Within care institutions, some residents whose directives indicate a desire for comfort-oriented care may still be given aggressive oral feedings by staff as part of "basic care" with the goal of providing physiologically adequate long-term nutrition and hydration.

In some cases, persons with advanced dementia may be coaxed or cajoled or even harassed or forced to eat or drink by caregiving staff (Aleccia 2017a). In the case of Nora Harris, a resident of a LTC facility in Oregon with advanced dementia, despite her surrogate decision-maker's belief that she would not have wanted assisted ONH in this situation, the facility's administrator argued successfully in court that she must be fed until she stops opening her mouth or begins to cough and choke on her feedings (Aleccia

2017b; Schwarz 2019). (See Chapter 10, Section 3.) People with dementia may move out of LTC facilities, or, more likely, their families may choose to move them out to avoid assisted feeding in the advanced stages of dementia, but people who lack financial resources or support from family and friends do not have that option.

Courts have typically concluded that unless cessation of ONH is specifically mentioned in an advance directive, the person whose directive calls for stopping nutrition and hydration was likely referring to *medically assisted* nutrition and hydration (Pope 2019; Schwarz 2019). As described in Chapter 10 (Sections 10.3, 10.8) in the case of Margot Bentley, a resident of a care facility in British Columbia with advanced dementia, the Supreme Court of British Columbia ruled that Ms. Bentley's advance directive was insufficiently clear. Her directive indicated that her surrogate decision-makers had authority to make health care decisions, but it was unclear whether they also had authority over personal care decisions (which according to the court included decisions about ONH). Ms. Bentley directed that she "not be kept alive by artificial means or heroic measures" and that "no nourishment or liquids" be given, but the court concluded that her directive did not specifically refer to stopping ONH. Additionally, because Ms. Bentley opened her mouth when offered food she was deemed to have given "current consent" to be given food and drink, thereby revoking her advance directive or making it non-applicable (Pope and West 2014; see Chapter 10, Section 10.3) On the second point, clinicians and legal scholars point out that capacity to give consent involves more than communicating a choice; it also involves the ability to understand relevant information, to reason about treatments and care options, and to appreciate the situation and the consequences of the available choices (Appelbaum 2007; Pope and West 2014).

As explored in greater depth in Chapter 9 (Section 9.2, "Change of Mind"), LTC facility staff may have various interpretations of what it means when a demented person opens her mouth to accept assisted hand-feeding. Is it a primitive reflex, or a sign of active interest in eating and drinking? For caregivers in any setting, it is challenging to know how to respond when a severely demented person has an advance directive that requests withholding ONH, but the resident seems to cooperate with attempts to feed. Concerns have been raised about interpreting apparent cooperation with feeding attempts as a sign of active interest in eating and drinking. Some experts point out that a severely demented person "no longer has enough mind to change," although in the moment she may experience a non-reflective desire to eat that does not constitute a relevant "change of mind" (Menzel 2019; Schwarz 2019).

11.4. Resistance to Implementation of Dementia Directives Limiting Oral Nutrition and Hydration in LTC Settings

Newer dementia-specific directives may increase the likelihood that a person's wish to discontinue assisted hand-feeding will be honored in the event of advanced dementia (Aleccia 2017a; Aleccia 2018). These directives describe specific circumstances that should trigger implementation of comfort-focused care, including CFO, or the withdrawal of ONH entirely (Volicer, Pope, and Steinberg 2019). These "triggering" clinical conditions might include loss of decision-making capacity, loss of ability to self-feed, and a physician determination that dementia is in an advanced or terminal stage. It is unknown whether certain triggering conditions would be more likely than other conditions to result in honoring an AD for SED, but it is reasonable to suppose that SED by AD in LTC settings would more commonly be supported when dementia is far advanced, such as with no intelligible vocabulary and complete dependence in all activities of daily living.

Dementia directives that specify withholding ONH such as the Washington and New York directives described earlier in this book (see Chapter 10, Section 10.3, and other such directives collected in Appendix B) have not been widely implemented in LTC facilities. LTC facility staff and administrators will need to become familiar with these new directives and develop policies and procedures to address requests to limit or discontinue ONH. Resistance to dementia directives that specifically call for SED in advanced dementia has arisen within the LTC community. Since March 2019, the policy of AMDA—The Society for Post-Acute and Long-Term Care Medicine—is that advance directives for stopping eating and drinking (AD for SED) should be universally rejected in LTC facilities (AMDA 2019).[1] Instead, the Society's Ethics Committee recommended that

---

[1] Formerly known as The American Medical Directors Association and referred to herein as "The Society," AMDA is a medical specialty society representing medical directors, physicians, nurse practitioners, physician assistants, and other practitioners working in various post-acute and long-term care (PALTC) settings (AMDA 2020). For simplicity and readability, "PALTC" and "LTC" are considered interchangeable in this chapter. The Society's members work in skilled nursing facilities, assisted living facilities, retirement communities, home care, hospice, and other settings. Its missions

"comfort feeding" (CFO, as defined previously) (Palecek et al. 2010) should be implemented or continued despite the existence of a patient's AD for SED.

The Society argues that no choice can be made in implementing an AD for SED in advanced dementia without practicing an injustice: if LTC staff refuses to implement the AD for SED, they violate the autonomy of the person who drew up the directive. If, on the other hand, staff refuses food and fluid to a patient who still accepts food, they practice an injustice against that person as they are now (AMDA 2019). The Society argues that LTC clinicians have a greater responsibility to the person as they are now—the "now-self"—than to the person who drew up the advance directive for stopping eating and drinking—the "then-self." The Society contends that all LTC residents have the right to receive comfort feeding until behaviors indicating distress or refusal develop. The Society bases this position in a belief in the value of life of persons living with advanced dementia, and a rejection of the "ageist" idea that life lived in dependency has less value.

The Society also expresses other concerns regarding implementing an AD for SED in advanced dementia, including perceptions (1) that residents undergoing such stopping of eating and drinking would need to be separated from other residents during mealtimes; (2) that staff and visitors would need instruction not to assist the resident with ONH; and (3) that sedation would be required in the event not assisting the resident resulted in agitation or discomfort (AMDA 2019).

11.5. Ethical Rationale for Dementia Directives Limiting Oral Nutrition and Hydration in LTC Settings

Other ethicists and experts on VSED and SED by AD argue that exercising the choice to implement an AD for SED in advanced dementia can be ethically justified. Schwarz acknowledges that directives that limit hand-feeding are a new concept for LTC staff, while pointing out that the now widely accepted practice of withdrawing medically assisted nutrition and hydration was at one time thought to be unethical, illegal, and possibly murder (Schwarz 2019). Similarly, Menzel notes that we accord patients (and surrogates acting on behalf of patients) the right to discontinue or withhold

include improving care quality in PALTC settings, professional development, clinical guidance, and advocacy (AMDA 2020).

unwanted ventilator support for respiration based on a clear advance directive, even though breathing is the most basic of necessities for life (Menzel 2019). Volicer and colleagues point out that adhering to the AMDA—Society for Post-Acute and Long-Term Care Medicine policy would not allow demented residents of a LTC facility with an AD for SED to avoid prolonged living with advanced dementia (Volicer, Pope, and Steinberg 2019).

Pope observes that when a person with end-stage dementia and an AD for SED opens her mouth and swallows when LTC facility staff place a spoonful of food in her mouth, she does not appreciate that consuming ONH will likely prolong her life in a condition she found intolerable. Thus, her "decision" to consume food and fluids lacks capacity, and it is argued that her directive remains valid (Pope 2019). Menzel argues for a "balanced" approach to determine when and whether to honor an AD for SED in dementia: as the evidence of subjective value in survival to the affected individual diminishes with advancing dementia, the weight given to a clearly stated advance directive and to a trustworthy health care agent should increase correspondingly (Menzel 2019).

Responding to the Society's concern that the AD for SED may no longer represent the interests of the person with advanced dementia as she is now, Volicer and colleagues critique the "then-self vs. now-self" dilemma as a false dichotomy (Volicer, Pope, and Steinberg 2019). Noting that decision-making capacity depends on the nature of the decision, they observe that people with advanced dementia may still be able to communicate choices nonverbally regarding whether they wish to eat or drink. In this view, consideration of the whole person and providing person-centered care involves careful interpretation of the wishes regarding ONH being communicated in the moment by the now-severely-demented person, in light of her prior expressed wishes. They also note that acceding to the Society's view, in which others' opinions regarding the "now-self's" best interests supersedes the individual's wishes as stated in the AD, is contrary to the purpose of advance care planning.

Regarding the Society's concerns that residents undergoing SED would need to be isolated from other residents during mealtimes and that sedation would be given to suppress the desire for food and drink, Volicer and colleagues observe that even severely demented residents may nonverbally or verbally express their preferences whether to eat and drink, and that if a resident indicates a desire for assisted ONH, then assistance should be offered (Volicer, Pope, and Steinberg 2019).

Volicer et al. (2019) propose a strategy to avoid the ethical and practical concerns raised by the Society: *assist with* eating and drinking only when requested. Comfort feeding would be provided until the condition specified in the AD occurs, then caregivers would continue to offer food and liquids within reach. Caregiver assistance with eating and drinking would be provided only if the person verbally or nonverbally indicated a desire for it, and residents no longer being assisted with ONH would continue to receive socialization with other residents as usual.

11.6. Conclusion—ADs for SED in Institutional LTC Settings

Disagreements in the LTC community regarding the acceptability of dementia-specific advance directives that limit hand-feeding are likely to continue. There may be opportunities to build consensus upon a shared understanding in several areas. First, even severely demented people may have the ability to communicate their preferences for ONH either verbally or nonverbally. Second, severely demented people living in LTC facilities must continue to have opportunities for socialization during mealtimes even as their desire or ability to ingest food and drink wanes. Finally, assisted feedings should be discontinued when both (1) a now-demented resident previously indicated a desire to hasten death rather than to live for long periods with advanced dementia, and (2) the burdens of assisted feeding now outweigh the benefits as evidenced by resident distress or complications such as coughing and choking on food and drink (and possibly apathy toward food and drink as well).

The decision to discontinue assisted feeding will be facilitated by a clearly worded directive specifying conditions under which feeding should be stopped, with decision-making support from a trustworthy and unconflicted surrogate working closely together with well-informed LTC facility staff and administrators who prioritize person-centered care at the end of life. The surrogate's task will be to determine when the affected person is suffering from advanced dementia or is now showing so little enjoyment and engagement in life that her previous wishes should now take precedence. Given that resistance to the implementation of an AD for SED may be present in LTC settings, individuals who have completed an AD for SED and their families should bring a copy of their directive with them when visiting prospective

LTC facilities and ask whether administrators and clinical staff will honor the directive at their facilities.

11.7. Case Comments from an Institutional Perspective

Consider for a moment how a situation similar to Case 7.2 might ultimately play out for a resident of a LTC facility. Steve's AD for SED calls for SED when he can no longer feed himself and has advanced dementia (FAST stage 6). Any requests he might make to resume ONH once SED has begun are to be ignored. He rejects comfort feeding as an alternative strategy, preferring to hasten his death by dehydration and to receive symptom management during SED including sedating medication if necessary, so that he does not suffer. His appointed health care agent and his primary care physician are to implement SED when the above criteria are met.

Note that Functional Assessment Staging Tool (FAST) Stage 6 is characterized by a loss of ability to perform basic activities of daily living, such as dressing, bathing, toileting, and continence of urine and feces (Reisberg 1988). For people with Alzheimer-type dementia, the rate of disease progression and survival prognosis varies widely, and the onset of functional impairments may be gradual, which may make it difficult to choose a time to initiate SED by AD. Persons with advancing "Stage 6" dementia may be relatively robust physically, especially early on, and may remain able to feed themselves to some extent even as other activities of daily living are lost.

The difficulty in enacting Steve's AD for SED at home was described in Case 7.2. Implementing his directive in an institutional LTC setting would likely be even more difficult. Most providers and caregivers in LTC facilities would likely recoil at the prospect of heavily sedating a robust-appearing and pleasantly demented person now lacking an understanding of the rationale and motivation to pursue SED. In fact, the prospect of heavily sedating a resident under these circumstances was one objection to implementing an AD for SED raised by AMDA—The Society for Post-Acute and Long-Term Care Medicine. Potentially sedating medications for management of behavioral symptoms are usually reserved for specific scenarios such as aggression or psychosis with risk of harm, and cases that do not respond to non-pharmacological management strategies (Gerlach and Kales 2018). Furthermore, no matter how clear the AD for SED, in many cases it may not be possible to enforce a requirement to withhold ONH (as in Cases 7.1 and

7.2) while patients are still nonverbally demonstrating desire and enjoyment. Even in the presence of a clear advance directive it would be challenging to implement for family members under this circumstance, much less professional caregivers who are trained to offer food and drink as a core feature of their responsibilities.

Additional Comments Regarding the Cases

In Case 7.4, SED by AD was successfully implemented for Charles in an institutional (inpatient hospice) setting. However, the attending hospice physician initially refused to honor the directive, acquiescing only after being presented with additional information, including (1) a written statement affirming the individual's decision-making capacity at the time he completed the AD; (2) an audio CD of his oral testimony discussing his values, his reasons for wishing to SED by AD, and his understanding of the alternatives, benefits, and burdens of his choice to SED by AD; and (3) an invitation to discuss the treatment options with the physician who counseled the individual for advance care planning.

Each of the cases presented in Chapter 7 illustrates a complex scenario of care planning, disease progression, and medical decision-making evolving over an extended time frame. Few LTC institutions are adequately resourced to optimally support these ongoing, iterative conversations and to guide the process to a mutually acceptable conclusion (whether resulting in SED by AD, comfort feeding only, or some other outcome). Support from hospice/palliative care or a highly engaged primary care provider would likely be necessary.

Bottom Line Points

- On top of the barriers to contemporaneous VSED in institutional settings described in Chapter 5, additional logistical and ethical hurdles are present with SED by AD in LTC facilities. All four cases in Chapter 7 are notable for the extent of advocacy of family members, and the intensive involvement of specialists with skills in conducting goals-of-care conversations, assessing the trajectory of dementia, and negotiating with professional caregivers and/or administrators.

- "Successful" implementation of SED by AD in a LTC institutional setting may require a combination of (1) pro-active selection of a LTC facility willing to consider SED by AD, (2) a detailed and compelling presentation of the individual's reasons for wanting to SED by AD, (3) ongoing advocacy for the individual's request to SED by AD by a capable and committed health care agent, (4) support from hospice/palliative care and possibly other consultants, and (5) the engagement of a provider at the LTC facility who is willing to support SED by AD.
- Residents of LTC facilities who wish to SED by AD but who lack one or more of the above elements for implementation of AD for SED may have no alternative but to accept CFO as their imperfect next-best option.

Disclaimer

This work was supported in part by the Department of Veterans Affairs. The views expressed herein are those of the author and do not necessarily reflect the views of the Department of Veterans Affairs or the U.S. Government.

References

Aleccia, JoNel. 2017a. "Despite Advance Directive, Dementia Patient Denied Last Wish, Says Spouse." *Kaiser Health News*, August 21, 2017. https://khn.org/news/despite-advance-directive-dementia-patient-denied-last-wish-says-spouse/.

Aleccia, JoNel. 2017b. "New Instructions Could Let Dementia Patients Refuse Spoon-Feeding." *Kaiser Health News*, November 3, 2017. https://khn.org/news/new-instructions-could-let-dementia-patients-refuse-spoon-feeding/.

Aleccia, JoNel. 2018. "Aggressive New Advance Directive Would Let Dementia Patients Refuse Food." *Kaiser Health News*, March 30, 2018. https://khn.org/news/aggressive-new-advance-directive-would-let-dementia-patients-refuse-food/.

Aleccia, JoNel. 2020. "Diagnosed with Dementia, She Documented Her Wishes for the End. Then Her Retirement Home Said No." *Washington Post*, January 18, 2020. https://www.washingtonpost.com/health/diagnosed-with-dementia-she-documented-her-wishes-for-the-end-then-her-retirement-home-said-no/2020/01/17/cf63eeaa-3189-11ea-9313-6cba89b1b9fb_story.html.

AMDA—The Society for Post-Acute and Long-Term Care Medicine. 2019. "Ethics Committee White Paper: Stopping Eating and Drinking by Advance Directives (SED by AD) in the ALF and PALTC Setting." https://paltc.org/amda-white-papers-and-resolution-position-statements/stopping-eating-and-drinking-advance-directives.

AMDA—The Society for Post-Acute and Long-Term Care Medicine. 2020. "About AMDA." https://paltc.org/about-amda.

Appelbaum, Paul S. 2007. "Assessment of Patients' Competence to Consent to Treatment." *New England Journal of Medicine* 357, no. 18: 1834–1840.

Cross, Sarah H., and Haider J. Warraich. 2019. "Changes in the Place of Death in the United States." *New England Journal of Medicine* 381, no. 24: 2369–2370.

Gaster, Barak, Eric B. Larson, and J. Randall Curtis. 2017. "Advance Directives for Dementia: Meeting a Unique Challenge." *JAMA* 318, no. 22: 3175–3176.

Gerlach, Lauren B., and Helen C. Kales. 2018. "Managing Behavioral and Psychological Symptoms of Dementia." *Psychiatric Clinics of North America* 41, no. 1: 127–139.

Menzel, Paul T. 2019. "Justifying a Surrogate's Request to Forego Oral Feeding." *American Journal of Bioethics* 19, no. 1: 92–94.

Palecek Eric J, Joan M. Teno, David J. Casarett, Laura C. Hanson, Ramona L. Rhodes, and Susan L. Mitchell. 2010. "Comfort Feeding Only: A Proposal to Bring Clarity to Decision-Making Regarding Difficulty with Eating for Persons with Advanced Dementia." *Journal of the American Geriatrics Society* 58: 580–584.

Pope, Thaddeus M. 2019. "Whether, When, and How to Honor Advance VSED Requests for End-Stage Dementia Patients." *American Journal of Bioethics* 19, no. 1: 90–92.

Pope, Thaddeus M., and Amanda West. 2014. "Legal Briefing: Voluntarily Stopping Eating and Drinking." *Journal of Clinical Ethics* 25, no. 1: 68–80.

Reisberg Barry. 1988. "Functional Assessment Staging (FAST)." *Psychopharmacology Bulletin* 24, no. 4: 653–659.

Schwarz, Judith K. 2019. "Lessons From New York's Dementia Directive and Applications to Withholding Oral Feedings." *American Journal of Bioethics* 19, no. 1: 95–97.

Volicer Ladislav, Thaddeus M. Pope, and Karl E. Steinberg. 2019. "Assistance with Eating and Drinking Only When Requested Can Prevent Living with Advanced Dementia." *Journal of the American Medical Directors Association* 20, no. 11: 1353–1355.

12

Best Practices, Enduring Challenges, and Opportunities for SED by AD

Timothy E. Quill, Paul T. Menzel, Thaddeus M. Pope, and Judith K. Schwarz

The previous four chapters explored SED by AD from clinical, ethical, legal, and institutional perspectives. In this chapter we offer key summary points in three sections. First, we recommend *best practices* when considering or implementing SED by AD. Second, we describe *enduring challenges* and suggest ways to overcome them. Third, we identify *opportunities* that SED by AD offers for patients and families.

12.1. Best Practices

Manage Comfort. Before AD for SED is activated, patients should have a skilled, committed clinician partner to manage any discomfort using various palliative measures, including proportionate sedation if needed.

Have Advance Directive Discussion, Planning, and Documentation. While the patient still has capacity, advance directive discussions should be strongly encouraged and perhaps even required among the patient, family members, treating clinicians, caregivers, and institutional administrators. These discussions should address the overall SED by AD plan including the patient's motivations and intentions. Such discussions are necessary for the parties to identify and potentially reconcile differences of opinion and approaches regarding both the advance directive's content and its prospective implementation.

Ensure Thorough Understanding. The patient must understand the risks, benefits, and alternatives to SED by AD. She must understand that the process, once initiated, may entail some short-term suffering, and that she may later request water without understanding it will prolong her dying process.

Clarify *Who* Should Be the Main Surrogate Decision-Maker If Capacity Is Lost. Patients will still make their own decisions in this regard while they retain capacity, but with whom should clinicians confer and make decisions if and when that capacity is lost? In addition to naming a proxy decision-maker, patients should have extended discussions with the named proxy about what kinds of treatment they would and would not want if they lose decision-making capacity.

Be Clear about *When* to Activate the Directive. Patients should clearly identify the clinical indications for activating their AD for SED, both to reflect their actual wishes and to remove as much of the burden of the timing of that final decision as possible from the patient's caregivers.

Be Precise about *What* to Forego. In addition to making clear the clinical indications for *when* food and drink are to be withheld, the AD for SED should make clear *what* kinds of feeding and drinking are to be provided or withheld: for example, (1) provide as much or as little as is compatible with comfort (as is standard of care for hospice); (2) provide the minimum amount still compatible with comfort; (3) forego all assisted hand-feeding; or (4) forego all assisted hand-feeding or even food and water when the patient can still self-feed. Even if the kind and amount of food and fluid to be withheld or provided are detailed in the AD, the patient should explicitly trust the eventual refinement of such decisions to the appointed health care proxy.

Specify *Where* the Patient Prefers to Receive Care when the AD for SED will likely be implemented. Many persons with advanced dementia will receive care in a long-term care facility, and many of those institutions will be unfamiliar with or opposed to following an AD to SED. When possible, the patient, while still decisionally capable, and family are encouraged to explore ahead of time which settings would most likely honor such completed directives.

Use Video Directives. The patient should be clear about "when to activate" and "what to forego" not only in a written advance directive but ideally also in a video supplement. This gives clinicians and future caregivers confidence that the patient understood and intended the options she chose.

12.2. Enduring Challenges

Uncertain Availability Once Capacity Is Lost. While VSED is legally available—not legally prohibited—in most jurisdictions, SED by AD is explicitly legal in only some. Consequently, many clinicians may be unable or unwilling to honor even a well-drafted AD for SED.

Possible Change of Mind. With an AD for SED, as with any AD, without the assurance of real time consent, the possibility cannot be eliminated that the patient might have changed her mind by the time of implementation. While not always a barrier to using ADs for SED, this uncertainty can pose special problems for the implementation of these ADs when a person's apparent willingness to eat and/or drink is present after the triggering conditions have been met. Deciding whether such apparent willingness constitutes a relevant change of mind can be difficult.

Family and Clinician Distress around Consent. Without real-time patient consent, family members and clinicians are likely to feel a substantial burden and moral distress from having to decide both (1) *when to initiate* the SED process and (2) *how to respond* to potential verbal and nonverbal requests for food and drink once the SED process has been initiated.

Symptom Management When Capacity Is Lost. The most difficult part of VSED (initiated by a patient with capacity) is counteracting the usually profound dry mouth and sense of thirst that emerges within a few days of beginning the process. Dry mouth and thirst will likely be even more difficult to evaluate and manage in SED by AD, where the patient is not clearly aware of being in control of the process with a clear endpoint in mind to help make sense of the associated discomfort which might not be easy to relieve.

Then-Self/Now-Self Problems. If an incapacitated patient for whom SED by AD has been initiated begins to demonstrate (verbally or nonverbally) a persistent desire to drink (or eat), should caregivers listen to instructions by the "then self" or the behavior of the "now self"? Appropriate distinctions can sometimes be made between cases where the desire appears to be less than intentional and those where there seems to be a relevant change of mind, but even when the patient's expressions are deemed not to be a relevant change of mind, the then-self/now-self problem can remain challenging.

Difficult Timing of Initiation. The most feasible point at which to start SED by AD is when the patient can no longer self-feed. For many who want to employ SED by AD to avoid living into years of severe dementia, however, this "feasible" point of initiating the process will come later than they would have preferred in protecting them from living into that condition. Identifying an earlier clear marker of when to initiate SED by AD is usually difficult.

Uncertain Gap between Contemplation and Activation. For example, in the state of Washington where MAID is legal, one in six terminally ill patients talk to their family about the option, and one in fifty talk to their doctors, yet MAID accounts for only about one in two hundred deaths (CDC 2019, Ganzini 2015, Oregon Department of Health 2020). There is clearly a difference between contemplation and initiation. The same phenomenon may be even more pronounced with ADs for SED, making it difficult for surrogates to decide whether or when to initiate SED on behalf of someone who had completed such a document but now lacks capacity to determine exact timing.

12.3. Opportunities

Potential to Live Longer by Not Acting Preemptively. An AD for SED can be attractive to patients who still find their lives meaningful but fear losing the mental capacity to control the time and circumstances of their death. It can potentially allow them to avoid having to act preemptively by initiating VSED or other immediate death-hastening measures while they still have the decision-making capacity to do so.

Consensus Building among Patients and Caregivers in Advance. If a patient is genuinely contemplating initiating SED by AD, it is incumbent on all concerned (patient, family, treating clinicians, supporting programs, involved institutions) to review the "enduring challenges" above and in Chapter 6 and make sure that they agree as much as possible on how to address them.

Comfort Feeding Only as a Standard Back-Up Measure. Patients who currently have decision-making capacity but anticipate the potential need to activate an AD for SED in their near future should be offered the potential to be managed in the interim with "comfort measures only" (CFO), so they may take advantage of an "opportunity to die" if an acute life-limiting event occurs before the conditions specified in their AD for SED are met. This would potentially protect them from having to count on SED by AD with its inherent challenges. Also, if no consensus can be reached about when to activate SED by AD for someone who had previously expressed that desire in an uncertain way, CFO or "minimum comfort feeding only" (MCFO), depending on the patient's prior preferences, should be the back-up plan.

Informed Consent Remains the Goal. Patients contemplating an AD for SED in their future should make themselves and their families aware of the full range of alternative "last resort" options to see if any would be preferable now or in their future. Counselors and caregivers can be immensely helpful in patients achieving such an understanding of their options in advance. A patient decision aid may also be valuable. A feasible and usually effective option that can easily go unnoticed is refusing basic lifesaving treatments (e.g., antibiotics) for relatively common conditions like pneumonia.

Life Closure Still Very Important. If a patient and his supporting team are seriously considering a future plan that includes SED by AD, they should try to make the most of their remaining time while the patient still has decision-making capacity, perhaps including activities with family and friends geared toward life closure.

Explore Backup Options When the Person's Condition Changes. If a patient with an AD for SED (or planning to execute one) experiences a deterioration in her quality of life that cannot be adequately treated with best possible palliative measures, then VSED and other potentially available concurrent "last resort" options should be revisited while the patient still has capacity to make his own decisions.

Ulysses Clauses. Only a few jurisdictions authorize Ulysses clauses in advance directives (see Chapter 10, Section 10.9). Because an incapacitated patient for whom SED by AD has been initiated may demonstrate (verbally or nonverbally) a desire to drink (or eat), Ulysses clauses can clarify the patient's preference when completing the initial advance directive document that family and clinicians should listen to the "then self" rather than the "now self." If the later desire to eat and drink is particularly strong, SED by AD may be too difficult to execute, and a back-up plan for MCFO can be considered.

Advance Directive Statutes. While SED by AD probably fits within the scope of decision-making authorized by advance directive laws, many family and professional caregivers are unsure. The legal validity of an AD for SED could be clarified by amending these statutes, by getting a judicial declaratory judgment, or by obtaining an Attorney General advisory opinion.

Institutional Policies. Most health care facilities have policies on withholding and withdrawing life-sustaining treatment. Facilities in MAID jurisdictions have policies on MAID. Yet, few health care facilities have policies on VSED or SED by AD. Without a policy, caregivers (especially hospice and long-term staff) may be uncertain whether and how to honor an AD for SED. Clear institutional policies could be a significant help not only to caregivers but also to patients and their proxies in making decisions among facilities.

Careful Discernment of the Value of Life. If the triggering conditions in an AD for SED have been met, but the person is not suffering (severe dementia, but otherwise appears to be enjoying life), proxies and caregivers may find it difficult to implement this aspect of the person's AD. Respect for the person who previously wrote the directive clashes with her current apparent interest in living. The difficulty can potentially be eased, however, by careful attention to the subjective value of life as expressed in the person's AD. If the person can no longer anticipate tomorrow and, when she gets there, cannot remember yesterday (conditions commonly met in very advanced dementia), and she clearly said in her AD that the value she would place on her own survival would greatly diminish in such circumstances, then following her directive becomes less problematic.

Dialogue. The trends toward (1) increasing numbers of older people with dementia, (2) increasing worry about its prospect, (3) lack of awareness of the option of VSED for those with decision-making capacity, and (4) general resistance to ADs for SED among many post-acute and LTC professionals all combine to suggest the need for ongoing dialogue and consensus-building around finding acceptable approaches to the associated dilemmas based on mutual respect and an attitude of open inquiry.

VSED is becoming a more widely recognized, legally available end-of-life option for those who experience unacceptable suffering or deterioration toward the end of their lives, or fear such suffering or deterioration in their future. An AD for SED is an important supplement to VSED for capacitated patients. SED by AD permits a patient to express her wishes about having VSED continued if she loses capacity late in the initiated process and, while confused, requests to resume drinking and eating.

SED backed up by a clear AD is not only an important supplement within VSED but can also be an important alternative of its own. It offers potential advantages for those who find their current situation acceptable and would prefer not to hasten their deaths preemptively before they lose decision-making capacity. These patients still want assurance that others would activate the SED process on their behalf once capacity is lost.

Initiating the stopping of eating and drinking by AD after decision-making capacity has been lost, however, is a far more complicated and controversial end-of-life option than when ADs for SED are used to supplement VSED that was initiated with real-time consent by a patient with full capacity. We have identified some pathways to address and potentially overcome significant clinical, ethical, legal, and institutional challenges associated with SED by AD, but a lot more work remains if those paths are to be predictably, reliably, and safely available.

Future prospects for SED by AD, however, should not be underestimated. ADs for refusing lifesaving treatment, now rather conventional, have come a long way since they were first suggested decades ago (including improvements in specificity, caregiver buy-in, legal support, and public knowledge), even though the same essential problems of possible change of mind and then-self/now-self conflicts still confront them, as well. As VSED becomes more widely recognized as a basic patient right and a compassionate option when properly managed, the realization is likely to grow that SED, too, should be available by a carefully articulated and communicated advance directive.

References

CDC. 2019. Deaths: Final Data for 2017. National Vital Statistics Reports 68:9. https://www.cdc.gov/nchs/data/nvsr/nvsr68/nvsr68_09-508.pdf.

Oregon Department of Health. 2020. Oregon Death with Dignity Act 2019 Data Summary. https://www.oregon.gov/oha/PH/PROVIDERPARTNERRESOURCES/EVALUATIONRESEARCH/DEATHWITHDIGNITYACT/Documents/year22.pdf.

Ganzini, Linda. 2015. "Legalized Physician Assisted Death in Oregon." *QUT Law Review* 16, no. 1: 76–83.

Appendices

Thaddeus M. Pope, Paul T. Menzel, Timothy E. Quill, and Judith K. Schwarz

Appendix A

Recommended Elements of an Advance Directive for Stopping Eating and Drinking (AD for SED)

Individuals with decision-making capacity who want to avoid current or imminent suffering or deterioration can voluntarily stop eating and drinking (VSED). But what about individuals who want to avoid suffering or deterioration in the future but are afraid of losing capacity, and thus the ability to act, by that time? An Advance Directive for Stopping Eating and Drinking (AD for SED) could help. It authorizes others to limit or stop a person's eating and drinking on the individual's behalf when she cannot contemporaneously authorize it. Furthermore, an AD for SED could even help individuals who initiate VSED while fully capacitated and want to ensure it is continued if they lose capacity during the process and thus also need to rely on others.

The essential elements to include in an AD for SED are:

- *What* food and drink to withhold
- *When* to withhold food and drink
- *Where* care is to be provided
- What to do if one seems to have desires contrary to the AD
- Desired intensity of palliative support during the process
- Central reasons and values motivating the AD for SED
- Verification of decision-making capacity at time of writing/recording
- Appointment of a health care agent (proxy)
- Discussion of AD's content with the appointed agent

What follows are the details of these most essential elements as well as other highly recommended ones, grouped into three stages: preparation, documentation, and follow-up.

I. Preparation

    A. **Learn Basic Options**. These include a written instructional advance directive (the "AD"), appointment of a health care agent (proxy), and possibly a video/audio recording of one's wishes. Ideally, information about these options would be provided by a person with experience in end-of-life counseling who has (1) some clinical understanding of the conditions that the person's AD would likely address, (2) some knowledge of the relevant state laws about completing an AD, and (3) some awareness of the psycho-social complexities involved in considering such documents.

    B. **Complete a Regular AD**. An AD for SED should always be either a part of, or a supplement to, a more encompassing "regular" AD covering other aspects of the person's future health care. Links to many good guides for ADs can be found at the American Bar Association's health decisions resources webpage (American Bar Association 2020).

C. **Discuss Options** with those whom one personally wants to consult (e.g., closest family and significant others), with particularly knowledgeable parties, and with one's primary physician and other clinicians who may be directly responsible for implementing one's directive. The discussion should include anticipated benefits and potential burdens of including SED as part of one's AD. Those considering an AD for SED should be prepared for lack of awareness and/or resistance by clinicians who are unfamiliar with such documents. But even if one particular hospice or LTC facility is ultimately unwilling to honor an AD for SED, others may be willing. Program or facility views and values on this subject might be explored before admission by those interested in this option.

D. **Confirm Decision-Making Capacity** to write such a directive. In most circumstances with most adults, such confirmation is routine, and testimony to it is part of the signed witnessed AD document itself. In some circumstances—for example, early to moderate dementia—additional professional assessment of decision-making capacity should be obtained, perhaps from a consulting neurologist or psychiatrist.

E. **Review and Update.** The person should understand that periodically reviewing, dating, and initialing the AD and agent (proxy) appointment is advisable. Long periods of time without such review and reiteration (or revision) may call into question whether the AD still expresses the person's wishes. Such review can also provide opportunities to meet with important parties such as one's health care agent, close family members, and primary physician to ensure that they are willing to support the choices one has expressed.

II. <u>Documentation</u>

A. The **Advance Directive for SED** (either part of one's general AD or a separate document).

The directive should address:

1. *What* food and drink is to be withheld, and *when* that process should be triggered (the "triggering" condition). There are three basic options:

a. <u>Minimum Comfort Feeding Only</u> (MCFO).

What: Provide only the minimum food and drink necessary for comfort, regardless of nutritional adequacy in sustaining life. The intent is simultaneously to maintain comfort while also hastening death. MCFO would typically apply to manually assisted feeding (hand-feeding), but it could also apply to self-feeding (see next option b).

When: The need for only a smaller amount of food and drink to achieve comfort than what is nutritionally adequate will often emerge naturally in the advanced stages of certain illnesses (e.g., Alzheimer's), when appetite and other functions often diminish. In the case of an AD for SED, because the person's instruction to minimize oral intake is part of his wish to hasten dying upon reaching the stipulated condition, the option here when appetite diminishes is the minimum necessary for comfort (MCFO).

In more standard "Comfort Feeding Only" (CFO) the person is provided neither more nor less food and drink than what is compatible with comfort, regardless of nutritional adequacy. The aim is to maintain comfort, and neither to extend life nor to hasten death. In hospice, where the person's best interest is already judged to be the maintenance of comfort and dignity while neither extending nor shortening life, CFO is typically regarded as "hospice standard of care." Where it is standard of care, CFO does not need to be specified in an AD. Because it is not the purpose of such CFO to hasten death, however, it is not one of the primary options for someone writing an AD for SED. MCFO, by contrast, is viable for those intending to simultaneously provide comfort and hasten death.

b. <u>Self-Feeding Only (SFO)</u>.

What: No manually assisted feeding. Food is offered only for self-feeding. In turn, by directive this could be further limited to only amounts necessary for comfort, presumably with the intention that life not be prolonged as much.

When: Only when someone is at least partially dependent on manually assisted feeding can "self-feeding only" constitute a real limit to the amount of food or fluid being ingested. In progressive dementia this dependence will often occur in DGS and FAST stages 6 and 7 (see Chapter 8, Section 8.1, Table 8.1). Individuals can pair a "self-feeding only" stipulation with other desired triggering conditions—for example, stop all manually assisted feeding when the person can no longer recognize friends and loved ones, or when any particular FAST or GDS stage of deterioration is reached, and regardless of whether the person is suffering at the time.

c. <u>No eating and drinking at all</u>.

What: Withhold all food and drink, even when the person can self-feed, based on the patient's clear prior written request.

When: Whenever the triggering condition the person specifies is reached—for example, inability to communicate orally or in writing, largely incontinent and unable to ambulate, continually distressed. The person may choose to refer to these by using one of the later stages of incapacity according to GDS or FAST scales and may want to be clear that they apply regardless of whether the person is suffering at the time.

It can be difficult, however, to implement an AD for SED with an earlier marker than "no longer being able to self-feed." When one has lost capacity but can still self-feed and seems to desire to do so, it is more feasible to implement one of the two previous options (MCFO or Self-Feeding Only) than to implement withholding *all* food and drink. Accordingly, it may be prudent to specify one of them as a "backup option" in case caregivers are legally, institutionally, or professionally not permitted or are personally unwilling to withhold *all* food and drink.

2. **What to Do in the Event of Contrary Expressions**. The most comprehensive AD for SED will address the potential circumstance in which, at the time one's directive is implemented, one may still express an apparent desire for food and drink contrary to the AD. By then, one will no longer have decision-making capacity to revise or revoke the directive, but such expressions can create moral and legal dilemmas for one's agent (proxy) and caregivers about whether to still follow the AD. A person may choose to address these directly in the AD. One could say that such expressions should take precedence over the directions about SED previously in the AD. Or, very differently, one could direct one's agent and caregivers to proceed with SED nonetheless—a "Ulysses clause" (Chapter 10, Section 10.9). This

typically requires more formalities like having an attorney confirm that the person understands she is authorizing her agent to follow the AD even if contradicted by her incapacitated future self. The legal status of such clauses can be complex and is sometimes addressed in state law (Vermont Medical Society 2007).

3. **Desired Palliative Support.** To maintain comfort at whatever level of restricted eating and drinking a person specifies in their AD, one should also convey, if possible, to what degree they request the use of medications such as anti-anxiety or anti-delirium drugs, analgesics, sedative medications, and their desired level of sedation.

Note: Maximal palliative measures, potentially including heavy sedation, may be able to render the process of dying by withholding all food and drink (II-A-1-c above) as comfortable for an incapacitated person as VSED can be made comfortable for a person with current decisional capacity. Being able to accomplish this would likely strengthen the argument for permitting SED by AD.

4. **Reasons and Values Motivating the Directive.** If such reasons and values are articulated, the directive will likely be easier for the agent, family, and caregivers to respect and interpret in making decisions about implementation. It also shows that the patient understood the risks, benefits, and alternatives to the decisions she made. If the reasons imply that suffering is not a necessary condition for implementing the AD, that should be made clear. Articulation of basic motivating reasons and values is often included in the main AD itself, and sometimes in a supplement, and can be included in a video recording.

5. **Other Directions about Life-Sustaining Treatment.** People writing ADs for SED may be so focused on the ability of SED to help them avoid living long into chronic conditions like dementia that they do not carefully attend to elements in a conventional directive to withhold lifesaving treatment that can also help accomplish the same goal. Whatever triggering conditions the person stipulates for withholding food and water in their AD, presumably they would want other potentially lifesaving treatment to be withheld, too. People may also request that "windows of opportunity" be seized for hastening death by refusing lifesaving treatments in advance of the specified triggering conditions, for such opportunity may not come along soon or ever again (e.g., refusing antibiotics for pneumonia).

B. **Verify Decision-making Capacity.** The decisional capacity of the directive's author should be explicitly verified at the time of writing. Usually this is attested to in the substantive Advance Directive document itself. For ADs with especially controversial directions such as withholding food and water by mouth *even when the person appears to want food or drink* (sometimes referred to as "Ulysses" clauses), a separate clinician assessment of capacity is recommended. (In some states, e.g. Vermont, it is required—Vermont Medical Society 2007, 4 and 8–11.)

C. **Audio or Video Recordings.** These can a strengthen the verification of decision-making capacity and provide powerful additional evidence that the person meant and understood what she was requesting to be withheld, the condition(s) when she wanted that to apply, and why she was making that decision.

D. **Appoint Health Care Agent.** Not only should an agent (proxy) and backup agent be named, but the patient should discuss their appointment with the agent, including the patient's preferences about CFO or MCFO under certain circumstances if desired. Some states require the written agreement of a health care agent in order to legally designate one. The person appointing them should also explicitly give them discretion to interpret the elements within the AD, choose the appropriate time for implementation, and fill in substantive gaps for conditions that the patient did not (or could not) expect, according to the agent's best judgment about what the person would have wanted ("substituted judgment"). Such explicit granting of discretion is especially important in an AD for SED if the agent is empowered to ignore/override requests of the incapacitated person for food or water.

III. Follow-up Discussion and Further Documentation
    A. **Communicate with Agent, Family, and Primary Physician.** Concerns and questions about the content and boundaries of an AD for SED should be shared by and with the person's agent, close family, and primary treating physician while the person is still able to participate. Among other benefits, such communication can help minimize later disagreements.
    B. **Copy and Share Primary Documents.** The patient should share copies of all primary documents and videos with their agent, alternate agent, and primary health care provider. The patient should also share these documents with other close family members and friends who may later be involved, directly or indirectly, in their care or end-of-life situation. In addition, many states have electronic registries that can securely store these materials.

References

American Bar Association. 2020. "Health Decisions Resources." https://www.americanbar.org/groups/law_aging/resources/health_care_decision_making/Advanceplanningresources/.
Vermont Medical Society. 2007. "Advance Directives: Legal and Clinical Issues FAQ" (October 2007). http://vtmd.org/sites/default/files/files/Registry%20FAQ%2010-07.pdf.

Appendix B

Sample Advance Directives for SED

A growing number of end-of-life advocacy organizations and individuals have developed tools and forms that facilitate the completion of an advance directive for stopping eating and drinking (AD for SED). While not all of these satisfy the recommended elements that we set forth in Appendix A, we collect cites and links to many below. Note that not all forms and tools called "dementia directives" are ADs for SED. We have not included dementia directives (like https://dementia-directive.org) that are not ADs for SED.

Bunnell, Megan E., Sarah M. Baranes, Colin H. McLeish, Charlotte E. Berry, and Robert B. Santulli. 2020. "The Dartmouth Dementia Directive: Experience with a Community-Based Workshop Pilot of a Novel Dementia-Specific Advance Directive." *Journal of Clinical Ethics* 31, no. 2: 126–135.

Cantor, Norman. 2017. "My Revised Advance Directive." https://blog.petrieflom.law.harvard.edu/2017/04/20/changing-the-paradigm-of-advance-directives/.

Caring Advocates. 2020. "Natural Dying Advance Directive." https://caringadvocates.org/.

Caring Advocates. 2018. "My Way Cards for Natural Dying." https://caringadvocates.org/.

Caring Advocates. 2020. "An Effective Living Will for Dementia: Plan Now, Die Later –To Live Longer." https://caringadvocates.org/.

Chabot, Boudewijn. 2008. *A Hastened Death by Self-Denial of Food and Drink.* Amsterdam: Chabot.

Chandler-Cramer, M. Colette. 2014. "The Advance Directive for Dementia of M. Colette Chandler-Cramer." Included in Menzel, Paul T., and M. Colette Chandler-Cramer. 2014. "Advance Directives, Dementia, and Withholding Food and Water by Mouth." *Hastings Center Report* 44, no. 3 (May-June): 23–37. https://onlinelibrary.wiley.com/doi/abs/10.1002/hast.313.

Compassion & Choices. 2020. "Dementia Healthcare Provision." https://compassionandchoices.org/end-of-life-planning/plan/dementia-provision/.

Dartmouth University Geisel School of Medicine at Dartmouth. 2020. "Dartmouth Dementia Directive." https://sites.dartmouth.edu/dementiadirective/.

End of Life Choices New York. 2020. "Advance Directive for Receiving Oral Food and Fluids in Dementia." https://endoflifechoicesny.org/directives/dementia-directive/.

End of Life Washington. 2020. "Dementia Directives." https://endoflifewa.org/choices-and-planning/dementia-directives/.

EXIT. 2020. "EXIT Living Will with Innovations." Nov. 23, https://exit.ch/artikel/exit-patientenverfuegung-mit-neuerungen/.

Final Exit Network. 2020. "Supplemental Advance Directive for Dementia (SADD)." https://finalexitnetwork.org/.

Hawkins, Lamar. 2020. "Elective Advance Directive for Dementia." https://www.thegooddeathsocietyblog.net/.

Hemlock Society of San Diego. 2019. "Draft Addendum to Advance Health Care Instructions." https://www.hemlocksocietysandiego.org/draft-addendum-to-advance-health- care-instructions-v-7/.

Hensel, William Arthur. 1996. "My Living Will." *JAMA* 275: 588.

Patient Choices Vermont. 2020. "Guide to Advance Care Planning for Dementia." https://www.patientchoices.org/guide-to-advance-care-planning-for-dementia.html.

Pflege Durch Angehorige. 2019. "Fasting to Death—Supplement to the Living Will." https://www.pflege-durch-angehoerige.de/sterbefasten/.

Appendix C

Cause of Death on Death Certificates

What clinicians write as the "cause of death" on a death certificate has potentially significant implications. For example, if a person's death is deemed a "suicide," that could create obstacles to receiving life insurance funds, problems with burial status in some religions, significant social stigma, and even immediate legal investigation by the medical examiner or police.

Nevertheless, the accuracy of death certifications in terms of identifying the actual cause of death is poor under the best of circumstances (McGivern et al. 2017; Schuppener, Olson, and Brooks 2020). Consequently, as long as there is no likelihood of nefarious activity, most medical examiners and investigating police officers are not overly concerned about that discrepancy, as the purpose of legal investigation is mainly to protect vulnerable patients.

Factors Determined by Death Certificates

Death certificates are utilized to determine several factors around death: (1) Was the cause of death natural, accidental, suicide, homicide, or undetermined? (2) What was the "immediate cause" of death? (3) What were the "underlying causes" of death (including time interval between their start and death)?

(1) **Was the cause of death natural, accidental, suicide, homicide, or undetermined?** Any cause other than natural will be referred to the medical examiner for investigation. Any death in this group is potentially followed by interviews of family, clinicians, police, and others with relevant information. A determination is quickly made if an autopsy is needed to clarify the cause of death. If Voluntarily Stopping Eating and Drinking (VSED) was admitted or discovered, what would happen next in terms of level of investigation can be very unpredictable, ranging from signing the death out as "natural" to an exhaustive exploration depending mainly on the views of the initial investigator.

(2) **What was the immediate cause of death?** The focus of this question is on the exact causal features that contributed to death occurring at the exact moment that it did. With VSED, a truthful answer would be "dehydration," which is a common final cause of death in many debilitated patients with severe underlying disease. However, dehydration from VSED would likely trigger a medical examiner evaluation, whereas dehydration from a coexistent underlying disease would be considered a natural cause and not trigger medical examiner review. The time interval between initiation of VSED and death would usually be 10–14 days, which would be similar in many "natural" deaths. Other conditions contributing to the immediate cause of death such as pneumonia or partial bowel obstruction might also be listed in either case.

(3) **What were the underlying causes of death (including time interval between their start and death)?** With VSED, the main underlying contributing causes listed would include diseases and conditions such as Alzheimer's disease, cancer, and/or heart disease.

This section of the death certification information would look the same whether or not VSED was a part of the immediate cause of death.

Approaches to Revealing Immediate Cause of Death

There are three potential approaches to answering the immediate cause of death where VSED was a significant factor in the timing of a patient's death: (1) open discussion before death, (2) open discussion after death, and (3) recording the death as natural.

(1) **Talk honestly in advance with patient, family, and medical examiner about how best to approach this challenge.** This is probably the best approach if patient and family agree. This works best if done while the patient still has full decision-making capacity and can confirm his consent in initiating the entire process. If one was considering SED by AD in the future, this approach would still be best, provided the patient had capacity at the time the inquiry was made, but there would be risk that the medical examiner would not agree to participate, potentially creating problems before or after initiation by involving unwanted others in the process at any stage.

(2) **The main treating clinician calls the medical examiner after the patient's death, honestly explains what happened, including VSED or SED by AD, and asks for advice about completing the death certificate and whether an investigation is needed.** A positive aspect of this approach is that it lets the investigators know that the clinician and family are not afraid of the truth and feel that nothing unethical (or illegal) has happened. If the process were SED by AD, the level of documentation of the patient's wishes would be very important. With either VSED or SED by AD, calling the medical examiner right after the patient's death instead of well before still risks an ambulance and police being called, and a small possibility of attempts at unwanted cardiopulmonary resuscitation and/or investigation as a crime scene.

(3) **The main treating clinician calls the medical examiner after death, explains that a seriously ill hospice patient died of "dehydration," and confirms that there were no suspicious circumstances and that the patient does not (or does) want an autopsy as they would with a routine death.** Death by dehydration is a half-truth that omits that the dehydration was by self-initiation to achieve an earlier death while the patient was still capable of eating and drinking. Unless there were other signs of irregularity, omitting this information would not raise any suspicion, and this is probably the most common approach in practice. It would seem to be a variant of "don't ask, don't tell," as there might be significant harm and likely nothing gained by a major investigation, but it does involve not telling the whole truth. In this circumstance does that amount to lying?

These are some of the underlying ethical ambiguities in reporting cause of death. They should continue to be considered seriously, and not get lost in such habitual, routine, uncritical acceptance of less than full honesty, that honesty itself ceases to be a virtue. While families and clinicians should be informed of the practices of medical examiners and police, those practices themselves undoubtedly warrant ethical assessment.

Comparison of VSED with MAID and RLST

The final approach above (omitting mention of VSED in cause of death certification) has wide support in both law and practice. For example, when patients die from medical aid in dying (MAID) or from refusing life-sustaining treatment (RLST), neither MAID nor RLST is listed as a cause of death (Aiken et al. 2015).

In the United States, four MAID statutes prohibit MAID from being listed as the cause of death on the patient's death certificate (Colorado, D.C., Hawaii, Washington). Instead, the death certificate must list the underlying terminal illness that led the person to use MAID. In four other states, even though the statute is silent, state agency guidance directs listing the underlying terminal illness (California, New Jersey, Oregon, Vermont). For example, the California Department of Public Health states: "Certifiers . . . report the underlying terminal disease as the cause of death on the death certificates. This approach . . . effectuates the California Legislature's intent to maintain the confidentiality of individuals' participation in the Act" California Department of Public Health 2020). Similarly, the New Jersey Department of Health "recommends that providers record the underlying terminal disease as the cause of death and mark the manner of death as 'natural'" (New Jersey Department of Health 2019).

Government public health agencies offer the same guidance with respect to RLST (Centers for Disease Control 2003, 23–24). For example, New York City Health offers this example: "A patient with Parkinson's disease is admitted for aspiration pneumonia and dies in the ICU after the family decides to withdraw ventilator support following a prolonged period of respiratory failure" (New York City Health 2020). The agency recommends listing "aspiration pneumonia" as the immediate cause of death and "Parkinson's disease" as the underlying cause. The withdrawal of mechanical ventilation is not noted on the death certificate. Moreover, most health care decisions statutes specifically prohibit the withholding or withdrawal of life-sustaining treatment to be construed as suicide (New Hampshire 2021).

On the other hand, some guidance documents recommend that deaths not solely due to disease should be reported to the local coroner or medical examiner (Hanzlick 2006, 81). Since death from VSED is caused by an intentional action directly connected to death and not generated exclusively by the main underlying disease, these guides suggest such deaths should be classified as "suicide" rather than as "natural." Some medico-legal commentators similarly argue that both "well-established practice (and sound logic)" require recording the terminal disease (e.g., pancreatic cancer) as the "underlying cause" of death and MAID or VSED as the subsequent antecedent cause of death (Downie & Oliver 2016).

Reasons, Conditions, and Causes

"Underlying" or "background" causes of a death are neither "proximate" nor "sufficient" causes. They are necessary conditions for what takes place, or they are causes only in the "but-for" sense. There are so many of those conditions for any particular event that we do not see them as the cause of the event. And they aren't really the "cause" *of the event*, but only a *condition* for it to have occurred. Having early signs of Alzheimer's disease was a condition for the action (VSED) that Mrs. H. took to hasten her death (Case 1.3 and 7.1), for example, but it was just that, a condition for her decision. When such conditions are pivotal for a decision intended to lead to death, as Alzheimer's was for Mrs. H., they become *reasons* for the decision.

That is the conceptual landscape. Practical considerations may stand in tension with this conceptual landscape when it comes to speaking and acting in actual situations. Alzheimer's is not what caused Mrs. H.'s death; her VSED did, yet in the practice of stating a "cause of death" in death certification, we pay attention to the purpose of the practice. If its practical purposes are those articulated in the sections above, there may be nothing wrong in listing "cancer," for example, as the cause of a person's death that was precipitated earlier by VSED than it otherwise would have occurred just from the cancer. We may take conditions or reasons to be tantamount to causes. There is nothing necessarily wrong with that. Words are used in contexts of cultural and professional understanding.

To be sure, an ethical case can often be made against lying. It can also be made for telling "the whole truth (and nothing but the truth)." Telling less than the full truth, however, is not necessarily "lying" or being "dishonest." Customary use of words in a way that is not literally accurate, like "cause of death," may similarly not be dishonest, particularly if those who hear the words do not expect full honesty and will not be deceived or misled when they are not used in their literal sense. There is more ethical room for practical clinical judgment on such matters than is sometimes acknowledged.

Nevertheless, in what to declare as the cause of death, such room is not unlimited. Parties involved in death certification should recognize the tensions and not bury them in a habitual, uncritical practice.

References

Aiken, Sally S., Elizabeth A. Bundock, Karen L. Gunson, and Katherine Aiken. 2015. "Death with Dignity Laws and the Medical Examiner." *Academic Forensic Pathology* 5, no. 3: 414–420.

California Department of Public Health. 2020. "California End of Life Option Act 2019 Data Report," 5 (2020). https://www.cdph.ca.gov/Programs/CHSI/CDPH%20 Document%20Library/CDPHEndofLifeOptionActReport2019%20_Final%20ADA. pdf.

Centers for Disease Control and Prevention. 2003. *Physician's Handbook on Medical Certification of Death.* Hyattsville, MD: DHHS.

Colorado End-of-life Options Act, Colo. Rev. Stat. § 25-48-109(2).

District of Columbia Death with Dignity Act, D.C. Code § 7-661.05(h).

Downie, Jocelyn, and Kacie Oliver. 2016. "Medical Certificates of Death: First Principles and Established Practices Provide Answers to New Questions." *Canadian Medical Association Journal* 188, no. 1: 49–52.

Hanzlick, Randy. 2006. *Cause of Death and the Death Certificate.* Northfield, IL: College of American Pathologists.

Hawaii Our Care, Our Choice Act, Haw. Rev. Stat. § 327L-4(b).

McGivern, Lauri, Leanne Shulman, Jan K. Carney, Steven Shapiro, and Elizabeth Bundock. 2017. "Death Certification Errors and the Effect on Mortality Statistics." *Public Health Reports* 132, no. 6: 669–675.

New Hampshire Statutes. 2021. N.H. Rev. Stat. Ann. § 137-J:10(III).

New Jersey Department of Health. 2019. "Medical Aid In Dying for the Terminally Ill Act Frequently Asked Questions," 3–4, July 31. https://www.state.nj.us/health/advancedirective/documents/maid/MAID_FAQ.pdf.

New York City Health Bureau of Vital Statistics. 2020. "Cause of Death Reporting Instructions." https://www1.nyc.gov/site/doh/data/data-sets/cause-of-death-reporting-instructions.page.

Oregon Health Authority. 2020. "Frequently Asked Questions: Oregon's Death with Dignity Act (DWDA)." https://www.oregon.gov/oha/PH/PROVIDERPARTNERRESOURCES/EVALUATIONRESEARCH/DEATHWITHDIGNITYACT/Pages/faqs.aspx#deathcert.

Schuppener, Leah M., Kelly Olson, and Erin G. Brooks. 2020. "Death Certification: Errors and Interventions." *Clinical Medicine and Research* 18, no. 1: 21–26.

Vermont Department of Health. 2018. "Report to The Vermont Legislature: Report Concerning Patient Choice at The End of Life," 4. https://legislature.vermont.gov/assets/Legislative-Reports/2018-Patient-Choice-Legislative-Report-12-14-17.pdf.

Washington Death with Dignity Act, Wash. Rev. Code § 70.245.040(2).

Appendix D

Position Statements and Clinical Guidance

This Appendix includes citations and links to professional society position statements and clinical guidance. These are grouped into four sections: (1) position statements by major organizations; (2) clinical guidance statements and articles; and (3) sample institutional policies and (4) measures of prevalence.

I. Position Statements by Major Organizations

Nearly a dozen national and international professional health care societies have issued position statements and policy statements on VSED. Many are new, having been issued within the past four years. We list these organizations alphabetically by name with citations or links to their position statements.

AMDA—The Society for Post-Acute and Long-Term Care

- Wright, James L., Peter M. Jaggard, Timothy Holahan, Ethics Subcommittee of AMDA—The Society for Post-Acute and Long-Term Care. 2019. "Stopping Eating and Drinking by Advance Directives (SED by AD) in Assisted Living and Nursing Homes." *JAMDA* 20: 1362–1366.
- Jaggard, Peter, and James Wright. "Stopping Eating and Drinking by Advance Directives: Choose Your Injustice." *Caring for the Ages* (April 2019): 12–13.

American Academy of Hospice and Palliative Medicine

- AAHPM. 2016. "Advisory Brief: Guidance on Responding to Requests for Physician-Assisted Dying." http://aahpm.org/positions/padbrief.

American Medical Women's Association

- American Medical Women's Association. 2018. "Position Statement on Medical Aid in Dying." https://www.amwa-doc.org/wp-content/uploads/2018/09/Medical-Aid-in-Dying-Position-Paper.pdf.

American Nurses Association

- ANA Center for Ethics and Human Rights. 2017. "Revised Position Statement: Nutrition and Hydration at the End of Life." https://www.nursingworld.org/~4af0ed/globalassets/docs/ana/ethics/ps_nutrition-and-hydration-at-the-end-of-life_2017june7.pdf.

American Society for Parenteral and Enteral Nutrition (ASPEN)

- Schwartz, Denise B, Albert Barrocas, Maria Giuseppina Annetta et al. 2021. "Ethical Aspects of Artificially Administered Nutrition and Hydration: An ASPEN Position Paper." Nutrition in Clinical Practice (forthcoming), DOI: 10.1002/ncp.10633.

Australian National Health and Medical Research Council

- ANHMRC. 2006. "Guidelines for a Palliative Approach in Residential Aged Care." https://www.caresearch.com.au/caresearch/tabid/3587/Default.aspx.

Austrian Palliative Society

- Feichtner, Angelika, Dietmar Weixler, and Alois Birklbauer. 2018. "Voluntary Refraining from Food and Fluids to Accelerate Death: A Statement from the Austrian Palliative Society (OPG)" ["Freiwilliger Verzicht auf Nahrung und Flüssigkeit umdas Sterben zu beschleunigen: Eine Stellungnahme der österreichischen Palliativgesellschaft (OPG)"]. *Vienna Medical Weekly* [*Wien Med Wochenschr*] 168: 168–176.

Christian Medical and Dental Associations

- CMDA. 2019. *CMDA Position Statements: Based on Scientific, Moral, and Biblical Principles.* https://cmda.org/position-statements/.

European Society for Clinical Nutrition and Metabolism

- Druml, Christiane, Peter E. Ballmer, Wilfred Druml, Frank Oehmichen, Alan Shenkin, Pierre Singer, Peter Soeters, Arved Weimann, and Stephan C. Bischoff. 2016. "ESPEN Guideline on Ethical Aspects of Artificial Nutrition and Hydration." *Clinical Nutrition* 35, no. 3: 545–556.

German Society of Palliative Medicine

- Nauk, Friedemann, Christoph Ostgathe, and Lukas Radbruch. 2014. "Physically Assisted Suicide: Help with Dying—No Help with Dying." *German Medical Journal* [*Dtsch Arztebl*] 111, no. 3: A67–A71.
- Radbruch, Lukas, Urs Münch, Bernd-Oliver Maier et al. 2019. "Position Paper of the German Society for Palliative Medicine to Voluntarily Refrain from Eating and Drinking," https://www.dgpalliativmedizin.de/category/167-stellungnahmen-2019.html.

Harvard Community Ethics Committee

- Harvard Community Ethics Committee. 2016. "Palliated and Assisted Voluntary Stopping of Eating and Drinking." https://bioethics.hms.harvard.edu/about/community-ethics-committee.

International Association for Hospice and Palliative Care

- De Lima, Liliana et al. 2017. "International Association for Hospice and Palliative Care Position Statement: Euthanasia and Physician-Assisted Suicide." *Journal of Palliative Medicine* 20: 8–14.
- Baracos, Vickie E. 2017. "International Association for Hospice and Palliative Care Endorses Volitional Death by Starvation and Dehydration." *Journal of Palliative Medicine* 20: 577.
- Radbruch, Lukas, and Liliana De Lima. 2017. "Response Regarding Voluntary Cessation of Food and Water." *Journal of Palliative Medicine* 20: 578–579.

Royal Dutch Medical Association [*Koninklijke Nederlandsche Maatschappij tot bevordering der Geneeskunst* (KNMG)]

- KNMG. 2011. "The Role of the Physician in the Voluntary Termination of Life." https://www.knmg.nl/actualiteit-opinie/nieuws/nieuwsbericht/euthanasia-in-the-netherlands.htm.

Swiss Academy of Medical Sciences (SAMS)

- Swiss Academy of Medical Sciences. 2018. "Management of Dying and Death." https://www.sams.ch/en/Publications/Medical-ethical-Guidelines.html.

United States Conference of Catholic Bishops

- USCCB. 2009. "Ethical and Religious Directives for Catholic Health Care Services (5th edition)." http://www.usccb.org/issues-and-action/human-life-and-dignity/ health-care/upload/Ethical-Religious-Directives-Catholic-Health-Care-Services- fifth-edition-2009.pdf.

World Medical Association.

- World Medical Association. 2016. "Declaration of Tokyo." https://www.wma.net/ policies-post/wma-declaration-of-tokyo-guidelines-for-physicians-concerning- torture-and-other-cruel-inhuman-or-degrading-treatment-or-punishment-in- relation-to-detention-and-imprisonment/.

II. Clinical Guidance Statements and Articles

Medical associations and peer-reviewed medical literature offer clinical guidance on how to counsel and assist patients to VSED. We collect citations and links to some of the more useful resources.

Beneker, Christian. 2020. "Assisted Suicide Allowed - What Will Become of the Alternative Fasting?" *Medscape*, Sept. 16, https://deutsch.medscape.com/artikelansicht/4909282.

Bolt, Eva. 2020. "Stop Eating and Drinking." *Pallium*, Nov. 20, https://www.palliumtotaal. nl/magazine-artikelen/stoppen-met-eten-en-drinken/.

Chabot, Boudewijn. 2017. "Informationen zum freiwilligen Verzicht auf Nahrung und Flüssigkeit: Was zu tun ist." In: *Ausweg am Lebensende: Selbstbestimmt sterben durch freiwilligen Verzicht auf Essen und Trinken* 59–80, edited by Boudewijn Chabot and Christian Walther. 5th ed. München: Reinhardt.

Chabot, Boudewijn. 2015. *Stopping Eating and Drinking, a Guide*. Amsterdam: self-published.

Chabot, Boudewijn, and Christian Walther. 2017. Way Out at the End of Life: Death Fasting—Self-Determined Death by Refraining from Eating and Drinking [*Ausweg am Lebensende: Sterbefasten—Selbstbestimmtes Sterben durch Verzicht auf Essen und Trinken*]. Munich: Reinhardt Ernst.

Chargot, Jane, Drew A. Rosielle, and Adam Marks. 2019. "Voluntary Stopping of Eating and Drinking in the Terminally Ill #379." *Journal of Palliative Medicine* 22, no. 10: 1281–1282.

Coors, Michael, Bernd Alt-epping, and Alfred Simon. 2019. *Voluntary Waiver of Food and Fluids Medical and Nursing Basics—Ethical and Legal Assessments* [*Freiwilliger Verzicht auf Nahrung und Flüssigkeit*]. Stuttgart: Kohlhammer.

Danis, Marion. 2021. "Stopping Nutrition and Hydration at the End of Life." In: UpToDate, Post, TW (Ed), UpToDate, Waltham, MA, https://www.uptodate.com/contents/ stopping-nutrition-and-hydration-at-the-end-of-life/print.

Eastman, Peter, Danielle Ko, and Brian H. Le. 2020. "Challenges in Advance Care Planning: the Interface between Explicit Instructional Directives and Palliative Care." *Medical Journal of Australia* 213, no. 2: 67–68.

Lowers, Jane, Sean Hughes, and Nancy J. Preston. 2021. "Experience of Caregivers Supporting a Patient through Voluntarily Stopping Eating and Drinking." *Journal of Palliative Medicine* 24, no. 3: 376–81.

Lowers, Jane, Sean Hughes, and Nancy J. Preston. 2021. "Overview of Voluntarily Stopping Eating and Drinking to Hasten Death." *Annals of Palliative Medicine* (forthcoming), https://apm.amegroups.com/article/view/44492.

Quill, Timothy E., Linda Ganzini, Robert D. Truog, and Thaddeus M. Pope. 2018. "Voluntarily Stopping Eating and Drinking Among Patients with Serious Advanced Illness—Clinical, Ethical, and Legal Aspects." *JAMA Internal Medicine* 178, no. 1: 123–127.

Royal Dutch Medical Association (KNMG) and Dutch Nurses' Association (V&VN). 2014. "Caring for People Who Consciously Choose Not to Eat and Drink So as to Hasten the End of Life." https://www.knmg.nl/advies-richtlijnen/knmg-publicaties/publications-in-english.htm.

Wax, John W., Amy W. An, Nicole Kosier, and Timothy E. Quill. 2018. "Voluntary Stopping Eating and Drinking." *Journal of American Geriatrics Society* 66, no. 3: 441–445.

III. Sample Institutional Policies

Hospices, hospitals, and long-term care facilities should have an institutional policy on VSED. Because providers typically start drafting a new policy by first reviewing sample policies from other institutions, we collect some of those here.

Benton Hospice Service [now Lumina Hospice & Palliative Care in Corvallis, Oregon]. 2015. "Voluntarily Stopping Eating and Drinking (VSED) Policy."

Post, Linda Farber, and Jeffrey Blustein. 2015. *Handbook for Health Care Ethics Committees 2nd edition.* Baltimore: Johns Hopkins University Press. https://www.press.jhu.edu/books/supplemental/Post_Handbook_Ch%2017_policies.pdf.

Visiting Nurse Service of New York. 2017. "VSED: Responding to a Patient's Desire to Voluntarily Stop Eating and Drinking."

IV. Measures of VSED Prevalence

Researchers across the globe have conducted empirical studies to measure the prevalence of VSED. We collect citations to some of these studies.

Chabot, Boudewin E., and A. Goedhart. 2009. "A Survey of Self-Directed Dying Attended by Proxies in the Dutch Population." *Social Science & Medicine* 68, no. 10: 1745–1751.

Bolt, Eva E., Martijn Hagens, Dick Willems, and Bregie D. Onwuteaka-Philipsen. 2015. "Primary Care Patients Hastening Death by Voluntarily Stopping Eating and Drinking." *Annals of Family Medicine* 13, no. 5: 421–428.

Fringer, André, and Sabrina Stängle. 2020. "Fasting for Death—Medical Nursing Science." In *Handbook of Dying and Death [Handbuch Sterben und Tod]* 409–412, edited by Héctor Wittwer, Daniel Schäfer, and Andreas Frewer. Berlin: J. B. Metzler.

Hoekstra, Nina Luisa, and Alfred Simon. 2019. "Empirical Data on Voluntary Waiver of Food and Liquid." In *Voluntary Waiver of Food and Fluids Medical and Nursing*

Basics—Ethical and Legal Assessments 94–105, edited by Michael Coors, Bernd Altepping, and Alfred Simon. Stuttgart: Kohlhammer.

Onwuteaka-Philipsen, Bregje D., Arianne Brinkman-Stoppelenburg, Corine Penning, Gwen J.F. de Jong-Krul, Johannes J.M. van Delden, and Agnes van der Heide. 2012. "Trends in End-of-Life Practices Before and after the Enactment of the Euthanasia Law in The Netherlands from 1990 to 2010: A Repeated Cross-Sectional Survey." *Lancet* 380, no. 9845: 908–915.

Shinjo, Takuya, Tatsuya Morita, Daisuke Kiuchi, Masayuki Ikenaga, Hirofumi Abo, Sayaka Maeda, Satoru Tsuneto, and Yoshiyuki Kizawa. 2019. "Japanese Physicians' Experiences of Terminally Ill Patients Voluntarily Stopping Eating and Drinking: A National Survey." *BMJ Supportive Palliative Care* 9, no. 2: 143–145.

Stängle, Sabrina, Wilfried Schnepp, Daniel Büche, Christian Häuptle, and André Fringer. 2020. "Long-term Care Nurses' Attitudes and the Incidence of Voluntary Stopping of Eating and Drinking: A Cross-Sectional Study." *Journal of Advanced Nursing* 76, no. 2: 526–533.

Stängle, Sabrina, Wilfried Schnepp, Daniel Büche, and André Fringer. 2020. "Voluntary Stopping of Eating and Drinking in Swiss Outpatient Care." *GeroPsych*, https://doi.org/10.1024/1662-9647/a000249.

Stängle, Sabrina, Wilfried Schnepp, Daniel Büche, Christian Häuptle, and André Fringer. 2020. "Family Physicians' Perspective on Voluntary Stopping of Eating and Drinking: A Cross-Sectional Study." *Journal of International Medical Research* 48, no. 8: 1–15.

Appendix E

Personal Narratives

Earlier in this book, we presented nine original, never-before-published cases. We included four VSED cases in Chapter 1 and one more in Chapter 2. We included four SED by AD cases in Chapter 7. But we are not alone. Many individuals have written about their experience or their family member's experience with either VSED or SED by AD. This Appendix includes citations and links to these personal narratives. These are grouped into four sections: (1) books, (2) articles, (3) video and audio recordings, and (4) collections of cases.

I. Books

Brewer, Colin O. 2019. *Let Me Not Get Alzheimer's, Sweet Heaven: Why Many People Prefer Death or Active Deliverance to Living with Dementia*. Bloxham: Skyscraper Publications.

Davidson, Sean. 2008. *Before We Say Goodbye*. Cape Town: Penguin.

Gross, Jane. 2011. *A Bittersweet Season: Caring for Our Aging Parents—and Ourselves*. New York: Alfred A. Knopf.

Jury, Mark, and Dan Jury. 1978. *Gramp*. New York: Penguin Books.

Kaufmann, Peter, A. Fringer, M. Trachsel, S. Stängle, J. Meichlinger, and C. Walther. 2020. *Sterbefasten—25 Fallbeispiele zur Diskussion über den freiwilligen Verzicht auf Nahrung und Flüssigkeit (FVNF)*. Stuttgart: Kohlhammer.

Lowers, Jane. 2020. *Caring for Someone Who Has Chosen to Stop Eating and Drinking to Hasten Death Lancaster University*. Doctoral dissertation, https://eprints.lancs.ac.uk/id/eprint/146437/1/2020lowersphd.pdf.

Mehne, Sabine. 2019. *I Die as I Want: My Decision to Fast at Death [Ich Sterbe, Wie Ich Will Meine Entscheidung zum Sterbefasten]*. Munich: Ernst Reinhardt Verlag.

Shacter, Phyllis. 2017. *Choosing to Die: A Personal Story: Elective Death by Voluntarily Stopping Eating and Drinking (VSED) in the Face of Degenerative Disease*. Scotts Valley, CA: CreateSpace.

Sutherland, Cassandra. 2018. *A 'Good' Death with Dementia: An Autoethnographic Exploration of Voluntary Stopping Eating and Drinking (VSED)*. University of Washington M.P.H. thesis, https://digital.lib.washington.edu/researchworks/handle/1773/42051.

Terman, Stanley A. 2007. *The Best Way to Say Goodbye: A Legal Peaceful Choice at the End of Life*. Carlsbad, CA: Life Transitions.

Zur Nieden, Christiane. 2016. *Fasting to Death. Voluntary Waiver of Food and Fluids—A Case Description*. Frankfurt: Mabuse-Verlag.

Zur Nieden, Christiane, and Hans-Christoph Zur Nieden. 2019. *Dealing with Fasting: Practical Cases*. Frankfurt: Mabuse-Verlag.

II. Articles

Many individuals have written about their experience or their family member's experience with VSED. The following sources are articles organized by the patient's name.

Anonymous

- Douglas, Carol, and Bill Lukin. 2016. "My Life—My Death." *Narrative Inquiry in Bioethics* 6, no. 2: 77–78.
- Marks, Adam. 2016. "'I'd Like to Choose my Own Way:' VSED in the Non–Terminal Patient." *Narrative Inquiry in Bioethics* 6, no. 2: 90–92.

Anonymous

- Henig, Robin Marantz. 2015. "Despite Sweeping Aid in Dying Law, Few Will Have that Option." *NPR*, October 7, https://www.npr.org/sections/health-shots/2015/10/07/ 446631786/despite-sweeping-death-with-dignity-law-few-will-have-that-option.

Beatrice Belopolsky

- Schaffer, Susan B. 2010. "Life, Death on Her Terms." *Philadelphia Inquirer,* July 25, https://www.inquirer.com/philly/opinion/currents/20100725_Life__death_on_ her_terms.html.

Margaret Bentley

- Hammond, Katherine. 2016. "Kept Alive—The Enduring Tragedy of Margot Bentley." *Narrative Inquiry in Bioethics* 6, no. 2: 80–82.

Bernard

- Dziedzic–Carroll, Julie. 2016. "The Less, the Better: One Patient's Journey with VSED." *Narrative Inquiry in Bioethics* 6, no. 2: 78–80.

Christine Bregnard

- Ita, Luisa. 2021· "I Want to Finally Redeem My Wife." *Blick,* Jan. 11, https://www.blick. ch/schweiz/bern/roger-bregnard-70-kaempft-dafuer-dass-seine-demenzkranke- christine-73-sterben-darf-ich-will-meine-frau-endlich-erloesen-id16285892.html.

Jeptha Carrell

- Menzel, Paul T. "Carpe Diem: The Death of Jeptha Carrell," based on interview of Carrell's surviving spouse, Demaris Carrell. 2010, updated 2013. https://sites.google. com/a/plu.edu/menzelpt/selected-unpublished-documents.   https://docs.google. com/viewer?a=v&pid=sites&srcid=cGx1LmVkdXxtZW56ZWxwdHxneneDphM2F mY2FlMWMwMzIwOGY.

Kate Christie

- Christie, Kate. 2017. "Let Me Tell You About My Mother." https://katejchristie.com/ 2020/03/05/let-me-tell-you-about-my-mother/.
- Christie, Kate. 2017. "Let Me Tell You About My Mother II." https://katejchristie. com/2020/03/05/let-me-tell-you-about-my-mother-ii/.

Alain Cocq

- AFP. 2020. "Alain Cocq Wants to Let Himself Die Again—He Announced That He Would Cease All Hydration, Diet and Treatment, Except Painkillers from Monday." *Le Monde,* October 10, https://www.lemonde.fr/sante/article/2020/10/10/alain-cocq-veut-a-nouveau-se-laisser-mourir_6055584_1651302.html.

Dorothy Stetson Conlon

- Seidman, Carrie. 2014. "The Traveler's Final Journey." http://finaljourney.heraldtribune.com/.

Virginia Eddy

- Eddy, David. 1994. "A Conversation with My Mother." *JAMA* 272: 179–181.
- Eddy, David. 2007. "I'm Still Telling Others How Well This Worked for My Mother." In *The Best Way to Say Goodbye: A Legal Peaceful Choice at the End of Life,* edited by Stanley A. Terman. Carlsbad, CA: Life Transitions.
- LaBarbera, Jennifer. 1994. "Editors of Medical Journals Wield Pens with the Deftness of Scalpels." *Physicians Financial News,* Sept. 30, at 26.

Grandpa

- Halpern, Scott D. 2020. "Learning about End-of-Life Care from Grandpa." *New England Journal of Medicine* 384, no. 5: 400–401.

Del Greenfield

- Span, Paula. 2016. "The VSED Exit: A Way to Speed Up Dying, Without Asking Permission." *New York Times,* October 21, https://www.nytimes.com/2016/10/25/health/voluntarily-stopping-eating-drinking.html.

Klaus Grosch

- Parth, Christian. 2019. "Deadly Means 'Only in Extreme Individual Cases.'" *Spiegel,* July 28, https://www.spiegel.de/panorama/sterbehilfe-bei-todkranken-im-extremen-einzelfall-a-1277361.html.
- Ebert, Sandra. 2019. "Fasting to Death: The Sad Story Behind Klaus Grosch's Obituary Notice." *Kölner Stadt-Anzeiger,* May 17, https://www.ksta.de/region/rhein-sieg-bonn/troisdorf/-ich-klage-an--die-traurige-geschichte-hinter-der-todesanzeige-von-klaus-grosch-32550778.

Estelle Gross

- Gross, Jane. 2008. "What an End-of-Life Adviser Could Have Told Me." *New York Times,* December 15, https://newoldage.blogs.nytimes.com/2008/12/15/what-an-end-of-life-advisor-could-have-told-me/.

Jo Ann Hallen

- MacWhyte, Marie. 2021. "Voluntary Stopping Eating and Drinking (VSED), an End-of-Life Alternative." *LinkedIn,* https://www.linkedin.com/pulse/voluntary-stopping-eating-drinking-vsed-end-of-life-marie-macwhyte.

William Arthur Hensel

- Hensel, William Arthur. 1996. "My Living Will." *JAMA* 275: 588.

Polly Jose

- Jose, Elizabeth Keller, and William S. Jose. 2016. "VSED at Home with Hospice: A Daughter's and Husband's Experience." *Narrative Inquiry in Bioethics* 6, no. 2: 82–88.

Ken

- Wolfe, Warren. 1994. "Three Lives, Three Journeys." *Star Tribune,* February 27, at 14A.

Margaret

- Henry, Blair. 2016. "Hunger Games." *Narrative Inquiry in Bioethics* 6, no. 2: E7–E9.

Michelle

- Jay Niver. 2020. "Alzheimer's: the Torture of Dementia." *Final Exit Network Newsletter* 19, no. 3: 1–2.

Mother

- Christie, Kate. 2017. "Let Me Tell You about My Mother." *Homodramatica,* Oct. 6, https://katejchristie.com/2017/10/06/let-me-tell-you-about-my-mother/.
- Christie, Kate. 2020. "Let Me Tell You about My Mother II." *Homodramatica,* Mar. 5, https://katejchristie.com/2020/03/05/let-me-tell-you-about-my-mother-ii/.

Mom

- Ann, Laurie. 2016. "Mom's VSED Journey." *Narrative Inquiry in Bioethics* 6, no. 2: E1–E4.
- Brown, David L. 2016. "She Never Met a Stranger—Death is No Stranger." *Narrative Inquiry in Bioethics* 6, no. 2: E4–E7.
- Webster, Deacon Gregory. 2016. "The Deacon's Mom Wants to Die." *Narrative Inquiry in Bioethics* 6, no. 2: 105–107.

David Muller

- Muller, David. 2012. "Physician-Assisted Death Is Illegal in Most States, So My Patient Made Another Choice." *Health Affairs* 31: 2343–2346.

Neta

- MacDonald, Richard. 2020. "Peace and Love: VSED Bests COVID for Neta." *Final Exit Network Newsletter* 19, no. 3: 4–5.

Margaret Page

- Chug, Kiran, Stacey Wood, and Tim Donoghue. 2010. "Margaret Page Dies in Rest Home after 16 Days." *Dominion Post,* March 31, https://www.stuff.co.nz/dominion-post/news/3531167/Margaret-Page-dies-in-rest-home-after-16-days.

Noa Pothoven

- Mackintosh, Eliza. 2019. "Teenager's Death Ignites Debate over Euthanasia." *CNN*, June 8, https://www.cnn.com/2019/06/08/europe/noa-pothoven-euthanasia-debate-intl/index.html.

Debbie Purdy

- BBC. 2014. "Debbie Purdy: Right-to-Die Campaigner Dies." *BBC News*, December 29, https://www.bbc.com/news/uk-england-leeds-25741005#:~:text=Right%2Dto%2Ddie%20campaigner%20Debbie,and%20had%20sometimes%20refused%20food.

Armond and Dorothy Rudolph

- Uyttebrouck, Olivier. 2011. "Couple Transported Out of Facility After Refusing Food." *Albuquerque Journal*, January 8, https://www.abqjournal.com/news/metro/08232859metro01-08-11.htm.

Sam

- Mitchell, Marilyn. 2016. "Sam's Final Story." *Narrative Inquiry in Bioethics* 6, no. 2: 92–94.

Sandra

- Terman, Stanley A. 2016. "To Live Long Enough to Warm the Hearts of Others: Reflections on Informing my Patient about a Peaceful Way to Die." *Narrative Inquiry in Bioethics* 6, no. 2: 101–105.

Sarah

- Schwarz, Judith K. 2016. "Sarah's Second Attempt to Stop Eating and Drinking: Success at Last." *Narrative Inquiry in Bioethics* 6, no. 2: 99–101.

Beatrice Schaffer

- Schaffer, Susan, Elliott Schaffer, and Janet Malek. 2016. "Life and Death on Her Own Terms." *Narrative Inquiry in Bioethics* 6, no. 2: 96–99.

Alan Shacter

- Shacter, Phyllis R. 2016. "Not Here by Choice: My Husband's Choice About How and When to Die." *Narrative Inquiry in Bioethics* 6 no. 2: 94–96.

Christina Symanski

- Kerwin, Jeanne. 2016. "The Art of Suffering: Christina's Story." *Journal of Pain & Symptom Management* 52, no. 5: 756-59.
- Symanski, Christina and James Morganti. 2012. Amazon Kindle.
- Symanski, Christina. 2012. *Life; Paralyzed*, lifeparalyzed.blogspot.com.

Mrs. T.

- Kohlhase, Wendy. 2016. "Voluntary Stopping of Eating and Drinking: A Patient's Right to Choose or an Act of Suicide?" *Narrative Inquiry in Bioethics* 6, no. 2: 88–90.

Avis Vermilye

- Hooks, Cody, and Morgan Timms, 2019. "A Remarkable Life, a Chosen Death." *Taos News,* February 21, https://www.taosnews.com/news/a-remarkable-life-a-chosen-death/article_dc01cb0e-e1c9-53cd-b58c-1d3a5cfa4071.html.

III. Video and Audio Recordings

Many individuals have recorded their experience or their family member's experience with VSED. The following sources are videos or podcasts organized by the patient's name.

Beatrice Belopolsky

- Schaffer, Susan, and Elliott Schaffer. 2019. "VSED (Voluntary Stopping of Eating and Drinking) Part 1." https://www.youtube.com/watch?v=-7k20b_h900.
- Schaffer, Susan, and Elliott Schaffer. 2019. "VSED (Voluntary Stopping of Eating and Drinking) Part 2." https://www.youtube.com/watch?v=9Lwz1VHlRuw.
- Schaffer, Susan, and Elliott Schaffer. 2020. "Voluntary Stopping of Eating and Drinking." https://www.youtube.com/watch?v=baaB9aDVVxg.

Margot Bentley

- Wells, Karin. 2015. "In the Presence of a Spoon." *CBC Sunday Edition,* https://www.cbc.ca/player/play/2669369280

Rosemary Bowen

- Bahrampour, Tara. 2019. "At 94, She Was Ready to Die by Fasting. Her Daughter Filmed It." *Washington Post,* November 3, https://www.washingtonpost.com/local/social-issues/at-94-she-was-ready-to-die-by-fasting-her-daughter-filmed-it/2019/11/03/41688230-fcd9-11e9-8190-6be4deb56e01_story.html.
- "Rosemary Bowen's Fast." https://youtu.be/FpEwH6AKeVA

J case

- Om, Jason. 2011. "Sounds of Summer: Angela's Last Wish." *World Today,* January 21. http://www.abc.net.au/worldtoday/content/2011/s3118110.htm.

Michael Miller

- "Dying Wish" https://www.dyingwishmedia.com/.
- Vetter, Pam. 2008. "Dying Wish Documents Death of Dr. Michael Miller with Conscious Choice to Stop Eating and Drinking." *American Chronicle,* July 28, https://www.dyingwishmedia.com/press/.
- Scheidt, Rick J. 2017. "Dying Wish." *The Gerontologist* 57: 1001–1003.

Diane Rehm

- PBS. 2016. "Diane Rehm Shares the Painful Story of Her Husband's Death." *PBS NewsHour,* March 3, https://www.pbs.org/video/diane-rehm-shares-the-painful-story-of-her-husband-s-death-1464310462/.

Jean Rough

- Hull, Rhonda. 2020. "Interview with Jim Rough: A Courageous Conversation about V.S.E.D." https://youtu.be/yS--RqHNOwU.

Herta Sturmann

- Sturmann, Jan. 2019. "It's My Right: The Handmade Death of Herta Sturmann." https://vimeo.com/359407878.

IV. Collections of Cases

Campaign for Dignity in Dying. 2019. *The Inescapable Truth*. https://features. dignityindying.org.uk/inescapable-truth/.

End of Life Washington. 2021. *Voluntary Stopping Eating and Drinking (VSED)*. https:// endoflifewa.org/end-life-choices/vsed/.

Kaufmann, Peter, Manuel Trachsel, and Christian Walther. 2020. *Sterbefasten: Fallbeispiele Zur Diskussion Uber Den Freiwilligen Verzicht Auf Nahrung Und Flussigkeit*. Stuttgart: Kohlhammer.

Palliacura. "Case Studies." https://sterbefasten.org/fallbeispiele.php.

Symposium. 2016. "Voluntarily Stopping Eating and Drinking." *Narrative Inquiry on Bioethics* 6, no. 2: 75–126.

Terman, Stanley A. 2007. *The Best Way to Say Goodbye: A Legal Peaceful Choice at the End of Life*. Carlsbad, CA: Life Transitions.

VSED Resources Northwest. 2020. "Personal Stories." http://vsedresources.com/ vsed-stories.

Western Australia Parliament. 2018. "Inquiry into the Need for Laws in Western Australia to Allow Citizens to Make Informed Decisions Regarding Their Own End of Life Choices." https://www.parliament.wa.gov.au/Parliament/commit.nsf/(EvidenceOnly)/ 702507C2CB8742824825818700247E53?opendocument

Appendix F

Glossary

Advance Care Planning (ACP): Process of preparing for health care in the future should one lose decision-making capacity, including: (a) getting information on the types of treatment available, (b) deciding who should speak on one's behalf, (c) deciding what types of treatment one would or would not want, (d) sharing one's values and preferences with family and clinicians, and (e) completing an advance directive.

Advance Directive (AD): Document completed by an individual with decision-making capacity that provides instructions to guide her health care (and sometimes personal care) if and when she loses capacity in the future. See also Living Will. Advance directives may also be used to appoint a health care agent/proxy to speak on the individual's behalf when she loses capacity in the future. See also Health Care Agent and Durable Power of Attorney for Health Care.

Advance Directive for Stopping Eating and Drinking (AD for SED): Special type of advance directive (or supplement to a traditional AD) that directs caregivers to withhold all or some food and fluids at a specified time or clinical circumstance if and when the individual loses capacity.

Agent: Usually a synonym for health care agent, health care proxy, or durable power of attorney for health care. A synonym for surrogate in some jurisdictions.

Artificial Nutrition and Hydration (ANH): Form of life-sustaining treatment (via feeding tubes or intravenously) that could be initiated, withheld (not started), or withdrawn (stopped) once already started with a patient who is likely unable to eat or drink enough to sustain herself in the near future. This is sometimes called "clinically-assisted nutrition and hydration." See ONH for contrast.

Advance Euthanasia: Method of hastening death where the clinician both provides and administers lethal medication to a seriously ill patient without decision-making capacity based on a patient's clearly expressed prior request.

Assisted Feeding: Action of one person feeding another person by mouth who cannot feed herself. Also called "hand feeding" or "oral feeding." See also ONH.

Capacity: Ability to understand the significant benefits, risks, and alternatives to proposed treatment or intervention and to make and communicate an informed health care decision.

Comfort Feeding Only (CFO): Offering as much or as little food and drink as the patient appears to enjoy without regard to the "adequate hydration and nutrition" (the latter would be required if the patient's goal also was long term survival). See also MCFO.

Decision-making Capacity: Synonym for capacity.

Do Not Intubate (DNI): Do not insert a breathing tube into the patient to provide assisted ventilation in the event the patient cannot adequately breathe on his own.

Do Not Resuscitate (DNR): Do not resuscitate in response to a cardiopulmonary arrest (heart stops effectively beating). Similar instruction: **Do Not Attempt Resuscitation (DNAR):** Do not *attempt* resuscitation in the same situation. (Preferred in some circles because successful resuscitation is relatively rare; DNAR articulates the point that the intervention *attempts* to resuscitate without suggesting that successful resuscitation is the expected outcome.)

Durable Power of Attorney for Health Care (DPAHC): Document by which an individual designates another (the Health Care Agent or Proxy) to make health care decisions when the individual loses capacity. A DPAHC is often included as one part of an advance directive.

Euthanasia: Means of hastening death where the clinician both provides and administers lethal medication at the request of a seriously ill patient with decision-making capacity at a time of the patient's own choosing. This practice is also known as "Voluntary Active Euthanasia." See MAID for contrast. The Netherlands also permits capacitated advance requests for euthanasia administered when the patient later lacks capacity.

Functional Assessment Staging Test (FAST): Well-validated functional scale designed to measure the progression of dementia. FAST divides dementia into seven stages.

Global Deterioration Scale (GDS): Measure of the stages of cognitive function for those suffering from dementia. Like the FAST scale, it divides dementia into seven different stages (overlapping but distinct from FAST).

Hand Feeding: Procedure where a patient is fed by another person who puts food into the patient's mouth. See also ONH and Assisted Feeding.

Health Care Agent: Someone an individual appoints to make health care (and sometimes personal care) decisions on his behalf if and when he loses decision-making capacity. The appointment is formally recorded in an advance directive or durable power of attorney for health care. See also Durable Power of Attorney for Health Care and Proxy.

Health Care Proxy (HCP): Usually a synonym for health care agent or durable power of attorney for health care. A synonym for surrogate in some jurisdictions.

Hospice: Supportive care provided in the final phase (last six months) of a terminal illness with a focus on comfort and quality of life, rather than cure. Hospice is also a Medicare, Medicaid, and private insurance benefit that pays for palliative medications and comfort-oriented supplies, intermittent nursing visits, and as much as two to four hours of home health aide support per week. Part of the hospice philosophy is to *neither hasten nor postpone death.*

Life-Sustaining Treatment: Interventions that, based on reasonable medical judgment, are intended to sustain the life of a patient and without which the patient will die. The term includes both life-sustaining medications and artificial life support, such as mechanical breathing machines, kidney dialysis treatment, and artificially administered nutrition and hydration.

Living Will: Less commonly used term for an advance directive that provides instructions to guide medical treatment if and when the patient loses decision-making capacity in the future.

Long Term Care (LTC): Institutional health care setting that includes a variety of services which help meet both the medical and non-medical needs of people with chronic illness or disability who cannot care for themselves for long periods.

Long Term Care Facility (LTC Facility): residential facilities that provide many or all of the LTC needs for people who need this level of help. These include skilled nursing facilities, assisted living facilities, continued care retirement communities and residential facilities. They rely on a variety of payment sources, including personal funds, government programs (Medicaid and Medicare), and private financing options.

Medical Aid in Dying (MAID): Method for hastening death where the clinician provides the patient with a prescription for lethal medication that the patient then takes (or potentially does not take) by her own hand at a time of her own choosing. MAID is also known as "physician assisted death," "physician aid-in-dying," and "aid in dying." The practice is also sometimes called "physician-assisted suicide," though this is not a preferred term because of suicide's association with mental illness. In Canada the term includes Euthanasia.

Minimum Comfort Feeding Only (MCFO): Modification of standard CFO in which the amount of food and fluid given (either offered for self-feeding or caregiver-assisted) is the "minimum amount needed for comfort" rather than "as much or as little as compatible with comfort." MCFO is triggered based on previously agreed upon criteria as a potential part of the patient's prior plan for VSED or SED by AD.

Oral Nutrition and Hydration (ONH): Food and liquids that are taken by mouth either through self-feeding or caregiver-assisted feeding. The goal could be (a) comfort only, (b) adequate hydration and nutrition, or (c) both. The term ONH does not include artificial hydration and nutrition (ANH) delivered through a nasogastric or gastric feeding tube.

Palliative Care: Type of health care that improves the quality of life of patients and their families by relieving the pain, symptoms, and stress of a serious or debilitating illness, and assistance with difficult medical decision-making. Palliative care can be provided alongside any and all desired disease-directed treatment, or it may be the sole purpose of treatment (as in hospice).

Palliative Sedation to Unconsciousness (PSU): Providing sedation to unconsciousness in one step in response to severe, acute suffering usually from a medical/palliative emergency that cannot be otherwise mitigated. Unlike proportionate palliative sedation (PPS), which is relatively common in palliative care (see below), PSU should be a relatively rare response to severe suffering that cannot be otherwise relieved.

Proportionate Palliative Sedation (PPS): Providing gradually increasing amounts of sedation as needed to relieve the suffering of a seriously ill patient (relatively common practice) while maintaining alertness if possible. The process might end up with palliative sedation to unconsciousness if lesser degrees of sedation are inadequate to provide relief.

Provider Orders for Life-Sustaining Treatment (POLST): Immediately actionable and portable medical order set usually covering the patient's preferences about cardio-pulmonary resuscitation, mechanical ventilation, dialysis, and other potentially life prolonging treatments. POLST directs treatments potentially received from the moment it is signed forward, while advance directives are only activated in the future when the patient loses capacity. Many jurisdictions use different acronyms such as MOLST (Medical Orders for Life Sustaining Treatment), COLST (Clinician Orders for Life Sustaining Treatment), or POST (Physician Orders for Scope of Treatment).

Proxy: Usually a synonym for health care proxy, health care agent, or durable power of attorney for health care. A synonym for surrogate in some jurisdictions.

Proxy Directive: Synonym for Durable Power of Attorney for Health Care. See also Advance Directive.

Refusing Life-Sustaining Treatment (RLST): Decision made by a seriously ill patient or by her surrogate decision-maker(s) to withhold or withdraw potentially effective life-sustaining therapies (mechanical ventilators, cardiopulmonary resuscitation, feeding tubes, dialysis, and others). This refusal can come before any such therapy is started, or it can be a decision to stop what has previously been started under different circumstances. In most circles and jurisdictions, RLST has come to be widely accepted legally, ethically, and in clinical practice.

Stopping Eating and Drinking by Advance Directive (SED by AD): Not providing any food or fluids to a person who has lost decision-making capacity based on the person's advance directive clearly stating that she would not want food or fluid under her current medical circumstances.

Self-Deliverance: In addition to medically supervised measures of hastening death, some individuals explore "do it yourself" methods using information from books, internet sites, or "exit guides." Self-deliverance involves various methods such as asphyxiation.

Stopping Manually Assisted Food and Liquids by Mouth: Not assisting a person to eat or drink who is unable to self-feed because of co-existing medical problems. In VSED, this would be based on clear knowledge of current wishes. In SED by AD, where capacity has been lost, this would be based on the patient's clearly expressed prior wishes.

Surrogate: Synonym for Surrogate Decision-Maker.

Surrogate Decision-Maker: Someone who makes health care decisions for an individual who has lost capacity. Most jurisdictions have default priority lists specifying who may speak for an incapacitated patient when the patient has no available agent or guardian. When the individual was officially appointed by the patient herself, he would then be designated as the patient's Health Care Agent/Proxy.

Ulysses Contract: Special provision an individual might include in an advance directive that is designed and intended to bind both them and caregivers in the future. When the individual later loses capacity, the Ulysses Contract directs care providers to listen to the individual's "past" self (as recorded in her AD) rather than her "now" self.

Voluntary Assisted Dying: Synonym for MAID. This term is primarily used in Australia where it includes Euthanasia only when the patient is unable to self-administer the medication.

Voluntary Active Euthanasia (VAE): Means of hastening death where the clinician both provides and administers lethal medication at the request of a seriously ill patient with decision-making capacity at a time of the patient's own choosing. This practice is also known simply as "Euthanasia." See MAID for contrast.

Voluntarily Stopping Eating and Drinking (VSED): Complete cessation of all oral intake (ONH) by a person with capacity who is physically able to eat and drink, with the intention of hastening his own death.

Index